§

I

THE DEMENTIAS

Diagnosis, Management, and Research

Second Edition

THE DEMENTIAS

Diagnosis, Management, and Research

Second Edition

Edited by

Myron F. Weiner, M.D.

Aradine S. Ard Chair and
Head of Geriatric Psychiatry
University of Texas Southwestern Medical Center
Dallas, Texas

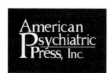

American
Psychiatric
Press, Inc.

Washington, DC
London, England

Copyright © 1996 American Psychiatric Press, Inc.
ALL RIGHTS RESERVED
Manufactured in the United States of America on acid-free paper
99   98   97   96   4   3   2   1

American Psychiatric Press, Inc.
1400 K Street, N.W., Washington, DC   20005

Library of Congress Cataloging-in-Publication Data
The dementias : diagnosis, management, and research / edited by Myron
   F. Weiner. — 2nd ed.
      p.   cm.
   Includes bibliographical references and index.
   ISBN 0-88048-718-6
   1. Dementia   I. Weiner, Myron F., 1934–   .
   [DNLM: 1. Dementia—diagnosis.   2. Dementia—theory.   WM220
D376391   1995]
RC521.D458   1996
616.8'3—dc20
DNLM/DLC
for Library of Congress   95-19191
                                                                        CIP

British Library Cataloguing in Publication Data
A CIP record is available from the British Library.

To persons with dementing illnesses
and their families, in the hope of
improving their quality of life

Contents

Contributors

Barton E. Bernstein, J.D., L.M.S.W.
Adjunct Professor of Psychiatry, University of Texas Southwestern
Medical Center at Dallas, Texas

Frederick J. Bonte, M.D.
Professor of Radiology and Director, Nuclear Medicine Center,
University of Texas Southwestern Medical Center at Dallas, Texas

Kathleen C. Buckwalter, Ph.D., R.N., F.A.A.N.
Professor, University of Iowa, College of Nursing, Iowa City, Iowa

Margaret P. Calkins, M.Arch.
Senior Fellow, Institute on Aging and Environment, School of
Architecture and Urban Planning, University of Wisconsin,
Milwaukee, Wisconsin

Paul K. Chafetz, Ph.D.
Assistant Professor of Gerontology and Geriatric Services, University
of Texas Southwestern Medical Center at Dallas, Texas

Kenneth L. Davis, M.D.
Professor of Psychiatry and Pharmacology and Chairman,
Department of Psychiatry, Mount Sinai School of Medicine,
New York, New York

Steven T. DeKosky, M.D.
Professor of Neurology, Psychiatry and Neurobiology, University of
Pittsburgh School of Medicine, Pittsburgh, Pennsylvania

Linda Garand, M.S., R.N., C.S.
University of Iowa, College of Nursing, Iowa City, Iowa

Linda A. Gerdner, M.A., R.N.
University of Iowa, College of Nursing, Iowa City, Iowa

Kevin F. Gray, M.D.
Assistant Professor of Psychiatry and Neurology, University of Texas
Southwestern Medical Center at Dallas, Texas

Geri Richards Hall, M.A., R.N., C.S.
Gerontology Clinical Nurse Specialist, University of Iowa Hospitals
and Clinics, Iowa City, Iowa

Zaven S. Khachaturian, Ph.D.
International Consultant on Alzheimer's Disease, Khachaturian,
Radebaugh, and Associates, Inc., Potomac, Maryland

Elisabeth Koss, Ph.D.
Assistant Professor of Neurology, Case Western Reserve University,
Cleveland, Ohio

William D. MacInnes, Ph.D.
Director of Neuropsychology, Mid-Michigan Regional Medical Center,
Midland, Michigan

Ronald G. Paulman, Ph.D.
Clinical Neuropsychologist, Timberlawn Psychiatric Center; Clinical
Associate Professor of Psychiatry, University of Texas Southwestern
Medical Center at Dallas, Texas

Lon S. Schneider, M.D.
Associate Professor of Psychiatry, University of Southern California,
Los Angeles, California

Valerie Stephenson, L.M.S.W.-A.C.P.
National Director of Alzheimer's Programs, Sunrise Health Care, Albu-
querque, New Mexico

Robert G. Stern, M.D.
Assistant Professor of Psychiatry, Mount Sinai School of Medicine,
New York, New York

Jacqueline M. Stolley, M.A., R.N.C.
University of Iowa, College of Nursing, Iowa City, Iowa

Doris Svetlik, B.S.N., R.N., M.S.
Administrative Director, Clinic for Alzheimer's and Related Diseases, University of Texas Southwestern Medical Center at Dallas, Texas

Linda Teri, Ph.D.
Professor of Psychiatry and Behavioral Science, University of Washington Medical School, Seattle, Washington

Ron Tintner, M.D., Ph.D.
Private Practice of Neurology, Monterey, California

Myron F. Weiner, M.D.
Aradine S. Ard Chair in Brain Science, Head of Geriatric Psychiatry and Vice-Chairman for Clinical Services, Department of Psychiatry, University of Texas Southwestern Medical Center at Dallas, Texas

Brent T. Williams, B.A., M.S.
Department of Psychology, University of Illinois, Urbana, Illinois

Foreword

This book, *The Dementias: Diagnosis, Management, and Research*, Second Edition, provides to physicians and other health care professionals much needed information about the growing public health problem of dementias in adulthood and old age and deals with critical issues concerning the diagnosis and management of persons with dementia. Alzheimer's disease (AD), the most common form of adult dementing illness, is estimated to affect nearly 4 million individuals. As the demographic trends of the past several decades continue into the early part of the next century, there will be nearly 17 million individuals affected by this devastating disease. At present, the annual cost of care for AD patients alone is nearly $100 billion. The individuals affected by this and other dementing illness, patients as well as family care providers, bear not only the financial costs of the illnesses but also the psychological and social stresses associated with the burdens of care.

During the past 15 years, scientific knowledge concerning AD has increased dramatically. At some of the specialized medical centers, it is possible to obtain an accurate and reliable diagnosis of AD. An important risk factor associated with the apolipoprotein E gene has been discovered and confirmed by many laboratories. The prospects of developing treatments, with both pharmacological and behavioral management approaches, are promising in delaying the onset of symptoms, slowing symptom progression, and reducing the intensity of the symptoms that emerge during the course of the disease. Despite the substantial progress made in many areas, the uncertainty of an early, accurate diagnosis poses a serious problem to physicians and other health care providers who come in contact with dementia patients early in the clinical course of their disease. Misdiagnosis is a serious problem, not only because of the unnecessary pain and suffering it can cause but also because of a missed opportunity to provide treatment. It has been reported that 10%–20% of the disorders presenting as dementia in older patients might respond to some form of treatment. In AD, the complexities of diagnosis and management are further exacerbated by the fact that this is a heterogeneous disease. So far, there are no positive biological markers for the disease or its subtypes. During the next few years, as we learn more about the neurobiology of AD and other dementias and as some of the national efforts to improve diagnostic procedures advance, we should be able to provide better tools to health care professionals.

This volume provides the best practical advice available with respect to diagnosis and management and reports on the progress that is being made in understanding and managing dementing illness.

Zaven S. Khachaturian, Ph.D.

Acknowledgments

My acknowledgements in the first edition of this book were to my department chairman, Kenneth Altshuler, who started me on my career in geriatric psychiatry, and to the John A. Hartford Foundation for its year of support for study with Robert Butler and Kenneth Davis at the Mount Sinai School of Medicine.

I owe much to my current and former colleagues at the University of Texas Southwestern Medical Center's Alzheimer's Disease Center (ADC), including Ron Tintner, Jim Hom, Charles White, III, Munro Cullum, Lawrence Honig, and Roger Rosenberg. The staff of our ADC Clinical Core, led by Doris Svetlik, and including Jackie Rabb, Robbin Peck, Shelly Daniels, Brent Williams, Lynn Shank, Carolyn Trimmer, and Teri Booty, have enabled me to study dementia patients in depth and from many perspectives. The generous support of Marsha Ard and the Ard Family has given me time to do so.

My fellow geriatric psychiatry faculty, Mustafa Husain and Kevin Gray, have also expanded my knowledge, as have the enthusiastic geriatric psychiatry trainees we have had since 1990. Affiliation of our ADC with the Consortium to Establish a Registry for Alzheimer's Disease, led by Albert Heyman, and the Alzheimer's Cooperative Studies Unit, directed by Leon Thal, has enabled me to be involved with skilled clinicians and researchers at the leading edge of clinical research in Alzheimer's disease.

I am grateful for the guidance of Richard Mohs and Steven DeKosky, both of whom have been advisors to our ADC. Creighton Phelps has also been an important source of advice, and Zaven Khachaturian, who kindly consented to do the foreword to this edition, is owed thanks from all who are touched by the specter of dementing illness for his role in promulgating dementia research.

Lawrence Honig kindly reviewed Chapter 4 and reviewed the material on HIV-1–associated dementia complex.

My colleagues and I are heavily indebted to the local and national Alzheimer's associations for their provision of information, support, and advocacy for our patients and their families and to the National Institute on Aging for funding and guiding our ADC and its satellite clinics. Thanks also to Carol Laabs for interfacing effectively with me and my word processor and helping to keep priorities straight and to the American Psychiatric Press for working with me this third time.

My wife Jeanette continues to be patient and understanding.

Myron F. Weiner, M.D.

Introduction

I can think of no better way to introduce this book than with the following words:

> My husband is most often kind, considerate, and understanding. I love him!
>
> But he does not understand my circumstances—
>
> He wants me to drive a strange car—little does he understand the danger involved. The synapses in my brain are not up to making quick decisions, such as a speeding trying to cut around me—or a need to push some crucial button on the dashboard—which takes a minute or 2 to find. In that minute the on coming car has hit me.
>
> (a synapse is the pount [point] where neurons in the brain touch & nerve impulses are transmitted from one to another).
>
> I am certainly sorry that you can't always handle the way I am.
>
> I will try to stay out of your way and be as little trouble to you as possible.
>
> Let me know if you want something!
>
> I love you!

The preceding words were penned by a woman with Alzheimer's disease, who was trying to say that she should not drive a strange car and why she should not. She handed the note to a man she did not recognize as her husband when she wrote it. She did not know that the strange car was the new family car. After all, it was strange to her! She points out that she reacts slowly and would have difficulty locating a "crucial button," and might thereby be a danger to herself and others. She can spell the word *synapse* and knows what it means, but at first she misspells the simple word *point*. She feels sorry for her husband having to put up with her, and writes that she will try not to be a bother. Then, finally recognizing him, she writes that she loves him.

We can see in this woman's words the confusion and fear that she experiences, her attempts to come to grips with her faulty synapses, the difficulty she is beginning to have in expressing herself, and her wish to maintain her loving relationship with her husband.

This is the human experience of Alzheimer's disease, and it is at the heart of the second edition of *The Dementias: Diagnosis, Management, and Research*. This edition, following the first by 4 years, has been revised, updated, and expanded. The revisions are based on critiques of the first edition. The updating and expansion are based on our changes in the classification, management, treatment, and research in dementing illness, and on the wish to include more of the accumulating body of information on dementing illness.

In DSM-IV, published in 1994, the designation of the dementias as organic mental disorders is no more. Instead, dementias are classified by etiology, and *organic* mental disorders are no longer separated from *functional* mental disorders. Also in 1994, formal criteria were proposed for the diagnosis of vascular dementia. Progress has been made in developing behavioral interventions for dementia-related symptoms, and many changes have come about in the pharmacological management of psychiatric symptoms, such as the virtual replacement in elders of tricyclic antidepressant use by selective serotonin reuptake inhibitors. The first FDA-approved cognitive enhancer has become available for prescription, and many others are in development. The genetic basis of Huntington's disease has been identified, and several genetic mutations that appear to be responsible for varieties of familial Alzheimer's disease (AD) have been found. Progress has also been made in unraveling the pathophysiology of AD, and a risk factor for late-onset AD has been identified. And, as will be detailed in Chapter 13, a potential animal model for AD has been developed.

In this book, which is addressed primarily to clinicians, we have attempted to present a broadly based approach to the diagnosis and management of the dementias and to convey some of the excitement of contemporary research. The book is divided into three sections; diagnosis, management, and research. A chapter on nursing issues has been added to the management section. A new research chapter has been added on the biology of AD.

Dementia is a diagnostic term that refers to global impairment of higher cognitive function sufficient to compromise social or work adaptation. Dementia may be accompanied by emotional, behavioral, ideational, perceptual, and vegetative disturbances in addition to impaired cognitive function. Although these cognitive, emotional, behavioral, ideational, perceptual, and vegetative disturbances occur in many different types of dementing illness, certain principles of management and treatment can be generalized.

As with all other physical and mental malfunctions, dementia occurs in a person. Unlike most of the dysfunctions that are classified as diseases, dementia directly attacks the personhood of its victims, robbing them of their ability to understand, communicate, fend for themselves, or do for others. This loss of personhood has been well-described in patients' own words in Cohen and Eisdorfer's *The Loss of Self: A Family Resource for the Care of Alzheimer's Disease and Related Disorders* (1986). Loss of personhood has been described by patients as a painful dismemberment, as drifting away, or as being enveloped by a hazy curtain. Ultimately, it is an alienation from self and others. Many individuals are unaware of their progressive loss of function and do not appear to struggle against it. Those who struggle against dementia, trying to remember what was once familiar or trying to grasp new situations, experience enormous emotional pain. Those of us who work with so-called neurotic patients know that failure to live up to an overinflated ideal self causes much psychological suffering. Surely, loss of the ability to be one's self must be several orders of magnitude more painful. Yet, such pain goes largely unnoticed by clinicians who deal with their inability to reverse many dementia syndromes by addressing themselves only to managing disturbing symptoms.

The pain is aggravated by clinicians addressing family members as though the dementia patient were not present. The perception of many who work with these patients is that the remnants of a person can often be detected through the distorting effects of perceptual and cognitive impairment. Such persons can often be reached, if not through spoken language, through tone of voice or physical contact. It is difficult to convey my experience, as a physician, of having momentarily touched another person, drifting out of contact with his or her world yet being able to experience me as an important point of contact in the world that is being lost. This experience, at once painful and gratifying, is the essence of the patient-physician relationship: maintaining both hope and human contact. Patients and their families are grateful to physicians or other clinicians who allow themselves to be "in touch" in this way and bond strongly with those who are willing to do so. For all health care providers, it is distressing to be unable to alleviate symptoms or cure disease. It is important to realize that, although patients have the same wishes as health care providers, they also see providers in the role of comforter and companion in dealing with the fading of their self-awareness and consciousness.

Having addressed briefly the impact of dementia on the person, let us now look at the larger picture.

Dementia is most common in elderly persons. Estimated conservatively, the prevalence of severe dementia approximates 4% in persons over the age of 65 years; approximately 1% of the elderly population develop dementia each year. The cumulative risk of developing severe dementia may reach 20% by age 80 years (Mortimer 1983). In a study

(Paykel et al. 1994) performed in England, incidence rates for dementia were 2.3% for persons age 75–79 years, 4.6% for age 80–84 years, and 8.5% for age 85–89 years, approximately doubling every 5 years. Twenty-five million Americans (11% of the total population) are now 65 years of age or older. By the 21st century, there will be approximately 31 million Americans 65 years of age or older, and 13 million will probably be older than 75 years (Rowe and Katzman 1992).

If we accept Khachaturian's estimate of 4 million present-day AD cases (see Foreword), we can anticipate 5 million AD cases by the year 2000 based on the population growth figures cited above. If AD (including mixed AD and vascular dementia) accounts for approximately 56% of dementia cases (Folstein et al. 1991), the total number of elderly dementia cases will swell by the year 2000 to nearly 9 million.

Dementing disorders are not confined to old age. Dementia is a common consequence of alcoholism in middle age, of head injury in youth and early adulthood, and of acquired immunodeficiency syndrome (AIDS) at all ages (Weiler et al. 1988).

Working with these patients, their families, and other caregivers requires a basis in medicine, pharmacology, cognitive and behavioral assessment, psychodynamics, family interaction, and systems management—an integration of biopsychosocial information that must be applied to address concomitantly the biological, psychological, and social spheres. Effective diagnosis and management call for collaborative interaction between primary care physicians, psychiatrists, neurologists, psychologists, nurses, social workers, physical and occupational therapists, lawyers, nursing home administrators, and other persons concerned with various aspects of family life, rehabilitation, and extended care.

Of utmost importance is the establishment of a diagnosis: whether cognitive decline is actually present (and, if so, determination of its etiology) and whether it is fixed, likely to progress, or reversible. On the other hand, diagnosis is never regarded as being fully established or as excluding other diagnoses. It is unwise to presume that an apparent progression of dementia is always due to the illness originally diagnosed. Various systemic illnesses aggravate preexisting dementias, and treating urinary tract infections, pneumonia, and congestive heart failure can alleviate these aggravating factors.

Management strategy depends on 1) whether the dementia is reversible, 2) the individual, 3) the individual's life situation, 4) the demands made on the individual, and 5) the amount and nature of support available. Management involves families and community resources as well. Complicated emotional, legal, and ethical decisions must often be faced at different points in the evolution of a dementing illness.

Early on, there are important role changes between child and parent or spouse and spouse; later, a decision may need to be made regarding nursing home placement that stirs up separation and abandonment issues in family members. Legal issues include power of attorney or guardianship. Ethical issues may involve decisions on, for example, the inclusion of a loved one in antemortem and postmortem scientific research or feeding by nasogastric tube or gastrostomy.

Health care professionals help to maintain patients' and families' hope while encouraging them to be realistic in terms of each patient's illness. Those who deal with dementia patients and their families need skill in working with individuals, families, and other professionals. Humane, effective care of dementia patients is one of the important challenges facing the next few generations of health care providers.

I hope this book conveys the enthusiasm of those of us who deal with dementia patients and their families daily. I have never found a more appreciative, cooperative, or responsible group of individuals.

CHAPTER 1

Diagnosis of Dementia

Myron F. Weiner, M.D.

The diagnosis of dementia is based on the appearance of certain signs and symptoms long associated with impairment of higher central nervous system (CNS) activity. The term *dementia* is derived from the Latin *de* (out of) + *mens* (mind) + *ia* (state of); its literal meaning is a state of being out of or deprived of one's mind. The historical origin of the term is unclear. Although attributed to Celsus in the first century A.D. (Lipowski 1980), the term does not appear in an English translation of Celsus's *De Medicina* (100/1756). The poet Juvenal, in the first or second century, is alleged to have used *dementia* in reference to the mental decrepitude of old age (Lipowski 1980). The term was used through the nineteenth century to designate mental impairment of many kinds (Thomas 1889). The first reference to *senile dementia* was made in the second century by Aretaeus, who used the term *dotage* to mean "a torpor of the senses and a stupefaction of the gnostic and intellectual faculties" (Aretaeus 200/1861, p. 301).

Pinel (1806/1962) used the term (in French, *demence*) to designate one of the five general classes of mental derangement. Although described as the derangement that abolishes the thinking faculty, dementia appeared to refer to what are called schizophrenia and the psychotic disorders in DSM-IV. Pinel's class of mental derangement that most closely corresponds to what we now call cognitive disorders or mental disorders due to a general medical condition was *idiotism*, which was defined as an "obliteration of the intellectual faculties and affections" (Pinel 1806/1962, p. 165). Pinel's student, Esquirol (1845/1965), used *dementia* to describe mental disorders that manifested by weakened sensibility, understanding, and will, with impaired recent memory, attention, reasoning, and abstracting ability. He described the dementias as acute, chronic, and senile and included end-stage psychoses and stuporous depression

1

in this category. Benjamin Rush (1812) used the term *fatuity* to designate the mental disorders characterized primarily by impaired reasoning and memory.

Prichard (1837) suggested that dementia might be primary or secondary to other disorders and described a four-stage natural history of dementia, beginning with loss of recent memory with preservation of remote memory. In the second stage, there was loss of reason; in the third, loss of comprehension; and in the fourth, loss of ability to care for vegetative functions. He did not regard dementia as a normal consequence of old age.

Kraepelin (1913) more effectively sorted out the functional psychoses from the consequences of obvious brain damage, calling the former the insanities and the latter varieties of imbecility. The two categories of imbecility were *acquired* imbecility (or dementia) and *congenital* (or ordinary) imbecility. The dementia category included apoplectic dementia due to vascular disease, old age (or senility), and epilepsy.

Bleuler (1924) defined an *organic psychosyndrome* as a set of behavioral manifestations of chronic, diffuse damage to the cerebral cortex. Its manifestations were impaired memory, judgment, perceptual discrimination, orientation, emotional stability, and impulse control. He recognized that all cognitive functions were not equally affected and that practiced (overlearned) abilities were the most resistant to deterioration. The current psychiatric nomenclature embodies the concepts of Bleuler and many earlier workers but attempts to be more precise.

DSM-IV Mental Disorders

Traditionally, dementia was classified as an "organic mental disorder," a constellation of cognitive, behavioral, and emotional symptoms resulting from "organic" factors (e.g., demonstrable changes in brain anatomy or physiology). Organic disorders were differentiated from "functional" disorders, in which no alteration in brain anatomy or physiology had been demonstrated or was thought to occur. It is clear that all mental disorders, whether classified as organic or functional, result from brain activity, making distinctions between organic and functional perhaps both superfluous and misleading. For these reasons, the American Psychiatric Association has deleted the diagnostic category of organic mental disorders from its newest *Diagnostic and Statistical Manual of Mental Disorders*, (DSM-IV; American Psychiatric Association 1994).

In DSM-IV, dementia is one of several mental disorders caused by or related to brain disease, general medical conditions, or substance use that result in transient or permanent brain dysfunction. The disorders listed under these three DSM-IV categories are shown in Table 1–1. They are 1) delirium, dementia, and amnestic and other cognitive disorders; 2) mental disorders due to a general medical condition; and 3) substance-related disorders.

Although these disorders are diagnosed as separate entities, they are overlapping symptom complexes. Most are associated with deficits in information registration, encoding, and retrieval. Despite their overlap, correctly diagnosing mental disorder subtype is important because of the differences in treatment and prognosis. In some cases, proper diagnosis is a life-or-death issue, such as differentiating barbiturate withdrawal or acute Wernicke's syndrome from an alcoholic dementia.

Diagnosis of Dementia

The clinical history and the mental status examination are the most important tools in making the diagnosis of dementia. The diagnosis of dementia cannot be made on the basis of radiological, biochemical, or psychological tests alone. Such tests serve to confirm the diagnosis of altered brain function and to help determine the cause of the dementia syndrome. Individuals with dementing illnesses such as Alzheimer's disease (AD) or acquired immunodeficiency syndrome (AIDS) may not meet formal criteria for dementia early in the illness.

Dementia may be defined as a reduction or impairment of multiple cognitive abilities, including memory, sufficient to interfere with self-maintenance, work, or social relationships. This intellectual impairment occurs without clouding of consciousness and may be temporary or permanent. The diagnosis is based on the history (usually supplied by informants other than the patient) and clinical examination. At times, the history and clinical examination will suggest the origin of the dementia, as in the case of a person who has suffered multiple strokes and subsequently demonstrated intellectual decline. At other times, extensive interdisciplinary evaluation and laboratory procedures are required. On rare occasions, brain biopsy is needed for a definitive diagnosis.

Translating the general definition of dementia into a precise clinical entity is difficult because of the enormous variation between individuals. For example, many persons who have declined intellectually may still be able to function at a level comparable to an average person their own age. Therefore, attempts at establishing a diagnosis of dementia are

Table 1–1.   DSM-IV classification

Delirium, Dementia, and Amnestic and Other Cognitive Disorders
Delirium
  Delirium Due to . . . *[Indicate the General Medical Condition]*
  Substance Intoxication Delirium
  Substance Withdrawal Delirium
  Delirium Due to Multiple Etiologies
  Delirium NOS

Dementia
  Dementia of the Alzheimer's Type, With Early Onset [if onset at age 65 or below]
    Uncomplicated
    With Delirium
    With Delusions
    With Depressed Mood
  Specify if: With Behavioral Disturbance

  Dementia of the Alzheimer's Type, With Late Onset [if onset after age 65]
    Uncomplicated
    With Delirium
    With Delusions
    With Depressed Mood
  Specify if: With Behavioral Disturbance

  Vascular Dementia
    Uncomplicated
    With Delirium
    With Delusions
    With Depressed Mood
  Specify if: With Behavioral Disturbance

  Dementia Due to HIV Disease

  Dementia Due to Head Trauma

  Dementia Due to Parkinson's Disease

  Dementia Due to Huntington's Disease

  Dementia Due to Pick's Disease

  Dementia Due to Creutzfeldt-Jakob Disease

  Dementia Due to . . . *[Indicate the General Medical Condition]*

  Substance-Induced Persisting Dementia

  Dementia Due to Multiple Etiologies

  Dementia NOS

Amnestic Disorders

  Amnestic Disorder Due to . . . *[Indicate the General Medical Condition]*
  Specify if: Transient/Chronic
  Substance-Induced Persisting Amnestic Disorder
  Amnestic Disorder NOS

(continued)

Table 1–1.   DSM-IV classification *(continued)*

Other Cognitive Disorders
Cognitive Disorder NOS

Mental Disorders Due to a General Medical Condition Not Elsewhere Classified

Catatonic Disorder Due to . . . *[Indicate the General Medical Condition]*

Personality Change Due to . . . *[Indicate the General Medical Condition]*
Specify if: Labile Type/Disinhibited Type/Aggressive Type/Apathetic Type/Paranoid
Type/Other Type/Combined Type/Unspecified Type

Mental Disorder NOS Due to . . . *[Indicate the General Medical Condition]*

Substance-Related Disorders
Alcohol-Related Disorders

Alcohol Use Disorders
Alcohol Dependence
Alcohol Abuse

Alcohol-Induced Disorders
Alcohol Intoxication
Alcohol Withdrawal
Specify if: With Perceptual Disturbances

Alcohol Intoxication Delirium

Alcohol Withdrawal Delirium

Alcohol-Induced Persisting Dementia

Alcohol-Induced Persisting Amnestic Disorder

Alcohol-Induced Psychotic Disorder
   With Delusions
   With Hallucinations

Alcohol-Induced Mood Disorder

Alcohol-Induced Anxiety Disorder

Alcohol-Induced Sexual Dysfunction

Alcohol-Induced Sleep Disorder

Alcohol-Related Disorder NOS

Amphetamine (or Amphetamine-Like)–Related Disorders

Amphetamine Use Disorders
Amphetamine Dependence
Amphetamine Abuse

Amphetamine-Induced Disorders
Amphetamine Intoxication
Specify if: With Perceptual Disturbances

Amphetamine Withdrawal

Amphetamine Intoxication Delirium

Amphetamine-Induced Psychotic Disorder
   With Delusions
   With Hallucinations

(continued)

Table 1–1. DSM-IV classification *(continued)*

Amphetamine-Induced Mood Disorder

Amphetamine-Induced Anxiety Disorder

Amphetamine-Induced Sexual Dysfunction

Amphetamine-Induced Sleep Disorder

Amphetamine-Related Disorder NOS

Caffeine-Related Disorders

Caffeine-Induced Disorders

Caffeine Intoxication

Caffeine-Induced Anxiety Disorder

Caffeine-Induced Sleep Disorder

Caffeine-Related Disorder NOS

Cannabis-Related Disorders

Cannabis Use Disorders

Cannabis Dependence

Cannabis Abuse

Cannabis-Induced Disorders

Cannabis Intoxication
Specify if: With Perceptual Disturbances

Cannabis Intoxication Delirium

Cannabis-Induced Psychotic Disorder
With Delusions
With Hallucinations

Cannabis-Induced Anxiety Disorder

Cannabis-Related Disorder NOS

Cocaine-Related Disorders

Cocaine Use Disorders

Cocaine Dependence

Cocaine Abuse

Cocaine-Induced Disorders

Cocaine Intoxication
Specify if: With Perceptual Disturbances

Cocaine Withdrawal

Cocaine Intoxication Delirium

Cocaine-Induced Psychotic Disorder
With Delusions
With Hallucinations

Cocaine-Induced Mood Disorder

Cocaine-Induced Anxiety Disorder

(continued)

Table 1–1.   DSM-IV classification *(continued)*

Cocaine-Induced Sexual Dysfunction

Cocaine-Induced Sleep Disorder

Cocaine-Related Disorder NOS

Hallucinogen-Related Disorders

Hallucinogen Use Disorders

Hallucinogen Dependence

Hallucinogen Abuse

Hallucinogen-Induced Disorders

Hallucinogen Intoxication

Hallucinogen Persisting Perception Disorder (Flashbacks)

Hallucinogen Intoxication Delirium

Hallucinogen-Induced Psychotic Disorder
  With Delusions
  With Hallucinations

Hallucinogen-Induced Mood Disorder

Hallucinogen-Induced Anxiety Disorder

Hallucinogen-Related Disorder NOS

Inhalant-Related Disorders

Inhalant Use Disorders

Inhalant Dependence

Inhalant Abuse

Inhalant-Induced Disorders

Inhalant Intoxication

Inhalant Intoxication Delirium

Inhalant-Induced Persisting Dementia

Inhalant-Induced Psychotic Disorder
  With Delusions
  With Hallucinations

Inhalant-Induced Mood Disorder

Inhalant-Induced Anxiety Disorder

Inhalant-Related Disorder NOS

Nicotine-Related Disorders

Nicotine Use Disorder

Nicotine Dependence

Nicotine-Induced Disorder

Nicotine Withdrawal

Nicotine-Related Disorder NOS

(continued)

Table 1–1.   DSM-IV classification *(continued)*

Opioid-Related Disorders

Opioid Use Disorder

  Opioid Dependence

  Opioid Abuse

Opioid-Induced Disorders

  Opioid Intoxication
  Specify if: With Perceptual Disturbances

  Opioid Withdrawal

  Opioid Intoxication Delirium

  Opioid-Induced Psychotic Disorder
    With Delusions
    With Hallucinations

  Opioid-Induced Mood Disorder

  Opioid-Induced Sexual Dysfunction

  Opioid-Induced Sleep Disorder

  Opioid-Related Disorder NOS

Phencyclidine (or Phencyclidine-Like)–Related Disorders

Phencyclidine Use Disorders

  Phencyclidine Dependence

  Phencyclidine Abuse

Phencyclidine-Induced Disorders

  Phencyclidine Intoxication
  Specify if: With Perceptual Disturbances

  Phencyclidine Intoxication Delirium

  Phencyclidine-Induced Psychotic Disorder
    With Delusions
    With Hallucinations

  Phencyclidine-Induced Mood Disorder

  Phencyclidine-Induced Anxiety Disorder

  Phencyclidine-Related Disorder NOS

Sedative-, Hypnotic-, or Anxiolytic-Related Disorders

Sedative, Hypnotic, or Anxiolytic Substance Use Disorders

  Sedative, Hypnotic, or Anxiolytic Dependence

  Sedative, Hypnotic, or Anxiolytic Abuse

Sedative-, Hypnotic-, or Anxiolytic-Induced Disorders

  Sedative, Hypnotic, or Anxiolytic Intoxication

  Sedative, Hypnotic, or Anxiolytic Withdrawal
  Specify if: With Perceptual Disturbances

(continued)

Table 1–1.   DSM-IV classification *(continued)*

Sedative, Hypnotic, or Anxiolytic Intoxication Delirium

Sedative, Hypnotic, or Anxiolytic Withdrawal Delirium

Sedative-, Hypnotic-, or Anxiolytic-Induced Persisting Dementia

Sedative-, Hypnotic-, or Anxiolytic-Induced Persisting Amnestic Disorder

Sedative-, Hypnotic-, or Anxiolytic-Induced Psychotic Disorder
    With Delusions
    With Hallucinations

Sedative-, Hypnotic-, or Anxiolytic-Induced Mood Disorder

Sedative-, Hypnotic-, or Anxiolytic-Induced Anxiety Disorder

Sedative-, Hypnotic-, or Anxiolytic-Induced Sexual Dysfunction

Sedative-, Hypnotic-, or Anxiolytic-Induced Sleep Disorder

Sedative-, Hypnotic-, or Anxiolytic-Related Disorder NOS

Polysubstance-Related Disorder

Polysubstance Dependence

Other (or Unknown) Substance-Related Use Disorders

Other (or Unknown) Substance Use Disorders

Other (or Unknown) Substance Dependence

Other (or Unknown) Substance Abuse

Other (or Unknown) Substance-Induced Disorders

Other (or Unknown) Substance Intoxication   *Specify if:*   With Perceptual Disturbances

Other (or Unknown) Substance Withdrawal   *Specify if:*   With Perceptual Disturbances

Other (or Unknown) Substance-Induced Delirium

Other (or Unknown) Substance-Induced Persisting Dementia

Other (or Unknown) Substance-Induced Persisting Amnestic Disorder

Other (or Unknown) Substance-Induced Psychotic Disorder
    With Delusions
    With Hallucinations

Other (or Unknown) Substance-Induced Mood Disorder

Other (or Unknown) Substance-Induced Anxiety Disorder

Other (or Unknown) Substance-Induced Sexual Dysfunction

Other (or Unknown) Substance-Induced Sleep Disorder

Other (or Unknown) Substance-Related Disorder NOS

Note.   NOS = not otherwise specified.
Source.   Reprinted with permission from American Psychiatric Association: *Diagnostic and Statistical Manual of Mental Disorders,* 4th Editon. Washington, DC, American Psychiatric Association, 1994

best made by comparing a person's present abilities with his or her own past abilities. However, this can usually be accomplished only by the retrospective accounts furnished by patients and their families—accounts that are subject to strong bias. For example, family members often minimize deficits by stating that a loved one who appears demented on clinical examination was never interested in reading or in current events. Individual family members' biases are minimized through the use of multiple informants, and studies show that, with the use of multiple informants and standardized instruments such as the Dementia Questionnaire (see Appendix 1), accurate data can be obtained (Silverman et al. 1986).

The fundamental DSM-IV criteria for dementia are presented in Table 1–2 and include the clinical means to elicit the diagnostic signs and symptoms. Table 1–3 indicates the criteria for diagnosing specific dementias. The DSM-III-R (American Psychiatric Association 1987) and DSM-IV definitions of dementia differ primarily from earlier definitions of the syndrome in that dementia symptoms are no longer regarded as irreversible.

Differential Diagnosis

The differential diagnosis of dementia includes

- Mental retardation
- Other cognitive disorders (delirium, amnestic disorder)
- Disorders due to general medical conditions
- Disorders brought about by the use of substances or exposure to toxins
- Psychiatric disorders

There are many instances in which several disorders affecting mental function coexist. For example, major depression may coexist with dementia. Patients with Down's syndrome often develop AD (Crapper et al. 1975). Also, a dementia may be engrafted on a preexisting psychiatric disorder such as schizophrenia or bipolar disorder.

There have been optimistic reports on the frequency of reversible conditions producing symptoms of dementia (Garcia et al. 1981; Marsden and Harrison 1972). Mild cognitive impairment, especially due to medications or metabolic disorders, is frequently reversible, but a full-blown dementia syndrome is rarely reversible.

Table 1–2. General diagnostic criteria for dementia based on DSM-IV criteria

A. The development of multiple cognitive deficits manifested by both

  (1) memory impairment (inability to learn new information and to recall previously learned information)

   (a) Primary memory can be assessed by digit span forward and in reverse, with a discrepancy of three digits or more suggesting impairment. Secondary memory can be tested by asking the examinee to recall three words presented by the examiner after an interval of 5 minutes. Secondary memory can also be tested by presenting three objects without naming them, covering them up, and asking the examinee to name them 5 minutes later. Another test of short-term memory is to read a short paragraph aloud to the examinee and then ask the examinee to tell what he or she recalls.

   (b) Long-term or tertiary memory is tested by asking for personal information that can be validated by the accompanying person (date of birth, graduation from high school, marriage, etc.) and by asking facts of common knowledge compatible with the examinee's education and cultural background, including questions such as the President of the United States, the immediate past presidents, the state capital, the location of the U.S. Capitol, etc.

  (2) one (or more) of the following cognitive disturbances:

   (a) aphasia (language disturbance) including, in addition to the classic aphasias, difficulty with word finding and confrontational naming. Word finding difficulty is evidenced in advanced dementia by empty speech devoid of nouns and verbs, with relative preservation of socially overlearned speech, such as "how are you?" Earlier, it can be demonstrated by asking the evaluee to name as many animals as possible in 1 minute. Dementia patients will typically name fewer than 10 animals and will often repeat names. They also have difficulty naming the parts of a watch (watch, band, stem, back, crystal), making paraphasic errors (such as strap for band or lens for crystal), or describing functions (for watch stem: it's how you set it) instead.

   (b) apraxia (inability to carry out motor activities despite intact motor function; e.g., strength and coordination), i.e., to draw the face of a clock and set the hands at 10 minutes after 11 (Sunderland et al. 1989)

   (c) agnosia (failure to recognize or identify objects despite intact sensory function)

   (d) disturbance in executive functioning (i.e., planning, organizing, sequencing, abstracting)

    1. Impaired planning, organizing and sequencing are indicated by inability to deal with interpersonal, family and employment-related issues and to describe logically how they might be dealt with. Changes in long-standing habits and personal hygiene may reflect executive dysfunction. The history is the best source of information about executive functioning, but it may also be evaluated by posing problems that individuals might encounter in daily life, such as an overdrawn bank account or a medical emergency. Executive func-

(continued)

Table 1–2.   General diagnostic criteria for dementia based on DSM-IV criteria *(continued)*

tioning can be additionally assessed by asking examinees to perform serial tasks, such as going through the steps of mailing a letter (i.e., folding the paper, inserting it into an envelope, addressing the envelope, placing a stamp on it, and sealing it).

2.   Impaired abstracting ability is evidenced by inability to abstractly categorize the similarity between objects such as a chair and a table, or a knife and a fork, or for highly educated persons, between a poem and a statue or praise and punishment. Impaired abstracting ability is also evidenced by inability to interpret abstractly common proverbs such as, "don't cry over spilled milk" or "the grass always looks greener on the other side of the street." (See Appendix 2 for detailed mental status examination.)

B.   The cognitive deficits in Criteria A1 and A2 each cause significant impairment in social or occupational functioning and represent a significant decline from a previous level of functioning.

C.   The deficits do not occur exclusively during the course of Delirium.

D.   The disturbance is not better accounted for by another Axis I disorder (e.g., Major Depressive Disorder, Schizophrenia)

In a review of 32 studies of 2,889 cognitively impaired patients with a mean age of 72 years, Clairfield (1988) found clinical diagnoses of AD in 56.8%, vascular dementia (VaD) in 13.3%, depression in 4.5%, alcohol-induced dementia in 4.2%, and drugs in 1.5% of the patients evaluated. Potentially reversible causes of dementia accounted for 13.2% of the cases, but not all cases of potentially reversible dementia were followed to see whether reversal actually occurred. In the 11 studies that provided follow-up, 8% of the dementias resolved partially, and only 3% resolved fully. Reversible causes of dementia included drugs (28%), depression (26%), and toxic-metabolic problems (15.5%). A relationship between potential reversibility and age has also been demonstrated.

Katzman (1992) suggested that *treatable* dementia-producing conditions account for about 10.5% of cases and include neurosyphilis, fungal infections, tumor, alcohol, subdural hematoma, normal-pressure hydrocephalus, and epilepsy. On the other hand, according to Katzman, *reversible* dementias, including drug toxicity, metabolic disorders, hyponatremia, vitamin B$_{12}$ deficiency, hypothyroidism, and hypoglycemia account for only 4.7% of cases. The relation of age to reversibility of dementia has not been established (reviewed by Clairfield 1988).

The most difficult diagnostic issue is the difference between early pathological cognitive decline and normal aging. This is important to many persons who are aware of changes in their cognitive functioning and seek assurance that they are not developing a dementing disease.

Table 1–3. DSM-IV diagnostic criteria for specific dementia syndromes

---

Dementia of the Alzheimer's Type

A. The development of multiple cognitive deficits manifested by both

    (1) memory impairment (inability to learn new information and to recall previously learned information)

    (2) one (or more) of the following cognitive disturbances:

        (a) aphasia (language disturbance)

        (b) apraxia (impaired ability to carry out motor activities despite intact motor function)

        (c) agnosia (failure to recognize or identify objects despite intact sensory function)

        (d) disturbance in executive functioning (i.e., planning, organizing, sequencing, abstracting)

B. The cognitive deficits in Criteria A1 and A2 each cause significant impairment in social or occupational functioning and represent a significant decline from a previous level of functioning.

C. The course is characterized by gradual onset and continuing cognitive decline.

D. The cognitive deficits in Criteria A1 and A2 are not due to any of the following:

    (1) central nervous system conditions that cause progressive deficits in memory and cognition (e.g., cerebrovascular disease, Parkinson's disease, Huntington's disease, subdural hematoma, normal-pressure hydrocephalus, brain tumor)

    (2) systemic conditions that are known to cause dementia (e.g., hypothyroidism, vitamin B_{12} or folic acid deficiency, niacin deficiency, hypercalcemia, neurosyphilis, HIV infection)

    (3) substance-induced conditions

E. The deficits do not occur exclusively during the course of a delirium.

F. The disturbance is not better accounted for by another Axis I disorder (e.g., Major Depressive Disorder, Schizophrenia).

Vascular Dementia

A.–B. See A and B in Dementia of the Alzheimer's Type.

C. Focal neurological signs and symptoms (e.g., exaggeration of deep tendon reflexes, extensor plantar response, pseudobulbar palsy, gait abnormalities, weakness of an extremity) or laboratory evidence indicative of cerebral vascular disease (e.g., multiple infarctions involving cortex and underlying white matter) that are judged to be etiologically related to the disturbance.

D. The deficits do not occur exclusively during the course of a delirium.

Dementia Due to Other General Medical Conditions

A.–B. See A and B in Dementia of the Alzheimer's Type.

C. There is evidence from the history, physical examination, or laboratory findings that the disturbance is the direct physiologic consequence of one of the conditions listed below.

◆ Dementia Due to HIV Disease

◆ Dementia Due to Head Trauma

◆ Dementia Due to Parkinson's Disease

(continued)

⌐ ₁–3. DSM-IV diagnostic criteria for specific dementia syndromes *(continued)*

◆ Dementia Due to Huntington's Disease

◆ Dementia Due to Pick's Disease

◆ Dementia Due to Creutzfeldt-Jakob Disease

◆ Dementia Due to . . . *[Indicate the General Medical Condition not listed above]*

For example, normal-pressure hydrocephalus, hypothyroidism, brain tumor, vitamin B_{12} deficiency, intracranial irradiation

D. The deficits do not occur exclusively during the course of a delirium.

Substance-Induced Persisting Dementia

A.–B. See A–B in Dementia of the Alzheimer's Type.

C. The deficits do not occur exclusively during the course of a delirium and persist beyond the usual duration of Substance Intoxication or Withdrawal.

D. There is evidence from the history, physical examination, or laboratory findings that the deficits are etiologically related to the persisting effects of substance use (e.g., a drug of abuse, a medication).

Dementia Due to Multiple Etiologies

A.–B. See A–B in Dementia of the Alzheimer's Type.

C. There is evidence from the history, physical examination, or laboratory tests that the disturbance has more than one etiology (e.g., head trauma plus chronic alcohol use, Dementia of the Alzheimer's type with the subsequent development of Vascular Dementia).

D. The deficits do not occur exclusively during the course of a delirium.

Dementia Not Otherwise Specified

This category should be used to diagnose a dementia that does not meet criteria for any of the specific types described in this section.

An example is a clinical presentation of dementia for which there is insufficient evidence to establish a specific etiology.

Source. Reprinted with permission from American Psychiatric Association: *Diagnostic and Statistical Manual of Mental Disorders*, 4th Edition. Washington, DC, American Psychiatric Press, 1994. Copyright 1994 American Psychiatric Association.

Normal Aging

Despite the wealth of material that is available on the cognitive changes of normal aging (see also Chapter 7), there is still no sharp distinction between the changes of normal aging and incipient dementia. The cognitive changes of aging vary from individual to individual, however, in general, younger and older adults perform differently on problem-solving tasks. On concept-identification tasks, older persons use less efficient strategies, are less successful at finding solutions, make more errors, and are less likely to change their strategy when their responses are incorrect. Older adults also use less sophisticated strategies on classification and categorization tasks (Reese and Rodeheaver 1985).

Older adults complain often of memory difficulties; 83% report forgetting names frequently, 60% report losing objects such as keys, and 57% report forgetting telephone numbers that were just checked (Bolla et al. 1991). Studies of memory function assessed by digit span show little change in immediate or primary memory with age (Drachman and Leavitt 1972). Encoding and retrieval from recent (secondary) memory appear to decline with normal aging, especially when the information seems irrelevant or nonsensical (Schludermann et al. 1983), but vocabulary, general information, and recall of past historical or personal events (tertiary memory) remain relatively intact (Poon 1985). Thus, healthy elders' memory is generally preserved for relevant, well-learned material, but the ability to process novel information declines. Memory impairment is sufficiently troublesome for many persons over 50 years of age that a specific syndrome of age-associated memory impairment (AAMI) has been described (Blackford and LaRue 1989; Crook et al. 1986). Criteria include complaints of gradual memory loss in tasks of daily life in person of greater than 50 years of age, objective evidence of impairment on a standardized memory test (as compared with the mean established for young adults), evidence of adequate intellectual function, and absence of dementia or any medical condition that could produce cognitive deterioration. AAMI is reported to have variable prevalence at different ages in elders. A Finnish study showed a prevalence of approximately 40% in persons age 60–70 years, with highest prevalence in the younger persons sampled (Koivisto et al. 1995). Although cholinergic and catecholaminergic mechanisms have been postulated (McEntee and Crook 1990), attempts to elucidate the common mechanisms underlying memory decline in old age await the development of cognitive norms for old age, a standardized battery of tests, and establishment of decline by longitudinal testing of individuals. A person with lifelong low scores on memory testing might well be diagnosed with AAMI unless earlier scores were available for comparison (G. Smith et al. 1991).

Slowing down the presentation of new information helps normal elders; cuing helps them retrieve more effectively from recent memory. Neither memory aid is greatly helpful in dementia. Thus, when asking for recall of three words—apple, table, penny—after a 5-minute period of distraction, mentioning fruit, furniture, and coins are associative memory aids that can help distinguish between normal aging changes and dementia. To differentiate "benign" from "malignant" senescent memory dysfunction, Kral (1959) suggested that the benign form involves intermittent inability to recall recent or remote events, whereas the malignant form involves prominent recent memory impairment and disorientation in time.

In my experience, the most sensitive tests for incipient dementia are impaired concentration, impaired recent and remote memory, and loss of the abstract attitude—the latter detected by the similarities and proverbs part of the mental status examination. Proverb interpretation is highly culture bound and may yield false-positive results in persons from other cultures. Performance on similarities, although not culture bound, is related strongly to education and premorbid intelligence. Early in the course of the illness, AD patients may also demonstrate difficulty with object naming (dysnomia) and drawing geometrical figures (constructional dyspraxia).

Mental Retardation

Mental retardation must be considered in the evaluation for dementia. Except when there are obvious stigmata of a syndrome ordinarily associated with mental retardation (such as in Down's syndrome), it is often impossible to distinguish clinically between mental retardation and dementia. The examiner must rely instead on the patient's history by an outside informant. That history usually includes academic failure with early dropout from school, or graduation from a special education program. Job history usually indicates limited skills and limited comprehension. In many instances, educational history can be deceptive. Graduation from an ungraded school, for example, while requiring 10–12 years, may be the equivalent of only a third- or fourth-grade education. In a study of an educationally and socially deprived population (Weiner and Lovitt 1984), there was a definite correlation of intelligence with educational level, but half the individuals with more than 12 years of education had full-scale IQs of less than 85; half the individuals with less than 12 years of education had IQs less than 75. A low level of schooling or limited intelligence markedly impairs performance in the fund of information, abstract reasoning, and judgment aspects of the mental status examination. Two important distinguishing features between developmental disorders and dementia are vocabulary and fund of information, which tend to be less impaired than other aspects of the mental status examination in dementia.

A significant problem for those dealing with mentally retarded persons is the issue of cognitive decline in Down's syndrome patients. Virtually all Down's syndrome patients who live past the age of 35 years demonstrate both the microscopic pathology of AD (reviewed by Mann 1988; Wisniewski et al. 1978) and cognitive deterioration, with severe deterioration of function occurring in 20%–30% (Ball 1987). It is important in this population, as in all others, to seek remediable causes of functional decline such as metabolic abnormalities and psychiatric disorders and to not assume that all cognitive decline seen in these patients is due to AD.

Delirium

Delirium is a state of altered consciousness and cognition, usually of acute onset (hours or days) and of brief duration (days or weeks). Delirium is very common in general hospital patients, with estimates of prevalence ranging from 30%–50% in patients 70 years of age or older (Lipowski 1987). Attention is markedly impaired. Sleep-wake disturbances are common, and there is often reduced or increased psychomotor activity. Visual hallucinations are common, as are tactile hallucinations and illusions. Delirium is usually characterized by generalized electroencephalogram (EEG) slowing, and the course of a delirium can be followed by serial EEGs (Engel and Romano 1959). The DSM-IV criteria for delirium are presented in Table 1–4.

Dementia and delirium frequently coexist, with dementia serving as a predisposing factor (Gustafson et al. 1988). In many individuals, the first sign of a dementing illness is postoperative delirium. Delirium differs from dementia in that delirium has a rapid onset and has a greater degree of personality disorganization and clouding of consciousness. Fluctuating cognitive ability occurs in dementia but not to the extent that it occurs in delirium. Dementia patients usually give their best cognitive performance early in the day when they are not fatigued, under circumstances in which they do not feel challenged or anxious. With the waning of sensory cues at night, many dementia patients become transiently delirious, a phenomenon often referred to as *sundowning*. The diagnosis of dementia cannot be made in the presence of delirium; the patient must be clear of the acute disturbance.

Amnestic Disorder

In this uncommon disorder, the primary manifestation is memory impairment. The DSM-IV diagnostic criteria for amnestic disorder are presented in Table 1–5. The most common cause is thiamine deficiency

Table 1–4. DSM-IV criteria for delirium

Delirium Due to . . . *[Indicate the General Medical Condition]*

A. Disturbance of consciousness (i.e., reduced clarity of awareness of the environment) with reduced ability to focus, sustain, or shift attention.

B. Change in cognition (such as memory deficit, disorientation, language disturbance disturbance) or the development of a perceptual disturbance that is not better accounted for by a preexisting, established, or evolving dementia.

C. The disturbance develops over a short period of time (usually hours to days) and tends to fluctuate during the course of the day.

D. There is evidence from the history, physical examination, or laboratory findings that the disturbance is caused by the direct physiological consequences of a general medical condition.

Substance Intoxication Delirium

A.–C. See A–C in Delirium Due to . . . *[Indicate the General Medical Condition]*

D. There is evidence from the history, physical examination, or laboratory findings of either (1) or (2):

(1) the symptoms in Criteria A and B developed during Substance Intoxication

(2) medication use is etiologically related to the disturbance

Substance Withdrawal Delirium

A.–C. See A–C in Delirium Due to . . . *[Indicate the General Medical Condition]*

D. There is evidence from the history, physical examination, or laboratory findings that the symptoms in Criteria A and B developed during, or shortly after, a withdrawal syndrome.

Delirium Due to Multiple Etiologies

A.–C. See A–C in Delirium Due to . . . *[Indicate the General Medical Condition]*

D. There is evidence from the history, physical examination, or laboratory findings that the delirium has more than one etiology (e.g., more than one etiological general medical condition, a general medical condition plus Substance Intoxication or medication side effect).

Delirium Not Otherwise Specified

Examples include

1. A clinical presentation of delirium that is suspected to be due to a general medical condition or substance use but for which there is insufficient evidence to establish specific etiology

2. Delirium due to causes not listed above (e.g., sensory deprivation)

Source. Reprinted with permission from American Psychiatric Association: *Diagnostic and Statistical Manual of Mental Disorders,* 4th Edition. Washington, DC, American Psychiatric Press, 1994. Copyright 1994 American Psychiatric Association.

associated with chronic alcohol abuse. Persons with Korsakoff's syndrome (in DSM-IV, Substance-Induced Persisting Amnestic Disorder due to Alcohol) differ from those with AD in that the former may recall rules and principles for organizing information and have access to previously acquired knowledge with impairment of recent memory, whereas the latter may have little access to previously acquired information and may

Table 1–5. DSM-IV criteria for amnestic disorder

Amnestic Disorder Due to . . . [Indicate the General Medical Condition]

A. The development of memory impairment as manifested by impairment in the ability to learn new information or the inability to recall previously learned information.

B. The memory disturbance causes significant impairment in social or occupational functioning and represents a significant decline from a previous level of functioning.

C. The memory disturbance does not occur exclusively during the course of a delirium or a dementia.

D. There is evidence from the history, physical examination, or laboratory findings that the disturbance is the direct physiological consequence of a general medical condition (including physical trauma).

Substance-Induced Persisting Amnestic Disorder

A.–B. See A–B in Amnestic Disorder Due to . . . [Indicate the General Medical Condition]

C. The memory disturbance does not occur exclusively during the course of a delirium or a dementia and persists beyond the usual duration of Substance Intoxication or Withdrawal.

D. There is evidence from the history, physical examination, or laboratory findings that the memory disturbance is etiologically related to the persisting effects of substance use (e.g., a drug of abuse, a medication).

Amnestic Disorder Not Otherwise Specified

An example is a clinical presentation of amnesia for which there is insufficient evidence to establish a specific etiology (i.e., dissociative, substance induced, or due to a general medical condition).

Source. Reprinted with permission from American Psychiatric Association: *Diagnostic and Statistical Manual of Mental Disorders,* 4th Edition. Washington, DC, American Psychiatric Press, 1994. Copyright 1994 American Psychiatric Association.

therefore have difficulty encoding ongoing events (Weingartner et al. 1983). Amnestic disorder patients often meet criteria for dementia, with the exception of patients with brief amnestic episodes that occur with the short-acting benzodiazepines lorazepam and triazolam. Bilateral lesions of the hippocampus appear to impair recent memory without impairing remote memory (Scoville and Milner 1957; Zola-Morgan et al. 1986). The importance of considering amnestic disorders in differential diagnosis is that they are reversible in the case of minor tranquilizers and partly reversible in thiamine deficiency–based Wernicke's encephalopathy seen in alcoholic patients or in nutritionally deprived persons.

Psychotic Disorder Due to a General Medical Condition

The DSM-IV diagnostic criteria for psychotic disorder due to a general medical condition are presented in Table 1–6. Hallucinations and delusions are the most common symptoms of this disorder. The following case, which is probably a combination of AD with other medical problems, is typical.

> Mrs. M. was an 84-year-old woman who had been delusional for 3 years. Her delusions seemingly began when her memory started to fail. She insisted that her husband was consorting with prostitutes and that he was trying to drive her crazy so that he could get rid of her.
>
> Mrs. M. had been jealous of her husband for nearly all of their 58-year marriage, beginning a year after the birth of their daughter, when he confessed a marital infidelity. He continued to be unfaithful, and she continued to accuse him of having affairs. In the 3 years prior to her evaluation, she developed increasing difficulty with her memory. Her emotions became increasingly labile, and at times she threatened her husband with physical harm. She was eating poorly and had reversed her sleep-wake cycle.
>
> She was hospitalized for evaluation, where physical examination revealed a cachectic woman with marked hearing impairment and marked visual impairment due to cataracts. Laboratory testing showed a macrocytic anemia, vitamin B_{12} level of 79 pg/ml, folic acid of 1.3 ng/ml, and low serum iron concentration. Mental status examination showed impaired concentration, impaired recent and remote memory, and markedly reduced fund of information. Her Mini-Mental State Exam score was 14. She became more tractable in a structured environment on an adequate diet, multiple vitamins with iron, and parenteral vitamin B_{12} but was transferred to a nursing home because it was believed that her husband could not manage her care adequately from a physical standpoint.

Mood Disorder Due to a General Medical Condition

Mood disorder due to a general medical condition and substance-induced mood disorder can be confused with dementia because of the many overlapping signs of both dementia and depression. The essential feature of this disorder is prominent and persistent mood alteration associated with a general medical condition. Carcinoma of the pancreas, viral illness, and stroke can cause depression. Hyper- and hypothyroidism and hyper- and hypoadrenocorticism can cause depression or mania. The DSM-IV criteria for mood disorder due to a general medical condition are listed in Table 1–6. The importance of this disorder is that it remits when the underlying cause is treated.

Table 1–6. DSM-IV criteria for mental disorders due to a general medical condition

Psychotic Disorder Due to . . . *Indicate the General Medical Condition*

A.   Prominent hallucinations or delusions.

B.   There is evidence from the history, physical examination, or laboratory findings that the disturbance is the direct physiological consequence of a general medical condition.

C.   The disturbance is not better accounted for by another mental disorder.

D.   The disturbance does not occur exclusively during the course of a delirium or dementia.

Mood Disorder
Due to . . . *[Indicate the General Medical Condition]*

A.   A prominent and persistent disturbance in mood predominates in the clinical picture and is characterized by either (or both) of the following:

(1)depressed mood or markedly diminished interest or pleasure in all, or almost all, activities
(2)elevated, expansive, or irritable mood

B.   There is evidence from the history, physical examination, or laboratory findings that the disturbance is the direct physiological consequence of a general medical condition.

C.   The disturbance is not better accounted for by another mental disorder (e.g., Adjustment Disorder With Depressed Mood in response to the stress of having a general medical condition).

D.   The disturbance does not occur exclusively during the course of a delirium.

E.   The symptoms cause clinically significant distress or impairment in social, occupational, or other important areas of functioning.

Anxiety Disorder Due to . . . *[Indicate the General Medical Condition]*

A.   Prominent anxiety, panic attacks, or obsessions or compulsions predominate in the clinical picture.

B.   See B in mood disorder due to . . . *[indicate the general medical condition].*

C.   The disturbance is not better accounted for by another mental disorder (e.g., Adjustment Disorder With Anxiety in which the stressor is a serious general medical condition).

D.–E.   See D–E in mood disorder due to . . . *[indicate the general medical condition].*

Catatonic Disorder Due to . . . *[Indicate the General Medical Condition]*

A.   The presence of catatonia as manifested by motoric immobility, excessive motor activity (that is apparently purposeless and not influenced by external stimuli), extreme negativism or mutism, peculiarities of voluntary movement, or echolalia or echopraxia.

B.   See B in mood disorder due to . . . *[indicate the general medical condition].*

C.   The disturbance is not better accounted for by another mental disorder (e.g., a Manic Episode).

D.   The disturbance does not occur exclusively during the course of a delirium.

(continued)

Table 1–6.   DSM-IV criteria for mental disorders due to a general
medical condition *(continued)*

Personality Change Due to . . . *[Indicate the General Medical Condition]*

A.   A persistent personality disturbance that represents a change from the individual's previous characteristic personality pattern. (In children, the disturbance involves a marked deviation from normal development or a significant change in the child's usual behavior patterns lasting at least 1 year).

B.   See B in mood disorder due to . . . *[indicate the general medical condition].*

C.   The disturbance is not better accounted for by another mental disorder (including other Mental Disorders Due to a General Medical Condition).

D.   The disturbance does not occur exclusively during the course of a delirium and does not meet criteria for a dementia.

E.   The disturbance causes clinically significant distress or impairment in social, occupational, or other important areas of functioning.

Mental Disorder Not Otherwise Specified Due to a General Medical Condition

This residual category should be used for situations in which it has been established that the disturbance is caused by the direct physiological effects of a general medical condition, but the criteria are not met for a specific Mental Disorder Due to a General Medical Condition (e.g., dissociative symptoms due to complex partial seizures).

Source.   Reprinted with permission from American Psychiatric Association: *Diagnostic and Statistical Manual of Mental Disorders,* 4th Edition. Washington, DC, American Psychiatric Press, 1994. Copyright 1994 American Psychiatric Association.

Substance-Induced Mood Disorder

This disorder is characterized by prominent and persistent mood alteration associated with substance use. Depressive symptoms may be caused by drugs such as reserpine, methyldopa, beta-blockers, and some of the hallucinogens. Exogenous steroids can cause depression or mania. This condition usually remits when the causative agent is withdrawn. The DSM-IV criteria for substance-induced mood disorder are listed in Table 1–7.

Anxiety Disorder Due to a General Medical Condition

Generalized anxiety or recurrent panic attacks are the chief characteristics of such anxiety disorders, which characteristically impair concentration. Endocrine disorders such as hyper- and hypothyroidism, pheochromocytoma, hypercortisolism, and fasting hypoglycemia are potential causative factors, along with a host of others. DSM-IV criteria for anxiety disorder due to a general medical condition are listed in Table 1–6.

Many persons with dementia become distressed or anxious when their cognitive and adaptive abilities are challenged. Often, the distress or anxiety is expressed through reiteration of physical complaints when intellectually challenged or emotionally stressed. Overt dysphoria is most common early in the course of a dementing illness. As dementia progresses, anxiety appears to diminish. This may occur because the ability to anticipate real or symbolic danger becomes impaired or because patients' ability to communicate anxiety diminishes.

Personality Change Due to a General Medical Condition

The greatest impact of a general medical condition may be exaggeration of preexisting personality traits or a change in personality instead of obvious intellectual impairment. There are many patterns, but emotional instability, recurrent outbursts of aggression or rage, impaired social judgment, apathy, suspiciousness, and paranoid ideation are frequent.

Table 1–7. DSM-IV diagnostic criteria for substance-induced mood disorder

---

A. A prominent and persistent disturbance in mood predominates in the clinical picture and is characterized by either (or both) of the following:

    (1) depressed mood or markedly diminished interest or pleasure in all, or almost all, activities

    (2) elevated, expansive, or irritable mood

B. There is evidence from the history, physical examination, or laboratory findings of either (1) or (2):

    (1) the symptoms in Criterion A developed during, or within a month of, Substance Intoxication or Withdrawal

    (2) medication use is etiologically related to the disturbance

C. The disturbance is not better accounted for by a Mood Disorder that is not substance induced. Evidence that the symptoms are better accounted for by a Mood Disorder that is not substance induced might include the following: the symptoms precede the onset of the substance use (or medication use); the symptoms persist for a substantial period of time (e.g., about a month) after the cessation of acute withdrawal or severe intoxication or are substantially in excess of what would be expected given the type or amount of the substance used or the duration of use; or there is other evidence that suggests the existence of an independent non-substance-induced Mood Disorder (e.g., a history of recurrent Major Depressive Episodes).

D. The disturbance does not occur exclusively during the course of a delirium.

E. The symptoms cause clinically significant distress or impairment in social, occupational, or other important areas of functioning.

Source. Reprinted with permission from American Psychiatric Association: *Diagnostic and Statistical Manual of Mental Disorders*, 4th Edition. Washington, DC, American Psychiatric Press, 1994. Copyright 1994 American Psychiatric Association.

Brain tumors, head trauma, multiple sclerosis, and strokes are common causes of personality changes. The above symptoms may also occur as interictal phenomena in temporal lobe epilepsy. The DSM-IV criteria for personality change due to a general medical condition are presented in Table 1–6.

Although many such cases do not meet criteria for dementia at first glance, detailed examination usually shows diffuse deficit, as the following case illustrates:

> Mr. M., a 69-year-old man, was referred for evaluation by his wife and son, who complained that he talked to himself, did "silly things," failed to maintain his personal hygiene, and didn't pay his bills on time. Mr. M. was a college graduate who had worked at a military installation until he contracted viral encephalitis at 44 years of age. He was comatose for a week and experienced residual weakness and slowness of motion. His personality changed. He became highly emotional and negativistic. At age 66 years, he suffered a right-hemisphere stroke that mildly weakened the left side of his body and impaired his speech for a short time.
>
> On psychiatric examination, Mr. M. was noted to be poorly groomed. His speech and language were normal, but he tended to engage in long diatribes. He laughed at inappropriate times during the interview. Difficulty with concentration was detected with serial subtraction. Recent and remote memory appeared intact. His construction ability was good. He was able to abstractly categorize the similarity between an egg and a seed but was unable to interpret simple proverbs. He was well versed on current events but had difficulty when asked to think of an appropriate course of action for dealing with a medical emergency.
>
> Neuropsychological testing revealed a verbal IQ of 117, a performance IQ of 94, and a full-scale score of 108—a performance surpassing 70% of his age peers. There was great scatter in his verbal intellectual abilities from below average to superior. He had difficulty with tasks requiring attention to verbally presented material. His perceptual motor abilities were much poorer, ranging from mentally defective to average. He had difficulty with sequencing social stimuli and with understanding part-whole relationships. He performed poorly on complex verbal problem solving and had mild to moderate difficulty with short- and long-term verbal memory. Language, communication, and constructional abilities were intact.

Other Cognitive Disorders

Cognitive disorder not otherwise specified (NOS) is a diagnosis for disorders that are characterized by cognitive dysfunction presumed to be due to the direct physiological effect of a general medical condition that do not meet criteria for any type of delirium, dementia, or amnestic disorder. Examples include impairment in cognitive functioning as evidenced by neuropsychological testing or quantified clinical assessment, accompanied by objective evidence of a systemic illness or central nervous system dysfunction; postconcussional disorder; and impairment in memory or attention with associated symptoms after a head trauma.

Major Depression

Major depression is the most important psychiatric disorder to be considered in the diagnostic evaluation of a person with a suspected dementia, either as a primary diagnosis or as a complication of an underlying disease. In my experience in a dementia clinic, depressive syndromes are a common cause of cognitive impairment in persons without demonstrable brain pathology, but major depression is a rare complication of AD. Of 317 consecutive cases in our dementia clinic, 19 (6%) had little or no evidence of brain disease or damage. In that group, 8 (42%) were thought to have depression-related cognitive impairment. In the 192 cases diagnosed as probable or possible AD, only 4 (2%) were thought to be depressed; of those, only 2 (1%) met DSM-III-R criteria for major depression (Weiner et al. 1991). By contrast, there is a 20%–25% prevalence of major depression in the first 2 years after stroke (Robinson and Forrester 1987), and depression is also frequent in Parkinson's disease (Mayeux et al. 1981).

It is clear that depressed patients suffer cognitive impairment, although the severity of their impairment does not always correspond with the severity of their depressive symptoms. Much attention has been paid to this phenomenon of *pseudodementia*, a term attributed by Bleuler (1924) to Wernicke in the 1880s and later resurrected by Kiloh (1961).

Cognitive processes susceptible to depression are attention, perception, speed of cognitive response, problem solving, memory, and learning. Depressed patients appear to use weak or incomplete strategies to encode events to be remembered. If depressed patients are provided organization and structure, memory deficits disappear (Weingartner et al. 1981). The cognitive and motor tasks most impaired are those requiring sustained effort (R. M. Cohen et al. 1982). Depressed patients tend to show impaired recent memory without impaired long-term memory. Short-term memory deficits are correctable by successfully treating the depression with antidepressants (Sternberg and Jarvik 1976). Scores on the Mini-Mental State Exam (Folstein et al. 1975) improved in depressed elders after successful treatment with antidepressants or electroconvulsive therapy (Greenwald et al. 1989). The response of both depressive and cognitive symptoms to antidepressant treatment does not firmly establish elderly patients' sole diagnosis as depression. Of 23 patients who had amelioration of cognitive symptoms with treatment of their depression, nearly half went on to develop a dementing illness (Alexopoulos et al. 1993).

DSM-IV criteria for a major depressive episode are presented in Table 1–8. The difference between the cognitive impairment of depression and that due to structural or metabolic brain disorder is based on the following:

1. Onset of depressive symptoms preceding cognitive impairment
2. Sudden, fairly recent (weeks or months), and often identifiable onset of cognitive impairment, both in terms of time and emotionally important life events (loss of job or spouse)
3. Patients stressing inability to think, concentrate, and remember
4. Signs and symptoms of depression
5. Objective cognitive testing showing patients' deficits to be less severe than their complaints, with performance improved by encouragement, cuing, and structure
6. Depressed patients more commonly giving "I don't know" answers in contrast to dementia patients, who make near misses, confabulate, or perseverate answers
7. Normal EEG
8. Absence of any condition known to affect brain function

Radiological evidence of mild generalized brain atrophy is not helpful in differentiating depression from dementia in elderly persons. The dexamethasone suppression test (DST) (Carroll et al. 1981) is also not useful in distinguishing depression from dementia. The DST is positive in 40%–70% of melancholic depressive patients (Rubin and Poland 1984), but it is also frequently positive in AD and VaD. Jenike and Albert (1984) and Greenwald et al. (1986) both found nonsuppression rates of approximately 27% in AD. Balldin et al. (1983) found nonsuppression in 57% of AD patients and 73% of VaD patients.

As indicated in Chapter 7, neuropsychological testing can be very helpful in distinguishing depression from structural or metabolic brain disorder and in identifying depression in a dementia patient.

Other Psychiatric Disorders

The Ganser syndrome is subsumed in DSM-IV under the heading of Dissociative Disorders NOS. In this syndrome, ludicrous approximate answers or responses are made to simple questions or commands, indicating that the questions are clearly understood and that deliber-

---

Table 1–8.   DSM-IV criteria for major depressive episode

Criteria for Major Depressive Episode

A.   Five (or more) of the following symptoms have been present during the same 2-week period and represent a change from previous functioning; at least one of the symptoms is either (1) depressed mood or (2) loss of interest or pleasure.

   Note: Do not include symptoms that are clearly due to a general medical condition, or mood-incongruent delusions or hallucinations.

   (1)   depressed mood most of the day, nearly every day, as indicated by either subjective report (e.g., feels sad or empty) or observation made by others (e.g., appears tearful).   **Note:** In children and adolescents, can be irritable mood.
   (2)   markedly diminished interest or pleasure in all, or almost all, activities most of the day, nearly every day (as indicated by either subjective account or observation made by others)
   (3)   significant weight loss when not dieting or weight gain (e.g., a change of more than 5% of body weight in a month), or decrease or increase in appetite nearly every day.   **Note:** In children, consider failure to make expected weight gains.
   (4)   insomnia or hypersomnia nearly every day
   (5)   psychomotor agitation or retardation nearly every day (observable by others, not merely subjective feelings of restlessness or being slowed down)
   (6)   fatigue or loss of energy nearly every day
   (7)   feelings of worthlessness or excessive or inappropriate guilt (which may be delusional) nearly every day (not merely self-reproach or guilt about being sick)
   (8)   diminished ability to think or concentrate, or indecisiveness, nearly every day (either by subjective account or as observed by others)
   (9)   recurrent thoughts of death (not just fear of dying), recurrent suicidal ideation without a specific plan, or a suicide attempt or a specific plan for committing suicide

B.   The symptoms do not meet criteria for a Mixed Episode.

C.   The symptoms cause clinically significant distress or impairment in social, occupational, or other important areas of functioning.

D.   The symptoms are not due to the direct physiological effects of a substance (e.g., a drug of abuse, a medication) or a general medical condition (e.g., hypothyroidism).

E.   The symptoms are not better accounted for by Bereavement, i.e., after the loss of a loved one, the symptoms persist for longer than 2 months or are characterized by marked functional impairment, morbid preoccupation with worthlessness, suicidal ideation, psychotic symptoms, or psychomotor retardation.

Source.   Reprinted with permission from American Psychiatric Association: *Diagnostic and Statistical Manual of Mental Disorders,* 4th Edition. Washington, DC, American Psychiatric Press, 1994. Copyright 1994 American Psychiatric Association.

ately incorrect responses are being given (Goldin and MacDonald 1955). When asked to add 2 and 2, the answer may be 5. The sum of 3 and 3 may be stated as 7. When asked to point upward, the patient may point down and then point up when asked to point down. The Ganser syndrome is frequently accompanied by complaints of auditory and visual hallucinations, circumscribed amnesia, and disorientation. These symptoms develop rapidly and usually occur in response to a severe environmental stressor, such as facing imprisonment. This syndrome is short-lived and requires essentially no active treatment.

Impaired cognition may also be malingered for various types of gain. The effects of trivial head injuries may be magnified to escape hard labor or to gain monetary compensation. Mental status examination and neuropsychological testing of the individual who is malingering impaired cognition show inconsistent deficits, with better performance on many items that call for high-level integration than on some items calling for lesser levels of cognitive function. For example, simple similarities will not be understood, whereas more complicated similarities will call forth an abstract response, or digit span, a simple test of attention, will be limited to three digits, whereas the patient can follow complicated directions to the rest room.

Schizophrenia and bipolar disorder are discussed in Chapter 4.

Language Disorders

Language disorders due to brain damage (aphasias) are easily confused with dementia. The categorization of aphasias is based on the language functions (i.e., fluency, comprehension, repetition, and naming) they impair. Global aphasia impairs all language functions and occurs in large left-hemisphere strokes. Anomic aphasia, by contrast, primarily affects word finding, may be related to lesions of the left angular or left posterior middle temporal gyrus, and is common in AD. Broca's (anterior, nonfluent) aphasia impairs verbal fluency, repetition, and naming and results from lesions of the posterior inferior portion of the left (or dominant) frontal lobe (Benson 1985). In Broca's aphasia, speech requires great effort, and the speaker omits word modifiers such as articles, prepositions, and conjunctions. For example, a person who wants to go to the bathroom might say, "Want . . . go . . . bath . . . room," with great effort and great relief after having expressed him- or herself. These patients generally understand what is said to them and can obey commands but have difficulty with repetition, reading aloud, and writing.

Although they have difficulty with naming, they are helped by prompting. Wernicke's (posterior, fluent) aphasia patients have fluent paraphasic, neologistic speech with poor comprehension, repetition, and naming. The naming difficulty is not usually aided by prompting. Reading and writing are also impaired. The sentence "I want to go to the bathroom" might be rendered by a posterior aphasic patient as "I wish to go to the you-know bath place now soon," with no awareness of the peculiarity of his or her speech. The brain damage in this syndrome is to the posterior superior portion of the first temporal gyrus of the dominant hemisphere. Other aphasia syndromes are transcortical motor (impaired fluency and naming), transcortical sensory (impaired comprehension and naming), conduction (impaired repetition and naming), and mixed transcortical aphasia—a combination of transcortical sensory and transcortical motor aphasias that leaves patients able only to echo speech (Cummings 1985).

The history of aphasia patients will usually reveal an obvious brain insult, most often stroke or head trauma. There are usually also neurological deficits such as hemiparesis (especially in the Broca type), unilateral hyperreflexia, and visual field deficits. On the other hand, there have been reports of slowly progressive aphasia without historical evidence of brain insult or localizing neurological signs Mesulam 1982). In addition, there have been reports of slowly progressive familial Morris et al. 1994) and nonfamilial (Mehler et al. 1987) aphasias leading to dementia. (For a more detailed discussion of the aphasias and their differentiation from dementia, see Benson 1985.)

Clinical Techniques and Tools

The clinical evaluation includes both history taking and direct examination of patients. History and mental status examination establish the presence of dementia; the neurological examination helps to determine its etiology. History taking involves not only the patient but also a knowledgeable informant and all pertinent medical information. Direct access to medical records is important because most lay informants do not know actual blood pressure values or the outcome of various laboratory tests. In the case of very elderly nursing home residents, there may be little information available from sources other than the nursing home staff and records.

In addition to eliciting information concerning patients' cognitive abilities, evidence is sought of emotional or interpersonal contributions to the presenting symptoms. Patients' emotional responses to their mental difficulties are evaluated, and an attempt is made to determine family strengths and weaknesses. Patients' personality patterns are also considered. This information helps shape the plan of management, even if treatment of the underlying brain disorder is not possible.

History Taking

Under ideal circumstances, medical records are gathered and reviewed in advance of examining the patient. My policy is to obtain a history from an outside informant over the telephone before the first visit. I also ask what medications are being taken. This information helps to focus the mental status examination. A trained interviewer may employ a dementia questionnaire such as the one modified from Breitner and Folstein (1984), shown in Appendix 1.

Personal and medical history are also elicited directly from the patient and accompanying friends or family members, if any, when I see them in person.

I first interview the patient in the presence of the accompanying person so that more accurate information can be obtained. I allow time to interview patients alone. I also allow time to interview the patients' accompanying friends or relatives alone because they often withhold information in the patients' presence out of concern that they may humiliate or anger them. Typical information withheld concerns patients' paranoid thinking, hallucinations, or incontinence. Having a friend or relative present during the psychiatric interview is a comfort to most cognitively impaired persons. Thus, history taking tends to be a three-way conversation rather than a formal interview. If patients object to an outside informant in the room at the time of the examination, I honor their request but still avail myself of the outside informant if one is available.

In the flow of the conversation, many clues emerge concerning the relationship between patients and significant others, the impact of patients on their families, and the impact of others on the patients. Husbands often resent their wives' diminished ability to maintain their household. Wives may resent having to be responsible for their formerly dominant husbands. In many cases, there is tension between spouses because one does not believe that the other truly cannot learn, remember, or understand. For example, a man who knew his wife had AD chided her for reading romance novels instead of the more substantial reading she had done earlier in her life. Examining one spouse in the

presence of the other can be helpful in breaching the intact spouse's denial and in demonstrating how to deal with defects in the other's ability
to remember, plan, and cooperate.

Mental Status Examination

The mental status examination can demonstrate the probable presence
or absence of a mental disorder. When the disorder is a dementia, information from the mental status examination can also suggest the nature
of the underlying brain disease. (For a highly detailed mental status examination, see Strub and Black 1993.)

The mental status examination contained in Appendix 2 is employed at
my clinic. It can ordinarily be accomplished in the course of a 60-minute visit
if historical and medical information have been gathered and reviewed in
advance.

Patients and their families are asked to bring all of the medications
in the family medicine chest. After the patient history has been taken, a
formal mental status examination is performed (with the patient's consent) in the presence of any accompanying persons. During this time,
tentative hypotheses are made as to how far patients can be pushed to
perform and how to best support their coping and defense mechanisms
while simultaneously obtaining the needed information. Hearing and
vision should be assessed. Hearing can be tested by whispering or by
using a tuning fork. Vision can be tested by asking patients to read a
standardized vision chart or to identify small objects.

Mental status examination is performed with consideration for patients' frustration tolerance and is also tailored to their level of cognitive
performance. For example, when it becomes obvious that the patient is
not oriented to year and month, I do not usually inquire about orientation to day and date. A patient who cannot perform well on the serial
subtraction of 3s is not asked to do serial subtraction of 7s. When the
patient is irritable or easily frustrated, I abbreviate each category of inquiry. All responses are treated as equally valid, whether correct or not,
and the patient is praised for effort by saying "good" or "that's fine" after
a series of responses. Exceptions to this general approach are in formal
testing of cognition for various studies, where completeness is important, or when I suspect that the patient is not making an effort to perform
the task, and I therefore withhold praise until the patient has made adequate effort.

Primary memory (attention) is tested by using digit span, forward
and in reverse. Secondary memory (recent memory, new learning, en-

coding) is tested by asking patients to recall three objects in 5 minutes. This test can be performed with objects presented verbally (verbal memory) or objects shown to the patient without naming them (visual memory). Response to cuing is also important, because it helps to distinguish forgetting from failure to encode.

A detailed examination of language function includes an assessment of articulation, fluency, comprehension, repetition, naming, reading, and the ability to write sentences.

Assessing language fluency includes delayed word finding, paraphasias, and neologisms. Word fluency (the ability to generate a list of words) is a very sensitive indicator of cognitive impairment. It can be tested by asking patients to name all the animals they can think of in 1 minute. The average score is 18 ± 6 (Goodglass and Kaplan 1972). Dementia patients tend to name few animals and to perseverate names they have already mentioned.

Comprehension tests begin with graded tasks, asking patients to point to one, two, and three objects in the room. This is followed by asking simple logic questions, as indicated in Appendix 2.

Naming tests should include the parts of objects, such as the parts of a watch (stem, watchband, back or case, face, crystal or glass) or the parts of a shirt. Reading ability should be considered in the context of patients' education. Writing ability is assessed by asking patients to write a dictated sentence and by then asking them to compose a sentence of their own. Calculating ability is tested with simple problems in addition, subtraction, multiplication, and division.

Praxis is evaluated by asking patients to imitate an action performed by the examiner, to perform simple motor acts in response to the examiner's request and to copy a set of simple geometric figures. For the figures, we employ intersecting rectangles, a Greek cross, and a cube (see p. 365). Drawing the cube is used to detect constructional dyspraxia in mildly impaired, well-educated persons. It is our experience that cognitively intact persons of 80 years of age or older cannot draw the cube well.

Fund of information is assessed by using a standard set of questions ranging from simple to difficult and by evaluating the responses in relation to patients' level of education and job performance. Patients with little formal education can be asked about current events that fall within their range of interest. This can be done most effectively by asking an outside informant about recent events in the patient's life.

The evaluation of the patient's ability to think abstractly requires detailed attention, and it is assessed by using similarities and proverbs. Assessment of abstract reasoning by the use of proverbs and similarities requires consideration of patients' education, cultural background, and native language.

Judgment can be estimated by asking patients questions on how they would manage certain life situations, such as, What would you do if you found a stamped, addressed, and sealed letter on the street? What would you do if you were in a church or theater and noticed a fire that nobody else saw? or What would you do if the electric company called and told you that the last check you wrote them was returned because of insufficient funds? However, judgment is probably best assessed from the patient's history.

Characterizing Dementias

Dementias can be characterized as *cortical* or *subcortical* (see also Chapter 7), based on the association of their characteristics with cortical or subcortical pathology. Cortical dementias present as one of two overlapping groups: *frontal* or *temporoparietal.* Frontal dementia is often found in Pick's disease or after anterior cerebral artery stroke. It occurs less frequently in AD. Frontal lobe degeneration is characterized by progressive personality change and breakdown in social conduct (Kumar and Gottlieb 1993), defective judgment, difficulty in focusing attention, apathy, disinhibition, silliness, echoing words, mirroring others' behavior, unawareness of deficit, difficulty in following instructions (often manifested as motor dyspraxia), and often with a slightly prancing gait. Neary (1990), for example, reported a patient who insisted on repeatedly changing into fresh clothes but refused to wash. Personality changes often antedate cognitive symptoms in frontal dementia; Miller et al. (1991) found social withdrawal and behavioral dysinhibition to be the earliest symptoms. Temporoparietal dementia, the most common presentation of AD, is accompanied by naming difficulties and constructional dyspraxia with relative preservation of personality. These patients are often painfully aware of their deficits.

Subcortical dementias, with primary pathology in the thalami, basal ganglia, rostral brain stem, and their frontal projections, overlap in symptomatology with frontal dementias but also usually have speech and motor abnormalities. The most prominent symptoms include overall slowing of movement and cognitive processing and deficits in social judgment and mood change. Causes of subcortical dementia include cerebrovascular disease, Parkinson's disease, Huntington's disease, Wilson's disease, and progressive supranuclear palsey (Cummings 1990).

The following case histories provide examples of each of these types of dementia:

Frontal Dementia

Mrs. H. was a 51-year old, right-handed housewife with 12 years of education. Her husband described her as exhibiting a pattern of decreasing initiative and increasing memory loss over 5 years. She at first compensated for her deteriorating memory function by leaving reminders around the house. She would leave the laundry basket by the door when she was doing her laundry. She had been giggling inappropriately for 3 years. She had not cooked in a year. Her husband reported that she had difficulty understanding verbal communication and that she often called different objects by the same name. He also said that she initiated no activity on her own.

There was no history of emotional disorder, head injury, or significant illness. The patient's maternal grandmother, mother, and three of her seven siblings had similar symptoms, as did several of her mother's siblings and their children. She was taking no medication.

Mental status examination revealed Mrs. H. to be alert and cooperative. She sat quietly, initiated little activity, and giggled. She knew the year and the month but not the day of the week, the date, or the season of the year. She knew the city, state, and her home address. She could not repeat the names of three objects, was unable to subtract serial 7s, could not name a watch or a pencil, and could not follow a three-stage command. She was able to compose and write a sentence but had moderate constructional dyspraxia. There was no evidence of thought or mood disorder. Neurological examination was within normal limits.

Neuropsychological testing revealed a Wechsler Adult Intelligence Scale (WAIS) verbal IQ of 53, a performance IQ of 58, and a full-scale IQ of 52. She was confused on the simplest tasks. Instructions needed to be repeatedly reinforced. She tended to echo questions and often responded, "I don't know." Neuropsychological testing suggested diffuse cerebral dysfunction with possible greater left and anterior involvement.

A computed tomography (CT) showed generalized cerebral atrophy, more prominent frontally. Magnetic resonance imaging showed generalized atrophy. An EEG was normal. No abnormality was detected in the blood, urine, or spinal fluid. A ^{133}Xe regional cerebral blood-flow study showed marked reduction of blood flow in the frontal lobes with no reduction of vascular reserve.

The frontal aspects of this woman's dementia were her lack of initiative, her inappropriate giggling, and her inability to concentrate and follow simple commands. At autopsy 3 years later, there was moderate frontal and temporal lobe atrophy with hydrocephalus ex vacuo. There was severe temporal lobe gliosis and loss of pyramidal cells. In addition, there was a striking loss of pigmented neurons in the substantia nigra and locus coeruleus with abundant free pigment and pigment contained in macrophages. The autopsy diagnosis was multiple systems atrophy because of the brain stem nuclei deterioration accompanying severe loss of cortical neurons.

Temporoparietal Dementia

Mr. F. was a 57-year-old, right-handed accountant with 17 years of education, who was still employed. He last seemed his old self 3–4 years earlier, when he began to hesitate in his speech. In the 2–3 years prior to examination, he had increasing difficulty with learning, concentrating, calculating, memory, and word finding. He needed a calculator to do simple mathematical problems. He continued to drive and to umpire softball games, which was his hobby. He had a concussion in his 20s and a hemorrhoidectomy in his 30s. His father, who died at age 86 years, and a paternal uncle suffered dementing illnesses. He was taking no medications.

On mental status examination, he was alert and cooperative. He was oriented in time, except for the date, and in space, except for the inability to name the place where he was being examined. He often failed to reach goal ideas and had frequent difficulty with naming. His attention and concentration were impaired. He could repeat only four digits forward and two in reverse. He was able to make only one correct subtraction on serial 7s. His language fluency and comprehension were good, but his repetition was impaired. His ability to think abstractly was impaired; he was able to do a few similarities and no proverbs. His ability to do simple calculations was impaired, as was his construction ability. He had difficulty with new learning. It took several tries to learn the names of three objects. He could recall three objects after a brief distraction but had marked impairment of remote memory and a diminished kind of information. There was no evidence of mood disorder or thought disorder.

Neurological examination was within normal limits. Neuropsychological testing revealed a verbal IQ of 91, a performance IQ of 84, and a full-scale IQ of 88. There was considerable scatter among subscales. He had moderate to severe impairment of recent and remote memory, dysgraphia, spelling dyspraxia, dyscalculia, ideomotor dyspraxia, right-left confusion, and perseveration. There was no difficulty with simple sensorimotor function but great difficulty with complex problem solving.

An EEG showed mild generalized slowing. A magnetic resonance imaging (MRI) scan was within normal limits. A ^{133}Xe regional cerebral blood-flow study showed bilateral reduction of flow in the lateral frontal and posterior temporoparietal areas bilaterally, without a significant change after the administration of acetazolamide. Cerebrospinal fluid, blood, and urine studies were all within normal limits.

The combination of memory impairment, impaired naming, and

constructional dyspraxia was suggestive of predominant temporo-parietal dysfunction. The clinical diagnosis was Alzheimer's disease. He died at 62 years of age; no autopsy was obtained.

Subcortical Dementia

Mr. L. was a 69-year-old, right-handed former salesman with 14 years of education. After undergoing a transurethral prostatectomy 7 years earlier, he experienced intermittent urinary dribbling to which he had been relatively indifferent. About 3 years previously, he became withdrawn and uncommunicative and seemed to have diminished recent memory. He was unable to drive his car because he lost his sense of direction. An avid worker and refinisher of old furniture, he could no longer complete tasks or construct furniture symmetrically but continued to work long hours at his hobby until 3 months prior to examination. At that time, he had an acute episode in which he was found incoherent and sprawled on the ground at his vacation home. His speech was slurred, he began to perseverate, and he developed a retropulsive gait. After that, he became incontinent of large amounts of urine and feces to which he was completely indifferent.

Medical history revealed a back injury treated with traction 30 years earlier, hernia surgery 5 years earlier, and the previously described prostatectomy. He experienced a concussion from a fall 30 years earlier and had suffered frequent headaches subsequently. He had a left bundle-branch block and had episodes of cardiac arrythmia over the years, for which he had intermittently taken quinidine. There was also a history of mild hearing loss. His medications were dipyridamole and aspirin.

The psychiatric examiner found that the patient required the assistance of a walker. His motor activity was slow. The right side of his face drooped. He was oriented to the year and month but not to the day of the week or date. He knew his street address, city, and state. He did not speak spontaneously, but language fluency and comprehension were good, as was his naming ability. He performed serial 7s well and had good abstracting ability but could not interpret proverbs. He gave the names of former presidents and vice-presidents of the United States and the governor of Texas. His remote memory was relatively intact, but his recent memory was markedly impaired. He had no awareness of his memory difficulty. He was able to write a sentence spontaneously and showed no constructional dyspraxia. There was no evidence of mood disorder or thought disorder.

Neurological examination revealed increased reflexes in the lower extremities, with bilateral positive Babinski reflexes. His gait was wide based and retropulsive, with turning en bloc. He had a great deal of difficulty sitting in and rising from a chair. His speech was slurred, and he made frequent paraphasic errors.

Neuropsychological testing indicated a WAIS verbal IQ of 113, performance IQ of 103, and full-scale IQ of 109. He had significant loss of perceptual-motor abilities, impaired short- and long-term memory, spelling dyspraxia, dysgraphia, and mild constructional dyspraxia. Right-hemisphere performance was reduced, as indicated by significant slowing of left-hand tapping speed and name writing, and pronounced weakening of left-hand grip strength.

An EEG showed left temporal slowing. A CT scan showed moderate generalized cerebral atrophy. An MRI scan showed mild cerebral atrophy with patchy areas of increased signal in the white matter on T_2-weighted images. A ^{133}Xe regional cerebral blood flow study showed a low-flow area in the deep and superficial areas of the left frontal lobe. After administration of acetazolamide, a vasodilator, flow reduced in both left and right frontal areas. A lumbar puncture was not performed. All other blood and urine tests were within normal limits except for mildly elevated blood glucose (113 mg/dl) and mildly reduced hemoglobin (13 g/dl). The working diagnosis was vascular dementia. This man had signs of motor involvement and had areas of excellent mental function, such as abstracting and mathematical ability together with areas of great impairment, such as recent memory.

At autopsy several years later, he was found to have an organized small infarct in the left basal ganglia, suggesting that his acute episode was probably due to a stroke. The most significant finding, however, was polyglucosan bodies throughout the white and gray matter in all areas of the brain. They were most prominent in the mid-frontal cortex, dentate nucleus of the cerebellum, and gray matter of the pons. They were also present in skeletal muscle fibers, myocardial fibers, endocardial cells, perivascular nerves in the heart and in hepatocytes. Peripheral nerve was not sampled. The diagnosis was adult polyglucosan body disease (see Chapter 4).

Quantifying Aspects of Dementia

Clinicians generally rely on impressionistic data to make diagnoses and to follow the course of an illness and its treatment. They also employ objective measures, such as pulse, temperature, blood pressure, hematocrit, and blood urea nitrogen concentration. Until recent years, there have been few tools available to clinicians for the office or bedside quantification of dementia-related symptoms and behaviors. Growing awareness of the potential reversibility of some dementias and the potential for palliative drug treatment of dementia-related symptoms (Reisberg et al. 1989) has led to developing means to quantify the phenomena associated with dementia, including overall functional ability, cognition, and behavioral, emotional, perceptual, and ideational symptoms.

The following are some commonly employed scales. In addition, I have included newer research scales for quantifying cognitive function and behavioral/emotional symptoms: the CERAD Battery, the CERAD Behavior Rating Scale for Dementia, and the Cohen-Mansfield Agitation Inventory.

Global Measures of Function

- Blessed Dementia Rating Scale (Blessed et al. 1968)
- Washington University Clinical Dementia Rating (CDR) (Hughes et al. 1982)

Measures of Cognitive Function

- Mini-Mental State Exam (MMSE) (Folstein et al. 1975)
- Alzheimer's Disease Assessment Scale (ADAS) (Rosen et al. 1984)
- The CERAD Battery (Morris et al. 1989)

Measures of Behavioral/Emotional Symptoms

- Brief Psychiatric Rating Scale (BPRS) (Overall and Gorham 1962, 1988)
- CERAD Behavior Rating Scale for Dementia (BRSD) (Tariot et al. 1992)
- Cohen-Mansfield Agitation Inventory (CMAI) (Cohen-Mansfield 1986)

Global measures of function.   The Blessed Dementia Rating Scale (see Appendix 4) is a 17-point, activities of daily living scale that includes a wide range of behaviors. It is administered to a knowledgeable informant—usually a person who spends 20 or more hours per week with the patient. This scale takes approximately 10 minutes to administer and is a useful complement to testing patients directly, a process that often does not expose many of the behavioral concomitants of dementia, such as lack of sphincter control or difficulty in eating or dressing. Its high degree of subjectivity and the use of an untrained observer make it less reliable than the MMSE and ADAS, but it encompasses a broader range of function and correlates well with MMSE and ADAS scores in AD patients.

The CDR (see Appendix 5) was designed for the assessment of AD outpatients. It grades on a scale ranging from 0 (normal) to 3 (severe) and is based on a structured interview that takes 30–40 minutes and involves interviewing an informant as well as the patient. Two additional stages have been added to the CDR (Heyman et al. 1987): stages 4 (profound) and 5 (terminal). In stage 4, speech is usually unintelligible or irrelevant, and patients are unable to follow simple instructions or understand commands. Patients occasionally recognize the spouse or caregiver, use fingers more than utensils, and require much assistance. They are able to walk a few steps with help (but usually are chairbound), often make purposeless movements, and are frequently incontinent. In stage 5, patients are unresponsive and neither comprehend communication or recognize others. Patients are bedridden and unable to sit or stand. They need to be fed, often by nasogastric tube, and may have difficulty swallowing.

Measures of cognitive function. The MMSE (see Appendix 6), administered directly to the patient, is probably the most widely used brief cognitive assessment tool. It requires 10–15 minutes to administer and samples orientation, attention, concentration, recent memory, naming, repetition, comprehension, ideomotor praxis, constructional praxis, and the ability to construct a sentence. A perfect score is 30 points. The MMSE is confounded by premorbid intelligence—higher intelligence making for better performance and lower intelligence for worse. The originators indicate that a score of 23 or below by someone with a high-school education is suggestive of dementia. A cutoff score of 18 or below is suggested for those with an eighth-grade education or less. A recent population-based study showed an inverse relationship between test score and education. The median score was 29 for unscreened individuals with at least 9 years of schooling, 26 for those with 5–8 years of schooling, and 22 for those with 0–4 years of education. The same study also showed an inverse relationship between age and test score, with a median of 29 for those 18–24 years of age and a median of 25 for those 80 years of age and older (Crum et al. 1993).

Although not a sensitive test, the brevity of the MMSE and the minimal training required in its administration make it especially useful as a screening test for dementia and for following the course of delirium in medical and surgical patients.

The ADAS (see Appendix 7) was designed to be sensitive to small changes in AD patients. It is heavily weighted toward the cognitive aspects of the disease and is based on the symptoms most commonly seen in 31 AD cases confirmed by brain biopsy (Mohs et al. 1983). The scale consists of 21 items, half of which are cognitive and half of which are noncognitive. Items are rated on a 6-point scale ranging from 0 (no impairment) to 5 (severe impairment). This test requires approximately 45 minutes and an outside informant, and needs to be administered by a person trained specifically in its use. The cognitive subtest items correlate well with other measures of dementia progression in AD. The noncognitive items such as depression, appetite, and pacing do not correlate well with dementia progression, but they do assess the major behavioral symptoms seen in AD. The cognitive portion of the ADAS has been used extensively in studies of cognitive enhancers for AD.

CERAD has developed a brief battery of tests that was administered to 350 probable AD patients and 275 healthy subjects. This battery detected deterioration of language, memory, praxis, and general intellectual status at 1-year follow-up (Morris et al. 1989). It includes tests of verbal fluency (name as many animals as you can in 1 minute); identification of 15 line drawings; the MMSE, tests of ability to learn, construction, recall; and word recognition. The battery is designed to be useful in epidemiological studies and treatment trials. It is available through CERAD Administrative Offices, Box 3203, Duke University Medical Center, Durham, NC 27710.

Measures of behavioral/emotional symptoms.   The BPRS (see Appendix 8) was designed to evaluate the treatment response of psychiatric inpatients, but it has been used successfully in drug studies in elderly patients (Kochansky 1979). Of the three scales described in this section, it is the only one that evaluates manic symptoms. There are few cognitive items on this scale. It involves direct observation and examination of patients with the conventional mental status examination. Each of the 18 points on the scale is rated on an 8-point continuum ranging from 0 (not present) to 7 (extremely severe). A descriptor for each item is contained on the scale. There is also a manual that provides more detailed instructions (Guy 1976).

The CERAD BRSD (see Appendix 9) is a 48-item caregiver questionnaire that assesses behaviors that occurred in the preceding month. Items are rated on a 5-point frequency scale ranging from 0 (has not occurred since illness began) to 4 (16 or more days in the past month). This scale can be scored by domains (depressive features, disturbed ideation/perception, executive dysfunction, irritability/agitation, vegetative features, apathy, aggression, and affective lability) or as a whole. The administration of the CERAD BRSD is facilitated by use of a response card on which the frequency of behaviors is indicated. A detailed administration and scoring manual is available from CERAD as above.

The CMAI (see Appendix 10) was designed to measure agitated behaviors in nursing home residents and has been well validated in that population (Miller et al. 1995). It has also been adapted for use in the community. It is a 36-item questionnaire administered to caregivers and is scored on a 7-point scale that rates frequency of occurrence of agitated, disruptive behaviors over the preceding 2 weeks. Cards to orient the informant are also used with the CMAI. These cards give key words for various behaviors in addition to a frequency scale. The CMAI is available from Jiska Cohen-Mansfield, Ph.D., Research Institute of the Hebrew Home of Greater Washington, 6121 Montrose Road, Rockville, MD 20852.

Summary

The diagnosis of dementia is becoming increasingly precise. As a result of this increasing precision, clinicians are able to better diagnose the underlying brain or systemic pathology. Along with greater precision in diagnosis has come greater awareness of the diversity of functions encompassed by dementing illness, including behavioral, emotional, vegetative, ideational, and perceptual disturbances. Many instruments have been developed to quantify the cognitive and noncognitive aspects of dementia. These instruments can help us to measure validly and reliably the effects of our interventions with dementia patients and to thereby aid in the process of developing effective treatment techniques.

CHAPTER 2

Dementia as a Psychobiological Process

Myron F. Weiner, M.D.

The syndrome of dementia is the psychobiological result of interacting social, psychological, and physical or chemical forces in persons with certain emotional, anatomic, metabolic, or genetic vulnerabilities. Dementia patients' emotional makeup and social environment determine their individual responses to impairment of cognitive functioning. The interaction of factors that both produce and aggravate the symptoms and functional impairment of dementia are illustrated in Figure 2–1.

Figure 2–1 indicates that the development of dementia symptoms depends on the relative weight of the factors that maintain psychological integrity in relation to the forces that impair adaptive functioning. Thus, an overt dementia may follow what appears to be a trivial brain insult, such as a mild episode of hypotension during spinal anesthesia for prostate surgery. The additional minor brain insult reduces the brain's overall integrative capacity to the point that the defect manifests. The same phenomenon may occur as the result of psychological factors in persons whose brain function is already compromised. Increasing the anxiety of such persons increases confusion because the brain is unable to deal simultaneously with intense emotion and multiple environmental stimuli. Another frequent occurrence is the increased confusion of persons whose compromised brain function is not apparent until they attempt adaptation to a new living situation, such as moving from one house to another.

Personality Function in Dementia

Although the mind is not independent of the brain, it is useful to conceive of the mind as having a dynamic structure of its own. To do this,

43

I have borrowed from the Freudian schema, which conceives of mental functioning as a balance of the mind's adaptive, coping, and defensive functions (the ego), the pressure of instinctual drives (the id), and internal standards of behavior (conscience, or superego). In dementia, adaptive or coping ability is reduced, which may result in the development of emotional symptoms, perceptual or ideational disturbances, or problem behaviors. The nature of the symptoms and behaviors are partly determined by a preexisting personality structure and the new relationship between individuals and their sense of what they ought to be (their ego ideal). For many people, their ego ideal may be the ability to nurture

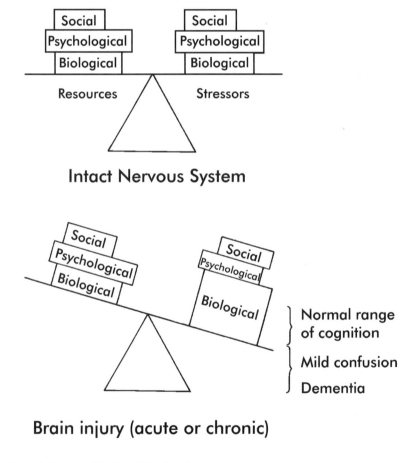

Figure 2–1.   A model of cognitive functioning.

others or to competently maintain a household; for others, it may be the ability to function at a paying job.

Coping Ability

The concept of adaptive or coping ability (ego strength, in Freudian terms) is important for a dynamic understanding of dementia. To cope adequately with the demands of everyday living, the personality must have sufficient ability to appropriately suppress, repress, or sublimate the demands of drives and conscience or to find an adequate substitute for meeting those demands. When lacking the ability to repress, suppress, sublimate, or substitute, the classic psychological defense mechanisms delineated by Anna Freud (1946) come into play.

Coping ability is related only in part to cognitive integrity. It is also related to the biological integrity of the person as a whole and to that person's ability to mobilize energy, make contact with others, control impulses, test reality, and assume responsibility. *Biological integrity* refers to the ability to perceive the environment through the sense organs, to perform motor behavior necessary for self-maintenance, and to have sufficient physical energy to attend to matters outside of maintaining the integrity of one's physical being. Thus, a person who has just suffered a massive myocardial infarction and is experiencing intense chest pain has little ability to deal effectively with other matters. The same is true of a person whose emphysema is so severe that breathing requires active concentration and deliberate effort.

Personality Structure

Personality refers to an individual's predominant patterns of coping mechanisms and defenses. Common patterns of personality structure are found in DSM-IV (American Psychiatric Association 1994) in their most exaggerated form—as personality disorders. A personality disorder differs from the traits that comprise more normal personality structure in the personality-disordered person's tendency to employ stereotyped patterns of dealing with the world. Thus, many persons enjoy self-display and being the center of attention, as do persons with a histrionic personality disorder. The person with a histrionic trait is still able to function when not the center of attention. The histrionic personality-disordered person is driven to seek attention through symptoms when not able to secure it through ordinary self-display. Personality styles include obsessive-compulsive, paranoid, avoidant, antisocial, schizoid, and others.

Premorbid personality has much to do with the ability to concentrate, make contact with others, test reality, and assume responsibility. It has been said that in old age we become more like ourselves. In other words, dementia (formerly attributed to aging, per se) uncovers aspects of the personality that were partially suppressed when the individual was biologically intact. Persons with pronounced dependent traits prior to the onset of dementia may become even less willing to do for themselves. Those who relish their autonomy may strive even harder to maintain that autonomy and refuse appropriate help. This is often seen in the case of widowed elders, independent for many years, who refuse the help of neighbors and the public health nurse in meeting their needs as their sight and hearing fail.

Through historical information provided by the patient and others, it is possible to determine which behaviors are temporary reactions and which are probably long standing and largely unalterable (Weiner 1984). This information also gives cues for managing patients. Knowing, for example, that a particular patient has had a lifelong inability to share, it would not be expected that this patient could comfortably tolerate a nursing home setting that involved sharing a room.

Dementia as a Psychological Process

A dynamic psychological view of dementia makes it easy to understand apparent minute-to-minute changes in cognitive ability, not only of dementia patients but also of persons who are cognitively intact. Emotionally healthy persons are kept alert and enabled to learn effectively by small increments of anxiety. Intense anxiety, on the other hand, impairs both concentration and learning. The greater the underlying cognitive impairment, the greater the detrimental effect of anxiety on cognition. Thus, small changes in a person's level of emotional tension during the course of a day can produce large fluctuations in cognitive ability. The same is true of sensory input. Adequate sensory input helps to maintain orientation in time and space; overwhelming input in the form of too novel or too many stimuli also increases confusion.

The psychology of dementia involves all of the coping mechanisms and defense mechanisms outlined in Tables 2–1 and 2–2. Table 2–1 indicates positive adaptive or coping mechanisms.

The capacity for positive adaptation involves the ability to make decisions and to mobilize sufficient will to enforce those decisions. Both decision making and mobilization of will involve the assumption of responsibility: owning one's actions as a product of one's own wishes or fears. Psychologically healthy persons tend to seek out novel stimuli and attempt to master and attribute meaning to their environment. They learn when they can trust their own judgment and the judgment of others, and they maintain hope that they can positively influence the world about them and derive a sense of satisfaction from their activities.

Five other coping mechanisms have been described by Vaillant (1977), based on a long-term study of healthy men. They are 1) sublimation, 2) suppression, 3) altruism, 4) anticipation, and 5) humor. *Sublimation* is converting one's physical and psychological drives into socially

Table 2–1.   Coping mechanisms

Decision making
Mobilization of will
Assumption of responsibility
Stimulus seeking
Mastery
Attribution of meaning
Trust of oneself and important others
Hope

Table 2–2.   Defense mechanisms

Neurotic
  Repression
  Intellectualization
  Isolation
  Displacement
  Reaction formation
  Dissociation
Immature
  Projection
  Fantasy
  Hypochondriasis
  Passive-aggressive behavior
  Acting out
Psychotic
  Denial of external reality
  Distortion
  Delusional projection

Source.   Adapted from Vaillant 1977.

acceptable thoughts and actions. *Suppression* is the act of willing one's self to wait for the best moment to express a thought or to act. *Altruism* is doing for others without the expectation of personal gain. *Anticipation* is the kind of thinking in advance that leads to constructive action. It differs from worry or rumination, which lead primarily to greater worry. *Humor* is the ability to enjoy surprise and uncertainty and to surprise others in a pleasant way.

In patients with dementia, coping mechanisms begin to fail. Because decision making and mobilizing will become difficult, such persons often blame others instead of assuming the primary responsibility. Instead of acknowledging an inability to remember, others are blamed when responsibilities are not met. New stimuli are avoided. Mastery and attribution of meaning become more difficult, leading to feelings of hopelessness and helplessness. Instead of sublimating, raw drives emerge, sometimes in the form of inappropriate aggression or inappropriate genital display. Lack of ability to suppress leads to impatience. Self-centeredness replaces altruism as impaired coping ability dampens the capacity for empathy, and anticipation is replaced by impulsiveness or inertness. Humor as a reaction to novel stimuli is replaced by easy startle and upsetness.

A positive strategy for coping with cognitive decline is acknowledging the deficit and consciously developing compensatory mechanisms such as making lists, avoiding unfamiliar places, and asking questions. Often, however, the dementing process involves the portions of the brain that enable self-awareness. Alzheimer's disease (AD) patients, for example, are frequently unaware of their memory deficits (Sevush and Leve 1993). Persons with frontal lobe disorders are unaware of the inappropriateness of their behavior. Without self-awareness, conscious compensatory mechanisms are less likely to be developed.

In psychological terms, normal aging depletes all aspects of the psychic apparatus equally. Thus, coping ability, standards for achievement, and drives remain in relative balance. In dementia, this balance may not be maintained and may result in various symptoms and behaviors. Inappropriate aggression or sexual activity in dementia can be seen as resulting from an imbalance between coping ability and those drives and wishes that are ordinarily repressed, suppressed, or shaped by the adaptive psychological functioning and expressed in appropriate ways at appropriate times. Persons with dementia whose coping mechanisms and self-awareness are intact may experience normal mourning for the loss of their former self (Bahro et al. 1995).

Many persons with early dementia experience self-criticism and lowering of self-esteem resulting from an imbalance between their ego ideal, their performance standards, and impaired coping ability. The person can no longer live up to an ego ideal that includes productive work. In addition, self-criticisms that would ordinarily be dismissed overwhelm the personality and flood it with guilt and self-recrimination.

The defenses shown in Table 2–2 represent failures of positive coping ability. They are mechanisms used to deal with its inadequate capacity to perceive, integrate, and act efficiently on stimuli that impinge on the organism from within and without. As originally formulated (Freud 1946), these mechanisms referred to defenses against awareness of unconscious wishes or conflict, but they can also defend against awareness of unpleasant or frightening aspects of reality. The defense mechanisms listed in Table 2–2 are classified by Vaillant (1977) into three groups: neurotic, immature, and psychotic, based on the frequency with which they are associated with various mental disorders and stages of development.

Many types of defense are adopted by dementia patients, depending on their premorbid personality, their environment, and the rapidity with which their dementing illness progresses. Rapidly progressive dementias may provoke more primitive defense mechanisms, with denial, distortion, and delusional projection being very common. Denial is found frequently in all forms of dementia but should not be confused with neglect syndromes, such as the syndrome of contralateral neglect that often accompanies right (nondominant)-hemisphere lesions (Denny-Brown et al. 1954). The apparent denial by many dementia patients of their defects in memory and judgment is often due to losing the neuronal substrate for self-observation.

Defenses from Vaillant's category of neurotic mechanisms are not prominent in dementing disorders. Some persons intellectualize about their deficits, appearing to accept their impairment, but then demonstrate by their behavior that they simultaneously do not recognize any impairment. Displacement is occasionally employed, as indicated in the following case of AD:

> A 67-year-old widow was being evaluated for symptoms of dementia that had progressed over a 4-year period. When asked if she had any difficulties, she replied that she had a painful ankle and showed her leather-braced ankle to the examiner. She said that since she had started wearing the brace, the arthritis in her ankle was considerably less troublesome. Later, the examiner began a formal inquiry into her cognitive state, asking questions to test her memory, concentration, and fund of information. When at a loss for an answer to a question, she would reply that her ankle was hurting and interfering with her concentration.

Other persons develop reaction formations against their impairment, putting in longer hours at work to compensate for their slowed thinking and impaired comprehension. On one occasion, it was necessary to hospitalize a man with an early dementia who had become delirious from working long hours and losing sleep in an effort to keep up with his work.

The catastrophic (Goldstein 1942) reactions that occasionally occur when dementia patients are faced with an intense emotional stimulus or unmanageable cognitive input may take the form of a confused state. The person suddenly becomes unable to recognize a familiar environment or undergoes a sudden emotional regression and begins calling for long-dead parents or other relatives as though they were still alive. This is illustrated in the following example:

> A 70-year-old man with dementia became frightened when unable to recognize his wife and began calling out for his mother. He remained in this excited state until calmed by his son, whom he was able to recognize.

Catastrophic reactions are usually self-limited and are best contained by distraction or by removing or making understandable the aggravating environmental stimulus.

Immature mechanisms of defense are often employed by dementia patients. Projection in the form of blaming (as opposed to delusional projection) often occurs early in the course of a dementing illness. A wife will exclaim with irritation that her husband did not tell her the children were coming to visit. An impaired husband will rage at his wife for hiding the car keys that he misplaced.

The potential use of fantasy as a defense mechanism is impaired because of attention and memory deficits, but somatic preoccupation is often encountered, with a host of physical complaints being offered as distractors from the potential awareness of decreased cognitive ability. Rather than passive opposition (which involves the ability to inhibit an impulse), dementia patients often express direct aggression in the form of blaming. Acting out is also common, precisely because these patients lack the ability to inhibit their behavior. Thus, inappropriate aggression or sexual display may sometimes occur. For example, a nursing home roommate is screamed at for intruding instead of being politely asked to leave, or open masturbation may occur in response to genital stimulation from tight clothes.

Psychotic defense mechanisms are seen frequently in dementia patients. The denial of impairment is common, as was previously noted. Distortion occurs when the dementia patient thinks that he or she is in a prison rather than a nursing home. Delusional projection may occur when a dementia patient who is unaware of having a defective memory attributes an inability to keep up with house keys to others deliberately removing them. Dementia patients occasionally develop a transient delusional system to support such contentions, as seen in the following example:

> Mrs. M., a woman with severe cognitive impairment who was unable to comprehend her environment, dealt with the problem by refusing to leave her house to venture into an unfamiliar environment. She responded to all visitors as intruders, calling them whores and attempting to drive them off in an effort to keep her environment simple and comprehensible.

Delusion formation also occurs without the element of projection, especially in those persons who develop prosopagnosia, the inability to identify faces. A man with prosopagnosia became very concerned when he failed to recognize his wife while on a trip. He became agitated and exclaimed that he was being kidnapped. Such delusion formation is usually transient and tends to occur when the environment becomes too demanding.

Regression is another prominent mechanism employed by dementia patients and is best defined as reverting to adaptive mechanisms appropriate to an earlier era of life, usually early childhood. Regression can take many forms. It may manifest as an infantile clinging to loved ones, avoidance of strangers, tantrums, inappropriate or unnecessary dependence, or attempts to obtain special attention from others. When regression takes the form of physical clinging to other persons, dolls or stuffed animals can often be substituted for the constant presence of another person, much as such transitional objects serve the emotional needs of young children who also lack object constancy—the ability to recognize that an object no longer in reach or in view can continue to exist (Piaget 1954). Whether such cognitive regression occurs in dementia has not been formally tested, but clinical experience suggests that it probably does. And, as with a young child, reassurances that one will return are often insufficient. A young child becomes upset by recalling the unpleasurable experience of loss; a dementia patient becomes upset in some measure because of inability to remember the promise to return.

The psychological mechanism of *splitting*, which is frequently evident in dementing illness, may be part of the regressive process. This mechanism, theorized by Klein (1957) to be characteristic of an early stage of personality development, involves the active separation of good from bad experiences, perceptions, and emotions linked to other persons. Thus, the frustrating aspects of an emotionally important person are split off from his or her caring aspects to form an entirely separate person. One is all good and the other is all bad, as seen in the following example:

> Mrs. T, a woman with Alzheimer's disease, was having increasing difficulty identifying her husband. One night, frustrated with her seemingly endless repetitiveness, the tone of her husband's voice became harsh. Mrs. T reacted with alarm. She perceived him as having become two persons, both of whom were claiming to be her husband. Frightened and unable to determine who was her real husband, she fled the house to the home of a neighbor and had the neighbor call the police. The following day, she was still not certain which of the two men was her husband.
>
> Mrs. T could not fathom how her real husband could be so unkind to her and resolved her psychological problem by splitting him in two.

The splitting process described in the preceding case may contribute to the development of the Capgras's syndrome.

Psychological, Behavioral, Ideational, and Perceptual Concomitants of Dementia

Certain frequent psychological and behavioral concomitants of dementing illness warrant individual discussion from a psychodynamic point of view. They are 1) depression; 2) delirium; 3) anxiety, agitation, and restlessness; 4) sleep-wake disturbances; 5) suspiciousness and delusion formation; 6) hallucinations; and 7) apathy and withdrawal. The catastrophic response has already been discussed.

Depression

Symptoms usually associated with depression are frequent in AD (Cummings et al. 1995), with agitation, motor restlessness, sleep disturbance, and tearful episodes occurring in 25%–50% of patients in one series (Reisberg et al. 1987). Major depression is less frequent, in some series occurring in 10%–20% of AD patients (Wragg and Jeste 1989). In our own dementia clinic, major depression was present in only 1% of AD patients at initial evaluation (Weiner et al. 1991), and there were no new cases of major depression in 153 patients followed for an average of 3 years (Weiner et al. 1994). However, our experience may not reflect the true prevalence of depression in AD because ours is a tertiary care clinic. Presumably, most cases of obvious depression would have been diagnosed and treated elsewhere.

Among other dementia-associated disorders, depression occurs in Parkinson's disease (Cummings 1992), Huntington's disease, multiple sclerosis, epilepsy, brain trauma, and stroke (Starkstein and Robinson 1993). The prevalence of depression is high during the first 2 years after a stroke (Robinson and Price 1982). The relation of stroke size, location, or cognitive impairment to depression is controversial (Robinson et al. 1983; Schwartz et al. 1993), but depression does appear to magnify the cognitive effects of the stroke.

There is evidence that depression occurring in old age may herald the onset of a dementing illness, whether the depressive episode is one of a lifelong pattern of depressive or manic-depressive episodes or arises de novo in old age. In one study, 57% of depressed nondemented elderly patients developed frank dementia within 3 years (Reding et al. 1985). In a study of 14 patients still alive at 15- to 47-month follow-up, 43% had developed dementia (Bulbena and Berrios 1986). Dhingra and Rabins (1991) found that of 25 bipolar patients 60 years of age or older followed for 5–7 years, 32% had developed significant cognitive impairment. It has been suggested that episodes of mood disorder may do damage to the brain, possibly caused by the accompanying hypersecretion of cortisol (Altshuler 1993). On the other hand, I do not have the impression of a high premorbid incidence of depression in AD patients.

Some element of underlying cognitive impairment usually accompanies depressive dementia and other pseudodementias. In one study, despite the fact that patients with reversible dementia did improve, only 3 of 92 patients recovered fully, and in 2 of those, the original cognitive abnormalities were subtle (Larson et al. 1984).

The bulk of contemporary evidence suggests that major depression is a psychosomatic-somatopsychic disorder in which a genetically determined vulnerability is triggered and reinforced by the interaction of psychological and physiological factors. In a study of poststroke depression, for example, 20% of the depressed patients had a history of depression (Schwartz et al. 1993). Norepinephrine deficiency has been proposed as an important physiological factor in the precipitation and maintenance of major depressive episodes (Schildkraut and Kety 1967). Although nor-epinephrine in the brain as a whole does not decrease significantly with age (Finch 1973), the locus coeruleus of the midbrain, which supplies most of the noradrenergic fibers to the forebrain (Foote et al. 1983), de-creases substantially in neurons (Vijayashankar and Brody 1979) and in norepinephrine content (D. S. Robinson 1975) with age. Bondareff et al. (1982) reported a locus coeruleus cell loss in AD far beyond that found in normal aging, and Gottfries et al. (1976) found decreased norepineph-rine content in the brains of AD patients. Zubenko and Moosy (1988) found that the best postmortem predictor of antemortem depression in AD was degeneration of both locus coeruleus and substantia nigra.

The diagnosis of a major depressive episode is phenomenological. It relies on the presence of the signs and symptoms indicated in Chapter 1. The phenomenology of depression can be explained on both physiologi-cal and psychological grounds. As the result of triggering by psychologi-cal or physiological stimuli, or as the result of a neuronal malfunction, an amotivational state appears. This state may result from catecholamine depletion (Cohen et al. 1982) or dysregulation (Siever and Davis 1985), or it may be an exaggerated phylogenetically determined reaction to a situation experienced as a type of overwhelming threat to psychological or physical survival. This state has been described as conservation with-drawal by Engel and Schmale (1972) and later suggested by Weiner and Lovitt (1979) as a possible physiological substrate of depression. The physiological reaction, once established, whether by psychological or physiological factors, becomes partially autonomous and unresponsive to changes in the precipitating psychological factors. Even so, it is useful to conceptualize depression psychodynamically. The utility of the psy-chodynamic conceptualization of depression is that it suggests a means for patients' psychological management.

Injury to or death of neurons depletes the capacity of the ego to deal effectively with the demands of the id, superego, ego ideal, and external reality. Subclinical impairment of cognitive functioning also interferes with the ability to live up to one's ego ideal and results in guilt and low-ering of self-esteem. There is an increased danger of id impulses erupt-ing or irrational superego demands increasing at the same time that the ego is having greater difficulty interpreting environmental stimuli. Given a biological vulnerability to depression, overt depression may manifest when triggered by stressors such as illness, brain damage, or aging. The most common of these stresses is loss, including loss of a loved one, loss of health, loss of meaningful occupation, and so on (Engel 1962). These losses may be real, but symbolic or threatened losses may be equally powerful precipitants of depression. Thus, the illness of a spouse (or other loved one) or a spouse's threat to leave can be as potent a trigger as the death of a spouse, as illustrated in the following example:

> Mr. A., an 82-year-old retired iron worker, became increasingly withdrawn and apathetic after his daughter's divorce and the near loss of a favorite grandson in a motorcycle accident. His sleep pattern was disturbed with initial, middle, and terminal insomnia. He reacted to his slowing of bowel function by refusing to eat, for fear that food would block his intestinal tract.
>
> This man had no history of emotional disorder before suffering a stroke some 10 years previously. This was his third episode of severe depression since that time. At the time of his first depressive episode, he developed the delusion that federal agents were pursuing him for tax evasion. He had previously responded well to electroconvulsive therapy; therefore, he was given five such treatments, since he was refractory to treatment with tricyclic antidepressants and because of the immediate danger of inanition. His mood responded well to that treatment, and his sleep disturbance was relieved with 25 mg of thioridazine hs.

Depression may not be accompanied by guilt (Harrow and Amdur 1971); in my experience, depression in the elderly is less often accompanied by guilt and self-derogation than depression in younger adults. It more commonly appears as apathy and listlessness out of proportion to that person's physical state. When pathological ideation is present, it may involve delusions of persecution for misdeeds, as indicated in the previous example. In the case of a 92-year-old nursing home patient with mild cognitive impairment, delusions centered on being possessed by the devil and the nursing home staff planning to get rid of her because she was too demanding.

Suicidal Behavior and Suicide

Suicidal behavior and completed suicide in dementia patients may be the result of depression or may result from a combination of factors including depression. Such factors may include other physical illness, social isolation, diminishing financial reserves, diminishing quality of life, and concern over burdening others. Suicidal ideation usually diminishes when depression is treated successfully. There is not great danger of suicide in dementia patients who are unaware of their deficits and who deny or do not comprehend their prognosis. On the other hand, persons with progressive dementing illnesses who are painfully aware of their cognitive deficits, their growing dependence on others, and the potential outcome of their disease (such as Huntington's disease or AD) may choose to end their own lives. They may make successful suicide attempts without being significantly depressed (Rohde et al. 1995).

Delirium

From the psychological standpoint, delirium may be seen as a result of rapidly developing impairment of coping or adaptive abilities, manifesting when the individual is acutely unable to understand the environment and suffers overload from internal or external stimuli. The cardinal features of delirium include reduced clarity of awareness of the environment; reduced ability to focus, sustain, and shift attention; and cognitive deficits, including memory disturbance and disorientation (see also Table 1–4). These symptoms develop acutely and often fluctuate in severity during the day, becoming most pronounced at night. There is often a prodromal stage of disturbed sleep, bad dreams, and increasing anxiety (Lipowski 1987). Delirium can occur in a person whose nervous system is intact if the precipitating organic process is of great magnitude and has a rapid onset. An example is the sudden onset of a pneumococcal pneumonia accompanied by high fever. More often, there is an antecedent vulnerability of the central nervous system, whether due to central nervous system immaturity or damage. Delirium that occurs in response to trivial insults is virtually pathognomonic of an underlying structural impairment of brain function.

From the Freudian perspective, when cognitively impaired persons experience a sudden further impairment, they become unable to adequately repress the contents of the unconscious part of the mind and to interpret environmental stimuli. Fragmented, repressed memories may come pouring forth, and persons in the environment are understandably confused with important personages from the past. Viewed from this perspective, it is easy to understand how a person with mild cognitive impairment can appear intact when admitted to a hospital in the company of a familiar loved one but can become delirious on awakening in the recovery room with no familiar person, no orienting cues, and with sensorium clouded by the aftereffects of an anesthetic and analgesic medication. Despite the ease of a psychological explanation, each case of delirium warrants medical investigation for conditions such as in an obvious stroke (Dunne et al. 1986). The following case is an illustration of delirium:

Mr. B., a 67-year-old man, had sought help for memory problems of 1–2 years' duration. He was treated for presumed normal-pressure hydrocephalus with a ventriculoperitoneal shunt. To Mr. B.'s disappointment (and that of his family), no change occurred in his cognitive state. In addition, he was very disturbed by a flare-up of his daughter's chronic illness. As a result, he became increasingly depressed. He was seen by a psychiatrist who elicited a history of weight loss, appetite loss, decreased energy, terminal insomnia, and crying spells. His mood was depressed, he had psychomotor retardation, and he cried during the interview. His concentration, attention, and recall were all markedly impaired. He saw himself as only a shadow of his former self. The psychiatrist prescribed 40 mg of imipramine qd in divided doses in addition to the 50 mg of diphenhydramine and 15 mg of flurazepam that he was already taking at bedtime to help him sleep. Because there was only slight amelioration of symptoms after 2 weeks, the imipramine dose was increased to 50 mg qd. Two weeks later, the psychiatrist received a call from the patient's internist, who said that Mr. B. had become psychotic. When interviewed at the hospital to which he had been admitted by the internist, Mr. B. was disoriented in time and space. He thought that his wife was trying to poison him. He insisted that he was in a brothel and that the nurses were trying to solicit him.

In this case, the patient was experiencing a delirium brought on by the three medications he was taking, two of which had strong anticholinergic effects. When his delirium cleared, his mood normalized, and there was no further need for the antidepressant medication.

Anxiety, Agitation, and Restlessness

Anxiety is often experienced in early dementia. Many dementia patients report fear of losing their mental capacities and a sense of helplessness to understand and deal with their environment. If the personality is totally overwhelmed by new or complex environmental demands, a catastrophic response or a delirium may occur.

As individuals become more compromised cognitively, the conscious experience of anxiety may no longer be communicated because of language compromise. Patients may also lose their conceptualization of what they are struggling against. Agitation and restlessness supervene as alarm responses and as preparation for fighting against or flight from an incomprehensible environment.

Sleep-Wake Disturbances

Sleep-wake disturbances are common among dementia patients and are an important factor in caregivers' decision to institutionalize them (Pollack and Perlick 1991). The most common sleep-wake disturbances are hypersomnia, insomnia, and reversal of the sleep-wake cycle. A study of demented and nondemented nursing home patients showed highly fragmented sleep, with patients averaging only 40 minutes of sleep per hour during the night (Ancoli-Israel et al. 1989). In a study comparing AD patients with age-matched control subjects, Bliwise et al. (1989) found no difference in the total amount of sleep, but AD patients had poorer quality of sleep, as evidenced by lower mean sleep efficiency, lower percentages of stages 3 and 4 sleep, and a higher percentage of stage 1 sleep.

Dementia patients who are not active frequently doze during the day because of boredom and are awake and restless at night because they have already obtained their required sleep during their naps. Elderly patients' sleep is often disturbed by pain, by the need to urinate, or by the need to take medications. Stimulants such as coffee, tea, or bronchodilators may contribute to the problem. In elderly patients with loosened pharyngeal tissue, sleep apnea due to mechanical obstruction may occur and may be responsible for frequent sleep interruption and poor quality of sleep, leading to daytime hypersomnolence (Guilleminault et al. 1973). These sleep-wake disturbances may be partly because of physiological, neurotransmitter, or metabolic changes that occur as a result of a dementia-causing disease or injury, but they are often of environmental or iatrogenic origin.

Hypersomnia

The most common medical cause of hypersomnia is overmedication with drugs to control agitation or help with sleep. Anticonvulsants and antihistamines are also strongly sedative. Somnolence is caused by metabolic disturbances such as hypercapnia due to chronic lung disease, uremia due to renal failure, or toxic levels of ammonia due to liver failure. From the environmental standpoint, the chief cause of daytime sleepiness is lack of engaging activities. Sleeping excessively is a way to deal with boredom and to evade the challenge of trying to understand the environment or to initiate behavior. Sometimes caregivers promote daytime sleeping to ease their burden. A sleeping person is easier to manage than a person who is restless and demanding and does not understand how or why certain things must be done, such as urinating or defecating in the toilet.

Insomnia

The inability of dementia patients to sleep the night through is a common complaint of caregivers. Home caregivers look forward to and need relief at night; nursing homes and other institutions are staffed lightly at night. Thus, both family and institutional caregivers bear an extra burden when their charges cannot sleep. Sleep is interrupted by anxiety, but the most common psychiatric syndrome leading to sleep loss is depression. Severely depressed persons have difficulty falling asleep and staying asleep, often waking 3–4 hours before their usual time and dreading the day ahead. Excessive stimulant intake in the form of caffeine in coffee, tea, or soft drinks or theophylline for bronchopulmonary disease adds to sleep difficulty. In addition, if there is little daytime physical activity, there is little physiological demand for rest.

Reversal of the Sleep-Wake Cycle

Daytime napping and nighttime awakening may lead to a reversal of the sleep-wake cycle. For elderly persons, getting to sleep and staying asleep are made difficult by painful arthritis and the need to urinate during the night, the latter being aggravated by diuretics to control blood pressure or to ameliorate heart failure. Sleep apnea, with its frequent interruptions of sleep, is also more common in elderly patients. More often than not, sleep difficulty is produced or aggravated by environmental factors, such as scheduling bedtime too early. When examined objectively, the dementia patient is found to be sleeping 6–8 hours, but sleep time begins at 8 P.M. and ends at 2–4 A.M.— with attempts at getting up and beginning the day. In many cases, dementia patients get sufficient sleep from napping during the day.

In a preliminary study (Satlin et al. 1992), exposure of 10 late-stage AD patients to 2,000 lux of light from 7–9 P.M. for 1 week increased evening wakefulness and reduced nighttime activity, with return to former levels 1 week after discontinuance of exposure to bright light.

Suspiciousness and Delusion Formation

Many persons attempt to compensate for their impairment with hyperalertness. In a hyperalert state, one becomes aware of many environmental stimuli that are not readily understood, so that the coping mechanism of hyperalertness leads to increasing confusion. Suspiciousness is a variant of the hyperalert or hypervigilant state in which stimuli are interpreted as dangerous. In a situation in which it is not possible to distinguish what is safe from what is dangerous, it makes sense to first view everything as dangerous.

It is also frustrating and aggravating to find so much that cannot be understood in a world that one could formerly grasp. What better explanation than that attempts are being made to deceive? In this way, defective perception and integration can be denied, and it is no longer necessary to explain every event individually or try to understand each confusing stimulus. The answer is that one is being deliberately deceived. For example, a man with dementia does not perceive himself as unable to identify his wife. Instead, he regards the woman who says she is married to him as an impostor. A final important aspect of delusional thinking is that it enables action. Perceiving danger as external enables one to avoid it or to attack it, thus reducing the unpleasant feeling of helplessness that comes from being confused. Anxiety is dealt with in the same way. No longer able to recognize that anxiety results from inner tension, the person with dementia experiences fear and attributes it to the external environment.

Common delusional beliefs include believing that others are in the house, that one is not in one's own home, that one's spouse is an impostor, and that deceased loved ones are still alive. The delusional beliefs of dementia patients can often be temporarily reduced by gentle confrontation with reality, in contrast to such beliefs of persons with a mental illness such as schizophrenia.

Delusional Syndromes

A number of delusional syndromes have been reported in dementia patients. They include Capgras's syndrome (Burns and Philpot 1987) and Cotard's syndrome. In the former, there is the fixed belief that there are doubles of others, and there may be the belief that there are doubles of one's self. Merriam et al. (1988) found Capgras-like symptoms to occur in 17% of AD patients. In Cotard's syndrome, individuals believe that parts of their bodies are missing, that they do not exist, or that the world about them does not exist. In dealing with Cotard's syndrome, the clinician must suspect major depression in addition to dementing illness. AD patients also often express the notion that an unseen person is living in the house; the so-called phantom boarder syndrome (Rubin et al. 1988). Patients unable to recognize themselves in a mirror may develop the delusion that another person is present. One of our patients became fearful of entering an automobile because he always saw the face of the same person in the window glass on entering a car.

Illusions occur commonly in dementia patients. An illusion is a mistaken perception: mistaking one thing for something else because of a real or imagined resemblance. For example, a man with dementia mistakes his wife for his mother. She resembles his mother in that she is roughly his mother's age when she was last alive, and the notion of "mother" is nurturing and comforting. An illusion that becomes a fixed belief is a delusion.

Hallucinations

Hallucinations are false perceptions; that is, they are reports of sensory impressions that cannot be consensually validated. Hallucinations are frequent in delirium and dementia. Delirious persons frequently envision animals crawling up the walls or feel ants crawling on their skin. Dementia patients often report children or small adults running in and out of their homes or airplanes flying overhead. They frequently watch in fascination but often become excited and upset.

Hallucinations can be explained psychologically in the same way as delusions. They are means to organize an otherwise incomprehensible environment and are often determined by personal needs or wishes, as exemplified by the frequent hallucination of loved ones who are no longer living. Hallucinations may also have a physiological component; that is, they may be stimulated by abnormal electrical discharges of the brain, as in partial complex seizures, which often have an olfactory aura of an unpleasant smell such as burning feathers or burning rubber. Just as it does with incomprehensible environmental stimuli, the mind can organize incomprehensible sensory stimuli from within the brain into perceptions that can be understood and reacted to (Weiner 1961).

The Charles Bonnet Syndrome

Patients with AD frequently experience a type of visual hallucinatory state or hallucinosis that may or may not be disturbing to them. Described as the *Charles Bonnet syndrome,* the state consists of seeing formed, complex, persistent ,or repetitive and stereotyped visual hallucinations. Patients often have the sense that they are not real. There are no accompanying delusions, and hallucinations are not present in other sensory modalities (Gold and Rabins 1989). One of our AD patients saw people in his house who had Xs for eyes. They were never the same people from day to day, and none was recognizable as anyone he knew.

He was mildly puzzled by the presence of these people, would talk to them (they did not reply), and was able to tolerate their presence very well. Another AD patient saw individuals with peculiarly colored hair. They seemed to appear in groups. They did not speak. Some of them had only half-bodies that they propelled with their hands.

Apathy and Withdrawal

Apathy, the inability or unwillingness to become involved with one's environment, can be a direct result of brain injury or a psychological consequence. Apathy is often associated with injury to frontal convexity (Cummings 1985). It can also be a psychological reaction to an environment perceived as hostile, unrewarding, or incomprehensible, and the last is frequently the case with dementia patients. As a result of feeling overwhelmed, dementia patients first withdraw into an environment that they can comprehend. When that fails, they may become apathetic and withdraw emotionally as well as physically.

Summary

Viewing dementia as the product of a dynamic interaction between biological and psychological forces enables clinicians to recognize that fluctuations in cognitive and coping abilities of persons with dementia are the norm. However, when confronted with increased disorientation in a brain-damaged person, clinicians must consider whether the increased disorientation results from progression of the underlying brain disease, metabolic factors, the onset of depression, change in the relationship between the dementia patient and others, or change in the physical environment.

The clinician's intervention will depend on which variable or group of variables predominates. Having made an adequate diagnosis of the disease underlying the dementia, and therefore having some sense of the normal progress of the disease with which they are dealing, clinicians will perform appropriate examinations, order appropriate tests, and assay the effects of interpersonal and environmental changes when the clinical course appears out of line with what is known of the general progress of the illness.

In some cases, cognitive function or behavioral dyscontrol will improve when cardiac function is improved, when a brain infection is treated, when the patient is better hydrated, when the environment is simplified by maintaining the same routine every day, or when the person is kept in a familiar environment. In other cases, there will be no change or the patient's status may actually worsen. The clinician will again investigate to determine whether there are any adverse effects from medication side effects or some unexpected reaction to interpersonal or environmental changes that was instituted. In all cases, the patient's level of functioning is the result of a delicate balance between factors that become increasingly difficult to evaluate as dementing diseases progress.

CHAPTER 3

The Dementia Workup

Myron F. Weiner, M.D.
Ron Tintner, M.D., Ph.D.
Frederick J. Bonte, M.D.

A medical evaluation is indicated for persons with subjective complaints of cognitive impairment, the objective development of cognitive impairment, or the sudden worsening of cognitive impairment or behavior in a well-diagnosed dementia patient. The extent of the evaluation depends on the physician's assessment of the problem, the facilities available to undertake a diagnostic workup, and the cost-benefit ratios of the various diagnostic procedures available. The most important reason for undertaking a medical workup is the possibility of finding a reversible cause of cognitive impairment. Fully reversible dementia syndromes are rare and are most often due to depression, drugs, or metabolic disorders. However, even if a dementia-producing illness is not fully reversible, partial reversal is still desirable.

A medical workup can also search for factors leading to "excess disability" (Barry and Moskowitz 1988), wherein frail elders or dementia patients experience worsening of their cognitive state by infection, cardiac decompensation, or even environmental changes. Younger persons suffering from head injury, acquired immunodeficiency syndrome (AIDS), or stroke may become more cognitively impaired as the result of depression. Barry and Moskowitz (1988) suggest that, in general, evaluation of (elderly) persons with cognitive impairment be undertaken with the goal of improving patient well-being rather than simply identifying disease. On the other hand, the number of untreatable diseases is shrinking, and precise diagnosis may be important in deciding which drugs to prescribe or not to prescribe. For example, strongly anticholinergic drugs may aggravate dementia symptoms in Alzheimer's disease (AD) patients by increasing the already-present cholinergic deficit.

We find that three main groups of patients present for cognitive status valuation. A few (usually self-referred) individuals seek evaluation because of a family history of AD or concern about the cognitive changes that normally begin in middle or advanced age. Most patients are brought in for evaluation by friends or family members because of concern over decreased cognitive function. Virtually all of these individuals have dementias. The third group is composed of individuals with cognitive impairment whose cognition is worsening. The families of these individuals have often been told that the cognitive change they noted in their loved ones was due to advanced age or that the patients may have AD. These families seek second opinions for various reasons, including the wish to explore every possibility of uncovering a treatable cause for dementia or a treatment for a dementing illness that had previously been described as untreatable. Also within this group are well-diagnosed nursing home residents whose cognitive state changes suddenly.

Different medical workups may be indicated for a subjective complaint of cognitive impairment, for the initial workup of a person whose friends and family have noted signs of cognitive impairment, and for the follow-up evaluation of sudden cognitive deterioration in an adequately diagnosed dementia patient.

A subjective complaint of cognitive impairment that is unsubstantiated by an outside informant requires a medical and psychiatric history, a formal mental status examination, and a general physical examination, including neurological examination and routine screening laboratory tests. If the history and mental status examinations do not confirm cognitive impairment and there is no sign of brain damage, psychiatric evaluation and psychological testing may be indicated. The complaint of cognitive impairment, like any other medical complaint, may be a means to deal with emotional issues and concerns (Weiner 1969). This is illustrated in the following case:

> A 60-year-old woman complained of impaired memory and concentration. Her medical history indicated that she had been worked up for several physical complaints with no definite findings. Her husband reported that he had not observed difficulty with her cognitive functioning. A complete battery of blood tests and a urinalysis were performed and were negative or within normal limits. A complete neurological workup, including a computed tomography (CT) and an electroencephalogram, was negative. Neuropsychological testing showed no clinically meaningful impairment, but personality testing using the

Minnesota Multiphasic Personality Inventory showed her to be highly anxious and highly preoccupied with physical symptoms. To the psychiatric examiner, she confided that her greatest problem was her husband's physical abuse, which she related to their chronic marital conflict. This patient was assured that she did not have a brain disorder and was helped to draw her husband into brief marital counseling.

The following material first describes the diagnostic procedures applicable in the medical workup of dementia symptoms and later describes minimal and optimal workups of patients with dementia syndromes. These guidelines are also useful in evaluating persons with known dementing illness in whom there has been a sudden decline in cognitive status.

Preparation

The evaluation process begins with gathering medical and psychological information. It is useful to obtain medical and psychological findings from other settings in advance to avoid duplication of tests and loss of information due to informants' lack of awareness or understanding of the diagnostic procedures that have already been employed or medications currently being prescribed. In all instances, we try to include a person with close knowledge of the patient in the diagnostic process. We also request that patients or family members bring in all prescribed or unprescribed medications to which the patient has access.

Setting

The medical evaluation of dementia symptoms is generally accomplished in an outpatient setting. Hospitalization is required only when behavioral symptoms make outpatient evaluation impossible or when it is suspected that an emergency medical or surgical procedure might be needed—such as the emergency treatment of lupus cerebritis with bolus intravenous steroids or evacuation of a rapidly expanding subdural hematoma. Otherwise, hospitalization may actually have transient deleterious effects. Some patients become more confused in a strange environment with a different daily routine (Etienne et al. 1981). A comprehensive multidisciplinary workup requires 1–3 days, depending on the efficiency of scheduling, the patient's tolerance, and the extensiveness of medical and neuropsychological testing. In this chapter, discussion is limited to the medical aspects of the workup.

History

The diagnostic process begins with history taking. An adequate evaluation also involves obtaining information from collateral sources. What is the chief complaint? A few persons report being unable to learn or to recall the names of persons and objects. Many do not report cognitive impairment but are brought for evaluation because others have noted lapses in memory or judgment and are concerned. Does the history specifically indicate difficulties characteristic of mental impairment? Have there been problems with memory, orientation, calculation, comprehension, word finding, carrying out simple tasks, reasoning, personality change, or judgment? Whether the history is obtained directly from patients or from outside informants, there are a number of key questions:

1. Were the symptoms acute, subacute, or gradual in onset?   An acute onset (within minutes or hours) suggests vascular, traumatic, or emotional origin. When vascular, the symptoms may be due to atherosclerotic thromboembolic disease, hemorrhage within a tumor, vasculitis (including systemic lupus), or embolization. In the case of suspected embolization, echocardiography is indicated if a cardiac origin is likely. In the case of patent foramen ovale with right-to-left shunt, angiography may be indicated to detect a venous source. In young adults developing schizophrenia, a catatonic episode may come on within hours. Malingered cognitive impairment and fugue states also develop suddenly, both usually occurring in the context of extreme environmental or interpersonal stress. Subacute onset (days to weeks) suggests infectious, toxic/metabolic, or neoplastic origin, whereas insidious onset is more typical of degenerative disorders.

It is often difficult to date the onset of cognitive difficulties. If the patient was employed, inquire about job performance. If he or she is retired, was retirement due in part to impaired performance? With a retired individual, ask about the person's usual activities (e.g., golf, bridge, reading). When was the first change in those activities or in other activities such as driving?

2. Have the symptoms progressed?   Lack of progression suggests a single insult, such as a vascular accident, trauma, or depression. Progression may be associated with infectious diseases (AIDS, Creutzfeldt-Jakob disease, neurosyphilis), trauma (subdural hematoma), and degenerative disorders. Degenerative disorders such as AD, Parkinson's disease,

Pick's disease, and multisystems degeneration tend to have a smooth downward course.

3. Have the symptoms diminished? Symptomatic improvement is associated with trauma, acute vascular disorders, and acute toxic/metabolic disorders. Fluctuations in cognitive dysfunction may occur in many types of dementing illness, including the degenerative disorders, but do not include a return to baseline. Paroxysmal deterioration with relatively full interepisode recovery occurs in alcoholic patients with encephalopathy due to liver disease. Transient global amnesia is a syndrome of intermittent confusion of diverse etiology, probably due in many cases to ischemia of the medial temporal lobes. Partial complex seizures can cause intermittent behavioral disruption with cumulative chronic deterioration, but the history also reveals motor stereotypy and postictal sleepiness. Porphyria can also cause transient cognitive impairment but usually is accompanied by disturbances of mood and thinking.

4. How have the symptoms progressed? Has the progress been stepwise or smooth? The former suggests vascular dementia (VaD) in older adults and multiple sclerosis (MS) in younger adults; the latter, AD. If symptoms have progressed rapidly, an acute or subacute process may be at work, including toxic and metabolic disorders, central nervous system infection, and subdural hematoma.

In the case of stepwise progression, sensory and motor changes accompany the cognitive change in VaD and MS. In most dementias, sensorial impairment fluctuates, depending on the complexity of the environment, emotional strain, fatigue, general physical health, and time of day. Symptoms are frequently worse in the evenings due to fatigue and loss of orienting sensory cues.

5. Are there symptoms related to noncognitive aspects of brain function? These symptoms include loss of consciousness, seizures, uncoordination, slowness of movement, weakness (generalized or localized), impairment of vision or hearing, and symptoms of other cranial nerve dysfunction. Loss of consciousness accompanies severe head trauma, lupus cerebritis, and toxic-metabolic disorders. Dysarthria and paralysis of gaze may suggest progressive supranuclear palsy. Seizures may point to a primary seizure disorder or to other conditions such as neoplasm, in which seizures are secondary. Slowness of movement may indicate depression, early Parkinson's disease, or a subcortical dementia; uncoordination and sensory and cranial nerve symptoms may indicate MS.

6. Is there a personal or family history of a disease or disorder associated with dementia?   The presence of diabetes, hypertension, and signs of generalized atherosclerosis point to possible VaD. Severe renal or hepatic disease may produce metabolic encephalopathy. Human immunodeficiency virus (HIV) positivity raises the possibility of AIDS encephalitis or brain infection due to opportunistic infection. Huntington's and Wilson's diseases exemplify familial diseases associated with dementia.

7. Is there a history of psychiatric disorder or severe environmental stress?   An episode of depression, whether mild or severe, can markedly impair cognitive functioning. Persons with long-standing schizophrenia frequently appear demented. Malingered cognitive impairment occurs in persons facing imprisonment (Ganser syndrome), and amnesias known as fugue states may develop in a variety of individuals who are seeking to escape the consequences of acts such as bigamy.

8. Are there behavioral or psychiatric symptoms?   Frequently, the first symptoms noted in a dementing illness are loss of initiative and loss of interest in activities that were formerly pleasurable. Individuals with impaired frontal lobe function may show either apathy or disinhibition. Suspiciousness and irritability may accompany early dementia as may depression or elation and grandiosity. Visual hallucinations unaccompanied by explanatory delusions are frequent in AD. Tactile hallucinations and illusions are common in delirium. Complex delusional systems are unusual in dementing illness, and auditory hallucinations tend to be those of familiar others rather than the accusatory or threatening voices speaking through the radio or television that are more characteristic of schizophrenia.

9. Has the person experienced the same or similar symptoms in the past?   Past experience of short confusional episodes may suggest a seizure disorder or transient ischemic attacks. Periods of cognitive dysfunction lasting days or weeks may be related to emotional disorders, metabolic disorders such as porphyria, or an autommimune disorder such as MS. Individuals who are malingering or in fugue states will often report similar previous episodes. Depressed persons may report similar episodes of cognitive impairment with past episodes of depression.

10. Are the symptoms constant or intermittent?   Intermittent symptomatology occurs with all disorders of brain function. Waxing and waning of symptoms over hours are typical of delirium. Dementing illnesses are also characterized by fluctuating symptomatology, but the fluctuations are less dramatic and are often more prolonged.

11. Does the person take any prescribed or unprescribed medications? Many medications have the ability to impair cognitive function, including benzodiazepine hypnotics and tranquilizers, barbiturates, anticonvulsants, propranolol, and cardiac glycosides. Episodes of porphyria may be induced by various medications, including barbiturates and chlordiazepoxide (Sack 1990). It is imperative that all the contents of the family medicine chest be brought in, especially in the case of older adults who may not be aware of the number or dosage of the medications they are taking.

12. Is there a history of abuse or heavy intake of alcohol or other substances? History of alcohol abuse may point to the origin of an amnestic disorder or dementia. Prolonged heavy alcohol use without evidence of intoxication can also cause significant cognitive impairment. In teenagers and young adults, evidence of glue or paint sniffing is important. Chronic marijuana use can lead to a syndrome of anergia, listlessness, and vacuousness.

13. Has there been exposure to environmental toxins? Arsenic, mercury, lead, organic solvents, and organophosphate insecticides can produce encephalopathies, usually accompanied by severe systemic symptoms.

14. Has there been exposure to HIV infection? Although the routes of potential infection that are most strongly suspect are intravenous drug abuse, transfusions, and unprotected anal sexual penetration, unprotected heterosexual contact is increasingly a risk factor, especially in young adults. HIV infection can also occur in older adults.

The history may suggest that the patient has a depressive disorder or that the patient is overreactive to the normal cognitive changes accompanying aging. In any case, a formal mental status examination should be performed. Even if there is no evidence of cognitive impairment in the clinician's estimation, it may still be wise to obtain a gross baseline measure of cognitive performance such as the Mini-Mental State Exam (Folstein et al. 1975) or the more sensitive Mattis Dementia Rating Scale (Mattis 1988).

Physical Examination

A general physical examination is an important part of the dementia workup. Diseases of many organ systems can produce the symptoms of dementia, cause brain changes leading to dementia, or contribute to excess morbidity from dementia.

Neurological Examination

A detailed neurological examination is performed on every patient (see Appendix 10). Posture and gait are observed. Gait tends to slow with aging, and tandem walking is difficult for elders. Gait disturbances are prominent in progressive supranuclear palsy and are frequent in individuals with Creutzfeldt-Jakob disease. A "magnetic" gait raises the possibility of normal-pressure hydrocephalus. Cranial nerve examination includes olfaction. Anosmia is a frequent concomitant of AD but also occurs in psychiatrically normal elders. Anosmia of sudden onset may point to a significant head injury. Visual and auditory acuity are tested. Pupillary abnormalities occur with neurosyphilis but may also result from cataract surgery. Examination of the interior of the eye may reveal damage from long-standing hypertension or diabetes. Pallor of the disk may point to optic neuritis from MS or choking of the disk to increased intracranial pressure from a space-occupying lesion. Impairment of downward gaze occurs in progressive supranuclear palsy.

Examination of the motor system includes muscle bulk and tone. Increased resistance to passive movement is common as AD progresses; increased muscle tone with cogwheeling occurs in Parkinson's disease and pseudoparkinsonism due to neuroleptic drugs. Patients are observed for involuntary movements, such as tremor, dyskinesia, or chorea. The sensory system is evaluated. Vibration sense in the lower extremities is frequently reduced in elders, but position sense is not. Sensory neuropathies occur in individuals with diabetes, syphilis, and pernicious anemia. Deep tendon reflexes are assessed, and the presence or absence of Babinski reflexes are observed. In the absence of radiculopathy or cord compression, asymmetric reflexes and the presence of Babinski reflexes suggest pathology involving upper motor neurons. The presence of primitive reflexes (palmomental, snout, grasp) substantiate gross cerebral impairment, but they are not generally useful in localizing brain pathology.

Data from the neurological examination, mental status examination, and history enable the clinician to differentiate dementias in one of the types described in Chapter 1: frontal, temporoparietal, and subcortical. The neurological examination allows the distinction of dementias into the categories of cortical, subcortical, or mixed. The distinctions between cortical and subcortical dementias include the relative predominance of behavioral over cognitive symptoms in subcortical dementias. Subcortical dementias may be typified by apathy or disinhibition. These dementias also tend to have motor signs that may be pyramidal or extrapyramidal. The anatomic loci for cortical dementias are the neocortical association areas and hippocampus; for subcortical dementias, they are the thalamus, basal ganglia, and rostral brain stem (M. C. Albert et al. 1974). Based on the foregoing criteria, the prototypical cortical dementias are Alzheimer's and Pick's diseases, but mild extrapyramidal signs, such as rigidity and bradykinesia, can occur in conjunction with AD. Typical subcortical dementias are Huntington's disease, Wilson's disease, AIDS dementia, and progressive supranuclear palsy. VaD, Creutzfeldt-Jakob disease, and trauma typically produce mixed cortical and subcortical signs.

Laboratory Studies

Unless specific evidence is present on clinical examination, we do not routinely perform tests to determine whether toxic substances have been ingested. If, on the other hand, there is a suspicion of covert or unreported drug use or of exposure to toxins such as lead or mercury, appropriate toxicological testing is performed. When it is known that digitalis, anticonvulsants, antidepressants, or other drugs that produce confusion when the therapeutic blood level is exceeded are present, we will determine their concentration in blood.

Blood

Recommended routine blood tests include evaluation of electrolytes; glucose, calcium, and phosphorus levels; liver and kidney function tests; thyroid function tests (TSH and T_4); erythrocyte sedimentation rate; antinuclear antibodies; serologic test for syphilis; and folic acid and vitamin B_{12} concentration. A complete blood count is also performed. Arterial blood gas concentrations are determined when severe pulmonary disease is present, and the serum ammonia level is determined when severe liver disease is detected.

Urine

In the case of frail elders, a urinalysis is indicated routinely. In many instances, a urinary tract infection will cause confusion (usually, a delirium), but in others it may present only as a worsening of cognitive state. Urine toxicological studies are indicated in persons with possible heavy-metal exposure and urinary porphyrins in suspected porphyria.

Spinal Fluid

Lumbar puncture is a relatively benign procedure that has produced virtually no complications in our hands, but in only 1 instance in more than 400 cases did our findings help in the differential diagnosis of patients evaluated for long-standing progressive dementia. Our experience is similar to that of Hammerstrom and Zimmer (1985), who reviewed the value of lumbar punctures in evaluating 80 dementia patients age 50 years or older. No diagnosis was made on the basis of the information derived from lumbar puncture in the 42 patients who underwent lumbar puncture. The only abnormalities found were 11 cases of nonspecific protein elevation and 1 case of increased cell count not due to bacterial infection. They reviewed an additional series of 422 cases from other series and found 4 patients whose diagnoses could have been made by lumbar puncture. One patient had neurosyphilis, and the other 3 were postencephalitic.

Nevertheless, lumbar puncture is justified, especially in the evaluation of young and middle-aged patients. It is indicated specifically in rapidly progressive dementia at any age, positive syphilis serology, and suspected central nervous system infection. It is also indicated in all cases of dementia occurring in patients with diagnosed or suspected AIDS and in dementia patients who have had a blood transfusion.

Special Diagnostic Procedures

Invasive Diagnostic Procedures

Cisternogram

Radionuclide cisternography is used to differentiate between communicating and noncommunicating hydrocephalus and helps establish the diagnosis of normal-pressure hydrocephalus by demonstrating reflux into the ventricles and delayed pericerebral diffusion.

Angiography

A radiopaque contrast medium injected percutaneously into a carotid, brachial, or femoral artery allows visualization of the entire circulation of the neck and brain. This technique is valuable for the diagnosis of aneurysms, vascular malformations, occluded arteries and veins, and mass lesions, such as hemorrhages, abscesses, and neoplasms. With this technique, there is danger of producing a frank ischemic lesion in the territory of the vessel or vessels being studied; high concentrations of contrast medium may cause spasm and occlusion. A clot formed on the catheter tip can embolize an artery. Because of the danger involved, direct arterial angiography should be performed only for specific indications.

Digital subtraction angiography, which produces computer-generated images of the major cervical and intracranial arteries, is a much more benign, less expensive, but somewhat less precise technique. This technique involves the intravenous injection of a small amount of contrast material.

Brain Biopsy

Although not associated with high morbidity, brain biopsy is reserved for situations in which a reversible dementia or a treatable illness is suspected or, in the case of Creutzfeldt-Jakob disease, to establish a diagnosis so that appropriate environmental precautions can be taken. We have reserved this procedure for suspected autoimmune cerebral vascular disease and suspected infectious brain disease that is not diagnosable by spinal fluid studies. We have requested brain biopsy four times. All instances were cases of rapidly progressive dementia. In one case, the biopsy report was normal brain tissue; in the other three, it was AD. Brain biopsy is of limited use in that only small amounts of tissue can be sampled, and the brain areas most affected by diseases such as AD are not readily accessible.

Noninvasive Diagnostic Procedures

Carotid Sonography

Evidence of generalized arteriosclerosis, neck bruits, transient ischemic attacks, or stroke warrants investigation by Doppler flow or ultrasound carotid sonography. Heyman et al. (1980) found that asymptomatic bruits in men (but not women) carry an increased risk of stroke but do not predict vascular locus or laterality. Adams and Victor (1989) recommend that surgery be undertaken only if the carotid vessel lumen is less than 2 mm. Our experience is that carotid obstruction does not often contribute to the development of dementia, but we have had one anecdotal report of a progressive dementia with pronounced bilateral carotid narrowing that improved dramatically after bilateral endarterectomy (R. Rosenberg, personal communication, October 3, 1989).

Electroencephalogram

Background EEG waveforms reflect the overall integrity of the cerebral cortex. Paroxysmal waveforms indicate specific events, such as seizures. Most AD patients have abnormal EEG studies (usually, diffuse slowing), Pick's disease patients tend to have normal EEGs, and Huntington's disease patients show low voltage (D. J. Robinson et al. 1994). Diffuse slowing occurs in delirium-producing toxic and metabolic disorders (Engel and Romano 1959). In patients with Creutzfeldt-Jakob disease, the EEG pattern is distinctive, with polyphasic sharp wave discharges superimposed on a slow background (Burger et al. 1972). Focal slow waves may suggest destructive lesions such as strokes and tumors. Because EEG recording is from surface electrodes, lesions deep within the brain may not be detected.

EEG-detected evoked cortical potentials such as the P300 do not seem to add to clinical diagnostic specificity in the dementias. Patterson et al. (1988), in a study of normal control elders, depressed patients, and AD patients, investigated auditory evoked potentials based on the detection of a target tone among a series of frequent nontarget tones. They found that none of the control or depressed persons was misclassified as demented; only 27% of individuals with dementia were classified correctly with P300 variability, and 13% were classified correctly with P300 latency.

Quantitative Electroencephalogram

Quantitative EEG replaces analog pen-and-ink recordings of brain electrical activity with digitized signals recorded on magnetic or optical media. Quantitative EEG pools and averages information from 20 or more EEG electrode placements, thus allowing the detection and depiction of patterns of electrical activity in the brain (Duffy et al. 1979). Breslau et al. (1989) compared topographic EEG in AD patients and in elderly and young normal control subjects. The elderly control subjects showed reduction in alpha, beta, delta, and theta rhythms when compared with their young counterparts. Further analysis showed the elderly control subjects to have increased midparietal and left midtemporal delta and theta rhythms as compared with the young control subjects. Also, the elderly control subjects showed less occipital and greater midparietal alpha and beta rhythms than the young control subjects. The only significant difference between elderly control subjects and the AD patients was a marked delta asymmetry in the temporal regions. Brenner et al. (1988) compared 35 AD patients, 23 patients with major depression, and 61 healthy elderly control subjects. Spectral analysis (transformation of data from amplitude versus frequency to energy versus frequency) afforded only modest advantages over visual EEG inspection in differentiating the three groups. Both EEG and spectral changes correlated with severity of dementia and identified essentially the same patients. The computer was not more sensitive than the eye in detecting mild cases.

A host of commercially packaged programs are available for this technique, but quantitative EEG is considered to be an adjunct to conventional EEG (American Psychiatric Association Task Force on Quantitative Electrophysiologic Assessment 1991). However, efforts are being made to translate images of surface-recorded brain activity into images with greater clinical relevance by comparing quantitative EEG recordings with various functional imaging techniques so as to determine the electrical equivalents of regional cerebral hypo- or hyperperfusion, and so on (Leuchter and Holschneider 1994).

Skull X Ray

Routine skull X rays are of little use in the evaluation of dementia patients because they show only the bony structures and the location of the falx and pineal gland, if either is calcified. Thus, only processes such as trauma or neoplasm that affect the skull or shift calcified midline structures are diagnosable with the help of a skull X ray. Skull X rays can also be helpful in detecting diseases such as toxoplasmosis that cause areas of intracerebral calcification, but more information is gained in almost every instance from CT.

Computed Tomography

Although more expensive than skull X rays, CT is an excellent means to visualize both the skull and the brain itself. The ventricles and cerebral gyri and sulci can be visualized well on CT. Areas of demyelinization, bleeding, and infarction are quite evident on CT scan, as are shifts in the midline structures and space-occupying lesions. Figure 3–1 shows an infarct; Figures 3–2 and 3–3 show malignancies. Despite the fact that CT does not visualize the posterior fossa well, this technique is the imaging procedure of choice in routine dementia evaluation. Loss of tissue in the caudate nucleus can be visualized in Huntington's disease, as seen in Figure 3–4. Lobar frontotemporal cortical atrophy can be seen often in Pick's disease. Generalized cortical atrophy and hydrocephalus ex vacuo are seen in AD, but a normal CT scan is not unusual. Enlarged ventricles are seen in both obstructive and normal-pressure hydrocephalus. Figure 3–5 shows the findings in normal-pressure hydrocephalus.

Magnetic Resonance Imaging

Magnetic resonance imaging (MRI) is based on the principle that the properties or structure of a tissue or substance can be determined by measuring changes that occur when the nuclei of atoms are placed in a strong magnetic field. Different types of imaging are possible depending on T_1 and T_2 relaxation time, which are tissue-specific longitudinal and transverse relaxation times following a radiofrequency signal deflection of the magnetic field induced in tissue atomic nuclei by the MR scanner magnets (Andreasen 1989).

Nuclear MRI surpasses CT as a procedure for studying the details of brain anatomy, but it is a poor means to study the skull. Gray and white matter are well delineated. The basal ganglia and even the hippocampus (Naidich et al. 1987) can be visualized in great detail, as can the cerebellum and brain stem. The principal drawbacks of this procedure are its greater expense in relation to CT, the extent of patient cooperation needed (lying still in a frightening environment for at least 30–40 minutes), our lack of knowledge of the significance of certain MRI findings, and the need for greater sophistication in interpreting the films obtained.

T_2-weighted MRI images frequently show areas of increased periventricular and deep white matter signal in elderly patients. This phenomenon, termed *leukoaraiosis* (Hachinski et al. 1987), is related to increasing age and cardiovascular risk factors (Erkinjuntti et al. 1994) and may be accompanied by subtle cognitive impairment (Austrom et al. 1990). Leukoaraiosis is shown in Figure 3–6.

T_1-weighted MRI images are best for delineating brain structure; T_2-weighted images are best for identifying lesions. Thus, T_1-weighted images are useful in detecting narrowing of the cortical ribbon in AD and

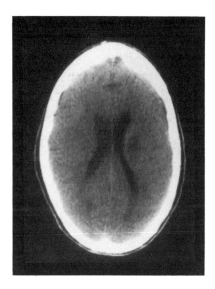

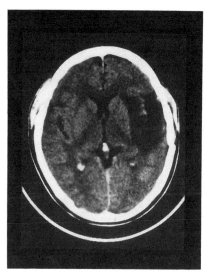

Figure 3–1. CT. Infarct, left corona radiata in distribution of middle cerebral artery (on viewer's right) (courtesy of Dr. Linda Judge).

Figure 3–2. CT. Recurrent fibrillary astrocytoma with extensive destruction of left temporal lobe (on viewer's right) (courtesy of Dr. Linda Judge).

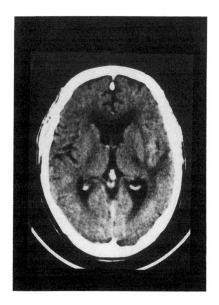

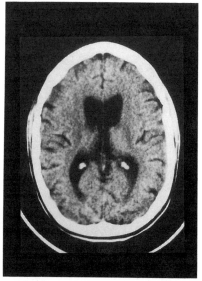

Figure 3–3. CT. Glioblastoma of left hemisphere (on viewer's right) (courtesy of Dr. Linda Judge).

Figure 3–4. CT. Huntington's disease. Destruction of head of caudate nucleus gives square appearance to ventricles (courtesy of Dr. Linda Judge).

shrinkage of the caudate nucleus in Huntington's disease. T_2-weighted images are more useful for detecting small strokes or demyelinization (Devous 1989). Figure 3–7 shows the lesions of MS; Figure 3–8 shows a large subdural hematoma; Figure 3–9 depicts a stroke involving cortex and deeper structures; Figure 3–10 shows a thalamic astrocytoma.

MRI can also be used to follow the course of treatment in brain infections. Figure 3–11 shows the changes characteristic of progressive multifocal leukoencephalopathy in an AIDS patient; Figure 3–12 shows the same patient after treatment with an antiviral agent.

MRI studies can be enhanced with the use of a gadolinium-containing compound that does not pass the intact blood-brain barrier (Niendorf et al. 1990). Such studies can help in the differential diagnosis of brain infections. Figure 3–13 shows multiple gray and white matter lesions of toxoplasmosis; Figure 3–14 shows enhancement of lesions by gadolinium. The lesions of progressive multifocal leukoencephalopathy, HIV, and cytomegalovirus are not enhanced.

Magnetic Resonance Spectroscopy

Magnetic resonance spectroscopy (MRS) generates spectra of the magnetic resonance signals of phosphorus, carbon, and hydrogen nuclei in-

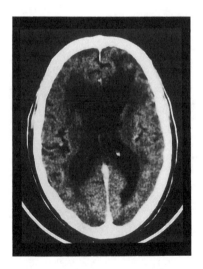

Figure 3–5. CT. Normal-pressure hydrocephalus with enormously dilated ventricles (courtesy of Dr. Linda Judge).

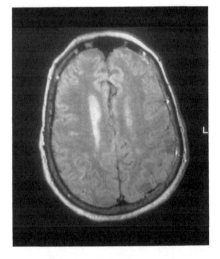

Figure 3–6. MRI. Leukoaraiosis. Increased periventricular signal with small areas of increased signal in corona radiata (courtesy of Dr. Dianne Mendelsohn).

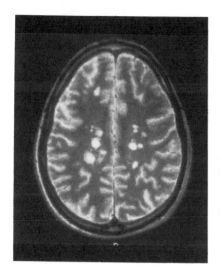

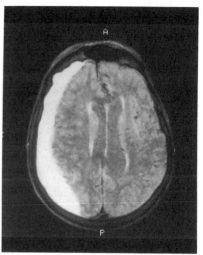

Figure 3–7. MRI. Multiple sclerosis; many discrete areas of increased signal throughout the white matter (courtesy of Dr. Dianne Mendelsohn).

Figure 3–8. MRI. Huge right subdural hematoma (on viewer's left) with shift of midline structures (courtesy of Dr. Dianne Mendelsohn).

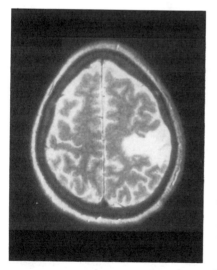

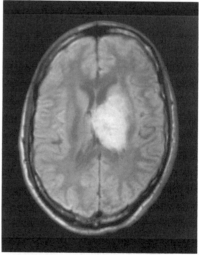

Figure 3–9. MRI. Old left middle cerebral artery distribution infarct (on viewer's right) involving cortex and deeper structures (on veiwer's right) (courtesy of Dr. Dianne Mendelsohn).

Figure 3–10. MRI. Left thalamic astrocytoma (on viewer's right) (courtesy of Dr. Dianne Mendelsohn).

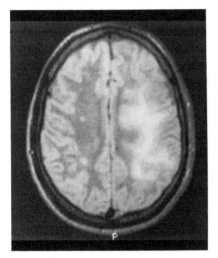

Figure 3–11. MRI. Progressive multifocal leukodystrophy with asymmetrical increase in white matter signal (courtesy of Dr. James L. Fleckenstein).

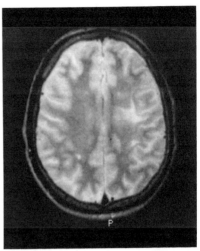

Figure 3–12. MRI. The same patient after treatment with antiviral agent (courtesy of Dr. James L. Fleckenstein).

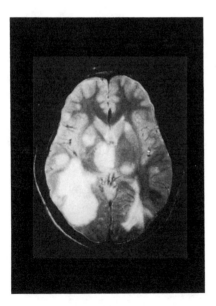

Figure 3–13. MRI. Multiple gray and white matter lesions of toxoplasmosis (courtesy of Dr. James L. Fleckenstein).

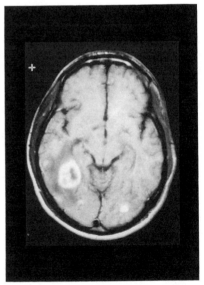

Figure 3–14. MRI with gadolinium contrast. Enhancement of toxoplasmosis lesions (courtesy of Dr. James L. Fleckenstein).

stead of generating images (Bottomley 1989). From the spectrum of ^{31}P, information can be obtained about concentrations of ^{31}P-containing substances. The ratio of phosphomonoesters to phosphodiesters can give information about cell membrane stability. Measures of adenosine triphosphate (ATP) can assess the energy metabolism of cells. In a study combining positron-emission tomography (PET) and MRS (Murphy et al. 1993), it was demonstrated that the low glucose metabolism evident on PET scan in AD was not due to rate limitation in glucose delivery, abnormal glucose metabolism, or abnormal coupling between oxidation and phosphorylation. Although this technique is still a research tool, it may soon find clinical application.

Single Photon Emission Computed Tomography[1]

Single photon emission computed tomography (SPECT) determination of regional cerebral blood flow (rCBF) is an important procedure in the differential diagnosis of dementia patients. Brain blood flow was first measured by Kety and Schmidt in 1948, using nitrous oxide. Their method has been adapted to the use of radionuclide diffusible indicators, principally ^{133}Xe, and external counting with scintillation multiprobe systems. The use of multiple probes permitted estimation of rCBF, which is an indirect measure of local brain physiological activity (Ingvar and Risberg 1967). Obrist et al. (1970), Simard et al. (1971), and Yamaguchi et al. (1980) used the washout of inhaled ^{133}Xe and scintillation multiprobe systems to identify blood flow patterns in AD. Because of serious limitations in the radioxenon multiprobe method, tomographic imaging is now used to provide three-dimensional images of altered brain physiology.

The first useful tomographic images of AD patients were made with PET. Metter et al. (1981), Benson et al. (1983), Foster et al. (1983), and Duara et al. (1986) used ^{18}F-labeled fluorodeoxyglucose ([^{18}F]FDG) to identify patterns of reduced [^{18}F]FDG uptake in posterior temporo-parietal regions and, occasionally, in frontal regions as well. Friedland et al. (1985) reported a correlation between regionally reduced uptake of [^{18}F]FDG and cell loss in AD patients. Although PET is a valuable research technique, it is too expensive to employ as a routine imaging procedure because it requires an on-site cyclotron, a costly imaging

---

[1] This section was written by Frederick J. Bonte, M.D.

device, and a sophisticated technical operating staff.

M. L. Cohen et al. (1983) showed that SPECT, with ^{235}I-labeled io-doamphetamine as a tracer, was of potential value in the differential diagnosis of dementia. Using a variety of SPECT techniques, many investigators (Bonte et al. 1986b, 1989; Derouesne et al. 1985; Gemmell et al. 1984; Hellman et al. 1989; Holman 1986; Jagust et al. 1987; K. A. Johnson et al. 1987; Sharp et al. 1986) identified patterns characteristic of AD, Pick's disease, progressive supranuclear palsy, multiinfarct dementia, and others. Derouesne et al. (1985) pointed out that the posterior flow defects of AD were often asymmetrical and were sometimes accompanied by asymmetrical frontal flow defects. All investigators observed the striking similarity between SPECT studies of rCBF and PET studies of regional brain physiology with [^{18}F]FDG, and they concluded that the former was a completely satisfactory substitute for the latter in evaluating dementia patients.

SPECT instruments and techniques are of two types: high sensitivity and high resolution. High-sensitivity (dynamic) SPECT is exemplified by ^{133}Xe tomography, in which the washout of inhaled ^{133}Xe from the subject's brain is recorded by a device such as the rotating four-detector scanner described by Stokely et al. (1980). The characteristics of the instrument and the means by which it measures rCBF have been described in detail (Bonte and Stokely 1981; Devous et al. 1986; Stokely et al. 1980). The advantage of the high-sensitivity method in dealing with dementia patients is the relatively short examination period of 4 minutes. The images produced, however, are of low resolution (on the order of 17–20 mm; see Figures 3–16 and 3–17). Three sections on 4-cm centers are generated. They are effectively 2 cm in thickness and are separated by 2 cm. They are usually placed 2, 6, and 10 cm above and parallel to the canthomeatal line (CML). All images in Figures 3–16 and 3–17 are at the 6-cm level.

Stokely et al. (1982) have devised a computer program in which cortical regions of interest (ROI) can be fitted to and superimposed on the images of transverse tomographic sections located 2 cm and 6 cm above and parallel to the CML (Figure 3–15).

Because the ^{133}Xe method yields quantitative data, the program can derive rCBF within each of the ROI in ml/min/100 g ± standard deviation. In each ROI, rCBF values can then be compared with a table of normal values (Devous et al. 1986). Devous et al. (1986) found that the ^{133}Xe washout rCBF study in 97 normal volunteers yielded quantitative flow values that were higher in women than in men, age for age, with flow values declining in both sexes with advancing age. These authors also found no significant differences in rCBF in second studies, which followed the first by intervals ranging from 30 minutes to 10 days. They also noted a slight tendency to overestimate gray matter flows in the ROI shown in Figure 3–15 and a greater tendency to overestimate white matter flows. Bonte et al. (1989) later added data on 16 normal volunteers ages 50–72, extending the observations of Devous et al. (1986) with respect to declining normal flow values, both in whole brain and in individual cortical ROI.

Initially, we interpreted brain blood flow studies by comparing rCBF in ml/min/100 g within a whole section (Bonte and Stokely 1981; Bonte et al. 1986b) and within individual ROI, identifying abnormal values as those that lay outside 2 standard deviations below or above the normal control mean value (Devous et al. 1986) for subjects in the same age decade and of the same sex. We found that visual interpretation yielded essentially the same results, and we now use the latter method almost exclusively.

Figure 3–16A is a transverse tomographic rCBF section made with inhaled ^{133}Xe and a high-sensitivity tomograph 6 cm above and parallel to the CML in a 58-year-old normal volunteer subject. In these images, the subject's left is to the reader's left, and the anterior direction is up. Quantitative rCBF in ml/min/100 g is shown in the color scale at the right,

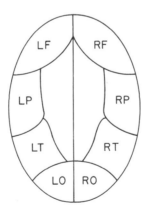

Figure 3–15. Map of cortical regions of interest generated within middle slice (6 cm above CML) of a high-sensitivity 133Xe SPECT rCBF study. F = frontal; P = parietal; T = temporal; O = occipital; L = left; R = right.
Source. Reprinted with permission from Bonte FJ, Devous MD, Reisch JS, et al: "The Effect of Acetazolamide on Regional Cerebral Blood Flow in Patients With Alzheimer's Disease or Stroke as Measured by Single-Photon Emission Computed Tomography." *Investigative Radiology* 24:99–103, 1989.

with lowest flows in blue and highest in red and white. There is an almost complete ring of higher cortical gray matter rCBF. The highest flow is often in the posterior midline because the subject is examined with eyes open in a dimly lighted room.

The pattern most commonly seen in AD is illustrated by Figure 3–16B, which shows symmetrical reduced flow in both posterior temporoparietal regions (corresponding to left and right in Figure 3–15). Another common pattern in AD patients is shown in Figure 3–16C, in which the posterior flow reductions are asymmetrical, with changes more marked on the patient's left side than on his right. There is also an area of frontal rCBF reduction, a finding often encountered in AD patients. The appearance of a lesion of vascular origin, a CT-confirmed stroke, is seen in Figure 3–16D, the study of a patient who developed dementia after his stroke. The left posterior temporoparietal rCBF deficit is wedge-shaped, and its apex points toward the midline. Flow reduction is much greater than in the lesions of AD. This is characteristic of a large stroke involving both gray and white matter.

When AD is present in patients with Parkinson's disease, the rCBF pattern is that of AD, as in Figure 3–17A, the study of a 75-year-old man with autopsy-confirmed evidence of both diseases. Characteristic patterns of rCBF abnormality have been identified in other dementing diseases, such as Pick's disease. Figure 3–17B is a 6-cm slice from a 54-year-old patient with autopsy-proved Pick's disease. There is characteristic bilateral frontal flow reduction, a pattern also seen with progressive supranuclear palsy in Figure 3–17C. One cannot objectively distinguish between the patterns seen in these two patients. We have had few opportunities to perform studies in patients with Creutzfeldt-Jakob disease, but the pattern has been an exaggeration of findings in AD (Figure 3–17D). Here, there is total posterior flow reduction.

We have studied high-sensitivity tomography prospectively in 122 patients who were referred to our Clinic for Alzheimer's and Related Diseases. This group assessed the clinical state of patients, using complete histories, neurological and psychiatric examinations, appropriate laboratory studies of blood and cerebrospinal fluid, EEG, and extensive batteries of neuropsychological tests. CT and/or MRI scans were obtained for all patients. The 122 patients included 48 men and 74 women ages 43–86 years. When a diagnosis of AD was made, it was based on the criteria of McKhann et al. (1984).

Using the working diagnosis of the clinical team as the diagnostic standard, we found good agreement between clinical diagnosis and SPECT. In our experience, AD patients who had first-degree relatives

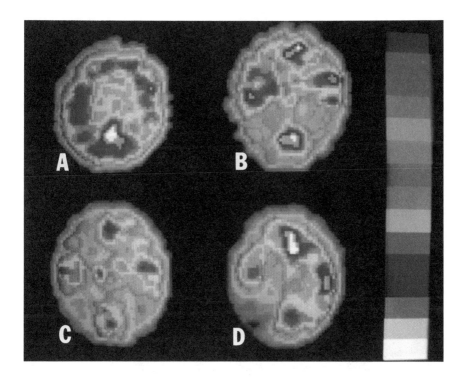

Figure 3–16.   High-sensitivity (^{133}Xe SPECT rCBF) studies. All images represent a trans-verse section 6 cm above the CML; rCBF in ml/min/100 g is seen on the linear scale at the right (low flows in blue and high flows in red and white). Subject's left is to reader's left; anterior is up.

Figure 3–16A.   Normal study in healthy volunteer, age 58 years; highest flow in posterior midline is in the visual cortex.

Figure 3–16B.   Patient, age 64 years, with a clinical diagnosis of probable AD. Symmetrical low-flow areas in the posterior temporoparietal regions bilaterally. This is a pattern com-monly seen in AD.

Figure 3–16C.   Patient, age 70 years, with a clinical diagnosis of probable AD. There are asymmetric posterior flow deficits, more marked on the patient's left. There is also a deficit in the left frontal region, which often accompanies AD.

Figure 3–16D.   Patient, age 59 years, with dementia after at least one known stroke. The wedge-shaped area of markedly reduced rCBF in left posterior temporoparietal region is characteristic of a stroke.

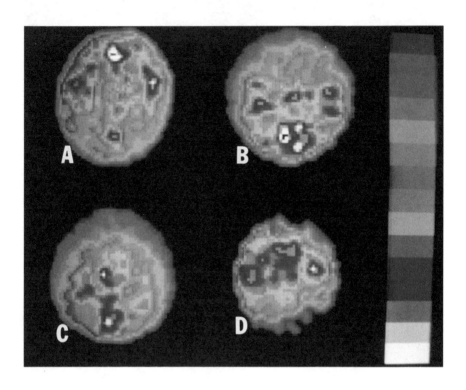

Figure 3–17.   Appearance of various dementias on high-sensitivity SPECT rCBF studies.
Figure 3–17A.   Patient, age 75 years, with autopsy-confirmed co-existing parkinsonism and AD. The rCBF pattern is that of AD, with symmetric posterior temporoparietal reduced rCBF.
Figure 3–17B.   Patient, age 54 years, with autopsy-proved diagnosis of Pick's disease, with characteristic bilateral frontal rCBF reduction.
Figure 3–17C.   Patient, age 61 years, with clinical diagnosis of progressive supranuclear palsy. Bilateral frontal flow reductions sometimes approach those of Pick's disease.
Figure 3–17D.   Patient, age 68 years, with autopsy-proved Creutzfeldt-Jakob disease. There is severe bilateral posterior flow reduction, including the visual cortex.

with dementia almost always had blood flow deficits on SPECT. Further-more, SPECT findings seemed unrelated to duration or severity of dis-ease. Significant flow deficits were detected in 11 of 14 patients with early AD (Mini-Mental State Exam score of 24 or greater). In 9 AD pa-tients restudied after 1- to 3-year intervals, there was further reduction of blood flow.

Triple-camera single-photon tomography units have now been de-veloped that provide high resolution, on the order of 7–9 mm, with sen-sitivity that permits acquisition of data from a three-dimensional volume in approximately 15 minutes with ^{99m}Tc- or ^{123}I-labeled rCBF radiophar-maceuticals (Devous and Bonte 1988). Unlike the high-sensitivity unit described above, which generates only three transverse sections with 2-cm gaps between, the modern high-resolution unit will provide 16 or more contiguous transverse sections, as well as coronal and sagittal sec-tions or any other sections that can be described to the instrument's com-puter.

Figure 3–18 shows representative transverse (Figure 3–18A), coronal (Figure 3–18B), and sagittal (Figure 3–18C) sections from the high reso-lution SPECT rCBF study of a 75-year-old normal volunteer subject. The subject's left is to the reader's right. This study was performed with a present-generation SPECT instrument with three scintillation camera detectors that rotate around the patient's head.

The rCBF tracer radiopharmaceutical employed was ^{99m}Tc-labeled hexamethylpropylene amine oxime (HMPAO). There is excellent gray-white separation, with good definition of the cortical ribbon and the ba-sal ganglia. Quantitatively, counts/pixel gray/white ratios are usually on the order of 1.5:1 or less, rather than 4:1, which approximates the real physiological value. With continuing evolution of rCBF tracers, the latter value should be approached. Figure 3–19 shows transverse (Figure 3–19A) and sagittal (Figure 3–19B) sections from the SPECT rCBF study of a patient, age 73 years, who had a clinical diagnosis of probable AD.

There is asymmetry in rCBF in the bases of the temporal lobes, with reduction on the left. Flow asymmetry continues from the temporal lobe into the posterior superior left parietal lobe on higher sections. Figure 3–19B, a series of sagittal sections, shows moderate diminution in flow in the right posterior superior parietal region (solid arrow, upper sections) and an even more marked and extensive parietal flow defect on the pa-tient's left (solid arrow, lower sections). There is relative deficit in flow in the left inferior temporal lobe compared with the right (open arrow). These are the classic AD findings on three-dimensional SPECT images of rCBF. An occasional finding is anteroinferior frontal flow reduction, usually asymmetrical, more often on the patient's left than on the right.

In a series of 127 patients, we had less agreement with clinical diagnosis than with high-sensitivity technique. Our results will probably improve with refinement in [99mTc]- or [123I]-rCBF radiopharmaceuticals.

Several groups (Hellman et al. 1989; Johnson et al. 1987) have attempted to improve the accuracy of their diagnosis of AD by establishing ratios of counts within appropriate cortical ROI, either to counts in an entire section or to counts in an ROI within cerebellar cortex. However, the use of cerebellar ROI might occasionally present a problem; for example, Akiyama et al. (1989) have described crossed cerebellar diaschisis in AD.

Currently, most SPECT rCBF studies are performed with a single-rotating camera SPECT system and either in [123I]- or [99mTc]-labeled, commercially available, or experimental rCBF radiopharmaceuticals. Although such systems are the forerunners of present-day high-resolution systems, they possess rather low sensitivity and quite modest reso-

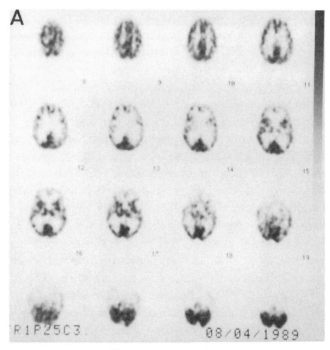

Figure 3–18. High-resolution [99mTc] HMPAO SPECT rCBF studies of a healthy volunteer, age 75 years.
Figure 3–18A. Transverse sections; subject's right is to the viewer's left, and anterior is up.

lution, often on the order of 12–20 mm. A representative study of a patient with moderately advanced probable AD is seen in Figure 3–20, in which selected transverse and sagittal sections are seen.

Flow abnormalities are readily visualized. We have not done a sufficient number of SPECT rCBF patient studies on dementia patients with a single-camera SPECT to determine the efficacy of this technique.

In our experience, as recounted above, the standard used to assess the accuracy of SPECT rCBF imaging was the clinical diagnosis. However, there is substantial variation in the accuracy of diagnosis of the various dementias by clinical means alone, even in the most experienced of clinical groups. Chui (1989) cited three series of patient groups, ranging in size from 58 to 776, in which pathological confirmation of the clinical diagnosis of AD varied from 69% to 87%. Sensitivity for multi-infarct dementia varied between 50% and 73%, whereas sensitivity for mixed vascular and AD was quite poor (17%–30%). Boller et al. (1989) reviewed a series of 54 of these patients with autopsy confirmation and found that

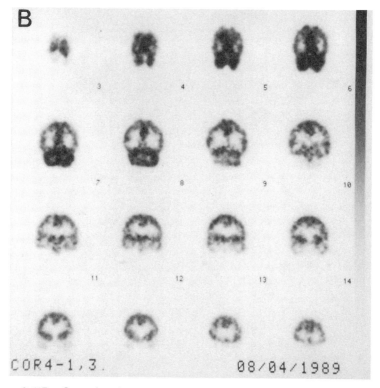

Figure 3–18B. Coronal sections.

two clinicians who reviewed the cases agreed on the correct diagnosis in only 63% of the cases. However, Forette et al. (1989) described an inter-institutional study in which 55 patients were seen at 1-year intervals and received the same clinical diagnosis in 95% of all cases.

We hope that SPECT rCBF imaging will augment the accuracy of clinical diagnosis. Thus far, 50 patients whom we had studied with SPECT have come to autopsy. In this small series, which contained mostly AD cases, there was good agreement between SPECT diagnosis, clinical diagnosis, and autopsy diagnosis. Our criteria for SPECT diagnosis of AD were unilateral or bilateral temporoparietal flow reductions whether or not accompanied by frontal flow reductions (Bonte et al. 1993). Our early experience with high-sensitivity rCBF studies in patients with a family history of dementia suggested that this procedure might be of value in screening persons at risk to AD. Our limited experience in studying patients with early AD indicates that a good deal of local physiological change accompanies clinical expression of AD, at least in some patients, because clear-cut flow deficits were already present in the majority of patients in the small group that we tested. Local brain blood flow is an epiphenomenon of local brain physiological activ-

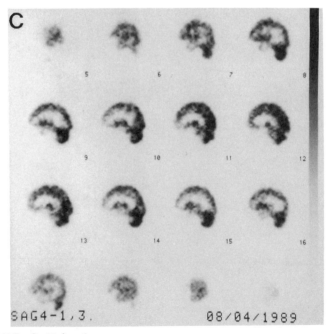

Figure 3–18C. Sagittal sections.

ity, but we do not currently know whether all flow deficits that characterize AD reflect cell death or whether there are remaining cortical cells that have lost function but are still viable and might be restored to normal activity by some pharmacological intervention. If the latter is true, then SPECT study of rCBF will furnish an important means of evaluating palliative drugs or, at some later time, drugs designed to reverse the course of AD.

SPECT rCBF imaging is capable of identifying entities among the dementing diseases other than AD. Figure 3–21 shows a SPECT study that confirmed a dementia involving the frontal lobes. SPECT may eventually be valuable in measuring the contribution of vascular disease to the dementing process in states ranging from VaD to dementia in which both AD and vascular disease are simultaneously active. Clinical diagnosis alone has low sensitivity for mixed AD and vascular disease (Chui 1989).

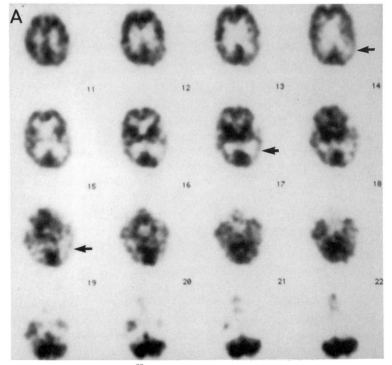

Figure 3–19.   High-resolution [^{99m}Tc]HMPAO SPECT rCBF studies of a patient, age 73 years, with a clinical diagnosis of probable AD.
Figure 3–19A.   Transverse sections show low flow that begins at the base of the left temporal lobe and extends superiorly into the posterior parietal lobe (solid arrows; second, third, and fourth rows).

To evaluate the role of a possible SPECT rCBF challenge test in identifying both degenerative and vascular components of dementing disease, we (Bonte et al. 1989) assessed rCBF in 35 patients with possible or
probable AD and 16 patients known to have had at least one stroke, using high-sensitivity SPECT rCBF determinations before and administering 1 g of acetazolamide (ACZ) 15 minutes after. ACZ, a carbonic
anhydrase inhibitor, is a cerebral vasodilator. We found that after ACZ,
rCBF rose in regions of low flow secondary to AD in proportion to flow
increases in the remainder of the less-involved brain. In patients with
vascular disease, low-flow areas, representing strokes, often responded
with a relative local reduction of flow due to abnormal vasculature in
that area. Although highly preliminary, this study suggests a possible
role for this sort of procedure in improving the diagnosis of possibly
treatable vascular disease in dementia patients.

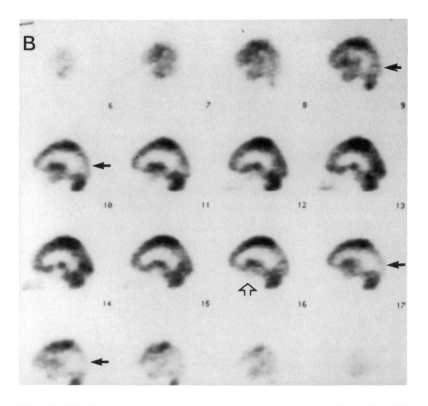

Figure 3–19B. Sagittal sections show posterior superior flow deficits bilaterally (solid arrows; upper and lower rows). Compare with paramedian sagittal sections in Figure
3–14C. Open arrow indicates reduced flow in the base of the left temporal lobe.

Positron-Emission Tomography

By means of PET, it is possible to measure the glucose and oxygen metabolism of the various brain regions and to measure various neurotransmitter systems and receptors with appropriate tracers. Using [^{18}F]FDG as a tracer, McGeer et al. (1986) found a correlation between areas of low glucose metabolism and areas of neuronal loss and gliosis in AD. Low glucose metabolism in parietal, temporal, and frontal cortex occurs early in the course of AD, at a time when patients do not yet meet criteria for dementia. This abnormality worsens as the disease progresses (Parks et al. 1993).

PET can also help to distinguish AD from depression—the former disease showing hypometabolism of the parietal lobes, the latter relatively high levels of glucose consumption (Buchsbaum et al. 1986). In Huntington's disease, the same technique showed losses in caudate nucleus glucose metabolism preceding CT-detectable tissue loss (Hayden et al. 1986).

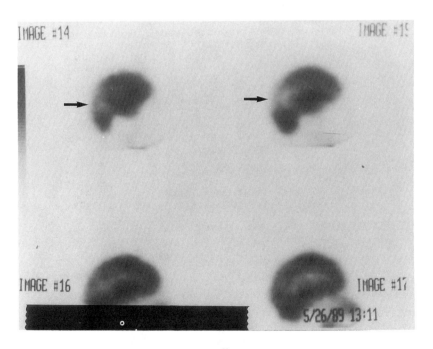

Figure 3–20.   Selected sagittal sections from [^{99m}Tc]HMPAO rotating-camera SPECT study of a patient, age 64 years, with probable AD. Solid arrow indicates posterior superior parietal flow defect, the most reliable diagnostic sign of AD on SPECT rCBF studies.

How Much Workup Is Enough?

There are considerable differences of opinion as to what is an adequate laboratory workup for dementing illness. The Canadian guidelines (Mohr et al. 1995) suggest that BUN, B_{12}, folic acid, serologic test for syphilis, urinalysis, and erythrocyte sedimentation rate be performed only if indicated by history or physical examination. They also suggest that neuroimaging is required only if the patient is less than 60 years of age, if there is use of anticoagulants or a history of bleeding disorder, recent head trauma, cancers that metastasize to brain, unexplained neurological symptoms, rapid progress of disease, dementia duration of less than 2 years, or urinary incontinence and gait disorder suggestive of normal-pressure hydrocephalus.

In our clinic, a minimum medical workup includes a history, physical and neurological examination, mental status examination, CT of the head, and the following laboratory studies: complete blood count, erythrocyte sedimentation rate, electrolytes, blood glucose, urea nitrogen, calcium, phosphorus, liver function tests, thyroid function tests, vitamin B_{12}

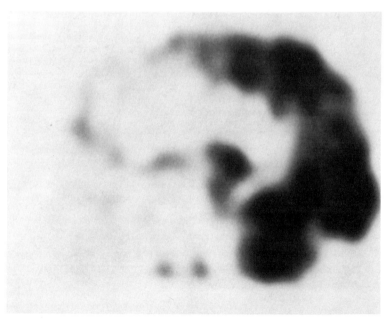

Figure 3–21. Sagittal section from [^{99m}Tc]HMPAO SPECT study showing marked frontal lobe blood flow reduction.

and folic acid level, and serologic test for syphilis. Lumbar puncture is indicated if an infectious, inflammatory, or autoimmune disorder is suspected. We use EEG if seizure disorder or Creutzfeldt-Jakob disease is suspected. MRI is useful for providing anatomic detail, for example, in estimating caudate nucleus size if Huntington's disease is suspected or in differentiating white matter loss occurring in subcortical dementias from the gray matter loss of cortical dementias. SPECT and PET supply indirect and direct evidence of the functional state of brain tissue, but the expense of SPECT and the greater expense and relative unavailability of PET suggest that both procedures should be reserved for the diagnosis of atypical dementias or for research. We have typically used SPECT to confirm frontal dementias and to differentiate dysphasic dementia from aphasia due to cerebrovascular disease. Jobst et al. (1994) combine temporal lobe CT with SPECT in AD and report a sensitivity of 90% and a specificity of 97%. Table 3–1 suggests minimal and optimal workups for dementia patients, depending on the resources available and the need for relative certainty of diagnosis.

Table 3–1. The dementia workup

Minimal	Optimal
History	History
Physical examination	Physical examation
Neurological examation	Neurological examation
Mental status examation	Mental status examation
	Neuropsychological testing
Blood tests:	Blood tests
CBC, sed rate	CBC, sed rate
Electrolytes	Electrolytes
Glucose, BUN	Glucose, BUN
Ca, P	Ca, P
Liver function	Liver function
B_{12} and folate	B_{12} and folate
Thyroid function	Thyroid function
Serology	Serology
	ANA, latex fixation
	Urine tests
	Urinalysis
	Heavy metals
	Lumbar puncture
CT	MRI
	EEG
	SPECT

How Often Are Evaluations Indicated?

Brief reevaluations should be done at least yearly. A minimum evaluation includes routine laboratory studies and sufficient evidence by history and direct physical and mental status examination of the correctness of the original diagnosis. More comprehensive evaluations are indicated when the clinician suspects a reversible component to the dementia, as in the following example:

> A 74-year-old widow with a 4-year history of progressive dementia was diagnosed as having AD after a comprehensive workup including a head CT scan. Six months later, a PET scan showed findings typical of AD. Six months after that, she returned with severe gait problems, marked urinary incontinence, and increasing ventricular size accompanied by diffuse white matter changes on an MRI. A diagnosis of normal-pressure hydrocephalus was made, a ventriculoperitoneal shunt was inserted. Over the next 2 years, the woman showed marked improvement in her cognitive status (Friedland 1989).

When Is a Workup No Longer Needed?

It is tempting to ascribe cognitive worsening in a dementia patient to progress of the originally diagnosed disease (frequently AD). It has been our experience that departures from the normal trajectory of a patient's diagnosed dementing illness are often worthy of investigation, particularly in frail elders. A minimum evaluation in these cases includes medication check, physical examination, chest X ray, all of the blood work indicated previously, and urinalysis. In cases of suspected falls, a head CT is also indicated. In suspected drug toxicity, blood levels can be determined.

Summary

The medical evaluation of cognitive impairment requires accurate history taking, mental status examination, physical and neurological evaluation, a relatively small number of blood tests, and a CT scan of the head. Dementias that progress rapidly or that have an atypical course warrant fuller investigation at a tertiary care center, even though the yield of treatable disorders is low. As the number of treatable disorders increases, the more sophisticated tests of brain function, such as SPECT and PET, may be used more frequently as means to detect those disorders and to monitor the course of treatment.

CHAPTER 4

Differential Diagnosis

Myron F. Weiner, M.D.
Kevin F. Gray, M.D.

In this chapter, we discuss the differential diagnosis of the most common causes of the dementia syndrome but not all causes of impaired brain function or all conditions that may worsen preexisting dementia or cause delirium. There are many causes of dementia symptoms, but they are fewer than the causes of delirium. For an exhaustive review of dementia-causing illnesses, the reader is referred to *The Dementias*, by Peter Whitehouse (1993). The causes of a dementia may be intrinsic to the central nervous system (CNS) or may be systemic processes, including various intoxications. Some are reversible; most are not. This chapter begins with a discussion of the reversible dementias, including drug-induced cognitive impairment, and concludes with a discussion of the dementias that are not yet reversible.

Reversible Dementias

The etiologies of potentially reversible dementias are listed in Table 4–1. Of the etiologies listed, the most often reversible are depression, drugs, and metabolic factors. It is important to realize that, in many instances, reversible does not mean fully reversible. Often, a reversible cause of dementia complicates an irreversible dementia. For example, an Alzheimer's disease (AD) patient who lives alone may not maintain nutrition or water intake after a febrile illness, greatly aggravating the preexisting cognitive impairment. With correction of the nutritional or metabolic abnormalities, the patient's cognition improves but does not return to normal.

Psychiatric

The primary psychiatric cause of the dementia syndrome seen in dementia clinics is major depression, which is discussed at length in Chapter 1. Although depression is reversible with antidepressant medication or electroconvulsive therapy, depressed patients with significant cognitive impairment deserve concomitant evaluation for other causes of dementia.

Table 4–1.   Etiologies of potentially reversible dementia

Psychiatric
  Depression
  Schizophrenia
  Ganser syndrome
  Malingering

Toxic
  Drugs (prescription or street)
  Alcohol
  Chemical poisoning (arsenic, mercury, lead, lithium and other metals; organic
    compounds and solvents)

Metabolic
  Azotemia/renal failure (diuretics, dehydration, obstruction, hypokalemia)
  Hyponatremia (diuretics, excess ADH, salt wasting, water intoxication)
  Volume depletion
  Hypo- or hyperglycemia
  Hepatic encephalopathy
  Hypo- or hyperthyroidism
  Hyperparathyroidism
  Cushing's syndrome
  Wilson's disease
  Acute intermittent porphyria

Infection and/or fever (in elders, pneumonia, urinary tract infection)

Anoxic
  Anemia
  Congestive heart failure
  Chronic obstructive pulmonary disease

Vitamin deficiencies (B_{12}, folic acid, thiamine, niacin)

Central nervous system disorders
  Vascular (ischemic or hemorrhagic stroke, ischemic-hypoxic brain lesions)
  Trauma (subdural hematoma, postconcussion syndrome)
  HIV and opportunistic infections
  Other infections (neurosyphilis, chronic meningitis, brain abscess, progressive multi-
    focal leukoencephalopathy)
  Neoplasm (primary or metastatic)
  Cerebral vasculitis
  Normal-pressure hydrocephalus
  Multiple sclerosis

Dementia may appear in long-standing schizophrenia (Granholm and Jeste 1994), hence Kraepelin's (1913) term *dementia praecox*. The dementia of chronic schizophrenia is nonprogressive (Hyde et al. 1994) and seems related to difficulty with concentration and organization of thought and to inability to avoid internal distractions that manifest as delusions and hallucinations. Perceptions are distorted, and information processing becomes disorganized. Communication may be characterized by echolalia, palilalia, and neologistic word salad and may be difficult to distinguish from fluent aphasia. Occasionally, patients are reduced to a state of near vegetation and mutism. Some patients with bipolar disorder will show cognitive deterioration. It seems likely that the cognitive deterioration in these illnesses is a combination of psychological and metabolic/anatomic factors. There is evidence of aberrant hippocampal neuronal organization (Altshuler et al. 1987) and decreased hippocampal pyramidal cell density in schizophrenia (Jeste and Lohr 1989), but further confirmation of these findings is needed.

Toxic

The classes of cognition-impairing drugs are listed in Table 4–2. Drugs of abuse are the most important toxins in young adults, prescription drugs in elders (Wilcox et al. 1994). In young adults, drug ingestion leads to delirium or acute psychosis rather than a dementia syndrome. In elders, dementia syndromes arise from use of long-acting benzodiazepines, barbiturates, meprobamate, and a host of others depending on their dose and the length of time they have been used. Drugs such as flurazepam, with a half-life of more than 120 hours, accumulate rapidly. Others accumulate more slowly or require relatively high doses for toxicity to develop.

Alcohol

Chronic alcohol abuse may be a direct cause of neurotoxicity but more important are the nutritional deficiencies that result from an inadequate diet. Thiamine deficiency is the most important, appearing to cause both Wernicke's and Korsakoff's syndromes. They are discussed under the section "Thiamine Deficiency."

Alcohol persisting dementia encompasses the signs and symptoms of dementia presented in Chapter 1; a case example is presented in Chapter 7. The exact relation of this condition to the Wernicke-Korsakoff complex is not clear, but it is likely that many cases of Korsakoff's syndrome, if examined closely, would meet DSM-IV criteria for dementia. The dementia syndrome is partially reversible if abstinence from alcohol can be achieved and an adequate diet maintained (Victor 1994).

We have followed seven persons referred to our clinic for evaluation of memory impairment who had a history of long-standing alcoholism or alcohol intake equivalent to four or more ounces of alcohol per day. All had good nutrition. Their cognitive impairment was mild but definite and primarily affected short-term memory and abstract reasoning. Follow-up of these cases over several years showed no progression for four of the seven who followed our advice to abstain from alcohol.

Chemical Poisoning

Chemical poisons that impair CNS function usually have their primary effects on other systems: gastrointestinal, renal, hepatic, blood-forming, and peripheral nervous systems.

Table 4–2.   Cognition-impairing drugs

Psychotropic	Nonpsychotropic
Sedative-hypnotics	Diuretics
	Cardiac glycosides
Benzodiazepines	Antiarrhythmics
Flurazepam	Calcium channel blockers
Diazepam	
Chlordiazepoxide	Antimanics
	Lithium
Barbiturates	Carbamazepine
Meprobamate	Antipsychotics
	Thioridazine
Antidepressants	Chlorpromazine
Imipramine	Clozapine
Amitriptyline	Antihypertensives
Doxepin	Rauwolfia alkaloids
Trazodone	Beta-blockers
	Alpha-methyldopa
Antihistamines	Analgesics
H₂ antagonists	Narcotic analgesics
Cimetidine	Propoxyphene
Ranitidine	
Anti-inflammatory agents	
Corticosteroids	
Nonsteroidals	

Metals

Metal poisonings often produce gastrointestinal symptoms and peripheral neuropathy. Cognitive changes tend to be more characteristic of delirium than dementia, with clouding of consciousness a prominent feature.

Lithium carbonate and lithium citrate are employed effectively in the management of bipolar affective disorder (manic-depressive illness). In the therapeutic range (0.8–1.2 mEq/L), lithium frequently produces a fine tremor and nausea (Vestergaard et al. 1980). Serious intoxication occurs at blood concentrations greater than 2 mEq/L, resulting in delirium, nystagmus, ataxia, and diffuse myoclonic twitching. In mild intoxications, treatment includes discontinuance of the drug and high-volume fluid intake, including ample sodium chloride. Hemodialysis is effective when life-threatening concentrations are present in blood.

The encephalopathy of arsenic poisoning occurs with chronic arsenic exposure or may be a sequel of acute arsenic poisoning. Its symptoms include headache, drowsiness, and confusion. Mercury poisoning results largely from industrial exposure. Tremors; extrapyramidal signs, including upper- and lower-extremity ataxia; depression; and confusion occur. Lead poisoning occurs in lead smelters and storage battery workers. The usual manifestations are abdominal cramps, anemia, and peripheral neuropathy. Encephalopathy is rare. Dimercaprol is used to treat arsenic poisoning; chelating agents, including ethylenediaminetetraacetic acid (EDTA) and penicillamine, are used to treat mercury and lead poisoning (Royce and Rosenberg 1993).

Manganese poisoning results from inhalation of manganese particles in miners and workers who sort manganese ore. The symptoms are predominantly extrapyramidal but may be accompanied by delirium. Levodopa (L-dopa) has been useful in treating the extrapyramidal symptoms in some of these cases.

Aluminum intoxication is the probable cause of so-called dialysis dementia (Frazer and Arieff 1994). It begins with myoclonus and speech disorders and is followed by seizures and cognitive impairment (Parkinson et al. 1981). Deionizing the water used in dialysis has essentially eliminated this disorder.

Other poisonous metals include thallium, iron, antimony, zinc, barium, bismuth, copper, silver, gold, and platinum (Dreisbach 1987).

Organic Compounds and Solvents

The list of potential organic toxins is long and includes carbon disulfide, halogenated hydrocarbons such as carbon tetrachloride, naphthalene, benzene and its derivatives, and many others. Neural and cognitive symptoms tend to occur preterminally. Toluene (methylbenzene), one of the toxins in glue and paint sniffing, causes extensive white matter damage (Filley et al. 1990) and profound cognitive impairment in addition to tremor, ataxia, and loss of vision and hearing (Fornazzari et al. 1983).

Metabolic Disorders

Azotemia

Uremic encephalopathy may develop slowly or acutely. If it develops slowly, it usually produces apathy, impaired concentration, and irritability. If it is acute, there is altered sensorium. Prerenal azotemia may be caused by diuretics, dehydration, and hypokalemia; postrenal azotemia may be caused by urinary tract obstruction.

Hyponatremia

Hyponatremia may be due to diuretics, inappropriate antidiuretic hormone (ADH) secretion, salt-wasting renal disease, and water intoxication. Serum sodium levels below 120 mEq/L are accompanied by impaired attention, drowsiness, and stupor. Diuretic abuse is common in young women preoccupied with losing weight, and hyponatremia occurs frequently in elders treated with diuretics for hypertension (Vieweg et al. 1994). Polyuria is common with lithium treatment. Inappropriate ADH secretion may occur with various brain lesions, lung tumors, chlorpromazine, carbamazepine, and fluoxetine (Vishwanath et al. 1991). Salt-wasting nephropathy may lead to hyponatremia. Water intoxication has been reported in subjects diagnosed with schizophrenia, mental retardation, depression, and alcoholism (Jose et al. 1979).

Volume Depletion

Volume depletion may occur as a result of diuretics, diarrhea, vomiting, bleeding, or inadequate fluid intake. With diuretics, vomiting, and diarrhea, there are also accompanying electrolyte abnormalities.

Hypoglycemia and Hyperglycemia

Hypoglycemia primarily appears as delirium (Fishbain and Rotundo 1988) but may manifest as sudden worsening of cognitive impairment, especially in elders. Oral hypoglycemic agents are the most common cause of hypoglycemia in patients over 60 years of age (Seltzer 1972). The oral hypoglycemic agent chlorpropamide is contraindicated in elders because of its 35-hour half-life. Other drugs may potentiate the action of sulfonylureas, including aspirin, dicumarol, lithium, and monoamine oxidase inhibitors. Other conditions leading to hypoglycemia in elders include alcoholism, sepsis, malnutrition, and myxedema. With rapid fall in blood glucose, symptoms may appear at blood sugar levels greater than 45 mg/dl. Hyperglycemia may cause impaired mentation in uncontrolled diabetic patients.

Hepatic Encephalopathy

Liver failure is usually accompanied by obvious clouding of sensorium, but intermittent mental dulling may be the primary symptom. Liver failure can aggravate preexisting dementia, which will improve as the blood ammonia level lowers. Diagnosis is by demonstration of arterial ammonia concentration of greater than 100 µg/dl (Cooper and Plum 1987). Borderline low serum albumin and increased prothrombin time should raise suspicion of liver failure and hepatic encephalopathy.

Thyroid Disease

Hypothyroidism is associated with lethargy, slowed thinking, slowed speech, and impaired recent memory (Haupt and Kurz 1993). It is more likely to be confused with depression than dementia. To the extent that it induces hypothyroidism, hypopituitarism may contribute to a dementia syndrome. Hyperthyroidism is associated with impaired attention and concentration and diminished short-term memory. The usual symptoms of tachycardia, increased sweating, and fine tremor may not be apparent in elders (Meneilly et al. 1988), who may present with apathy.

Hyperparathyroidism and Hypercalcemia

Hyperparathyroidism is most often due to parathyroid adenoma. Demineralization of bone and kidney stones is the most common clinical indicator. Blood calcium is increased, as is parathyroid hormone level. The predominant mental symptoms are depression and lassitude, but both delirium and dementia syndromes may occur (Alarcon and Franceschini 1984).

Hypercalcemia itself can cause mental dulling. In one case, a woman with multiple myeloma had been given calcium supplementation to minimize pathological fractures that were occurring in the course of her illness. Over a period of months, she became increasingly dull and lethargic. When she was found to have an elevated serum calcium concentration, her calcium supplementation was discontinued, and her mentation improved considerably.

Although hypoparathyroidism with its accompanying neuromuscular irritability and paresthesias has been suggested as a cause of dementia (Sier et al. 1984), there is little to support this contention.

Cushing's Syndrome

Cushing's syndrome is caused by a chronic excess of circulating cortisol, whether endogenous or exogenous. Its clinical features include facial and truncal obesity, flushed facies, purplish abdominal striae, hypertension, diabetes, and osteoporosis. Depression and delirium are the most common associated mental states, although neuropsychological testing shows diffuse bilateral cerebral dysfunction, with impairment more frequent and severe in nonverbal, visual ideational, visual memory, and spatial-constructional abilities than in language or verbal reasoning (Whelan et al. 1980).

Wilson's Disease

Wilson's disease is a recessively inherited disorder of copper metabolism. Its onset is in the second or third decade of life, and its first manifestations are usually related to impaired liver function, including jaundice and hepatosplenomegaly. Neurological symptoms begin with head or limb tremor, slowed movement, dysarthria, dysphagia, and choreic movements or dystonia (Dening 1991). As many as 20% of Wilson's disease patients develop prominent emotional symptoms before the diagnosis is made, but cognitive impairment is not a prominent feature early in the disease (Dening and Berrios 1989). As the disease progresses, patients drool and become dysphagic; have rigid, slow-moving limbs; develop a fixed, vacuous smile; and develop a wing-beating tremor when their limbs are outstretched.

The disease is diagnosed by the findings of low serum ceruloplasmin (< 20 mg/dl) and confirmed by Keyser-Fleischer rings on slit lamp examination. Liver biopsy shows high copper content. The pathogenesis of the disease seems related to the toxic effects of excessive copper deposition in the liver and the lentiform nuclei. Treatment is reduction of dietary copper intake and the copper-chelating agent D-penicillamine.

Acute Intermittent Porphyria
(Pyrroloporphyria, Swedish Type)

Inherited as an autosomal dominant, this type of porphyria is not associated with photosensitivity. It is caused by a metabolic defect in the liver that causes increased production and urinary excretion of porphobilinogen and of the porphyrin precursor, δ-aminolevulinic acid. The physical signs and symptoms of porphyria are bouts of abdominal pain, peripheral neuropathy, altered mental state (usually delirium), and intermittently wine-colored urine (Massey 1980). Attacks are frequently induced by barbiturates, sulfonamides, estrogen, phenytoin, griseofulvin, and succinimide anticonvulsants. The diagnosis is confirmed by finding large quantities of porphobilinogen and δ-aminolevulinic acid in urine. The urine of such patients turns dark on standing due to the oxidation of porphobilinogen to porphobilin. There is usually good remission of symptoms between acute episodes (Adams and Victor 1989).

Infection and/or Fever

Severe or systemic infections and fever often cause delirium. In frail elders, febrile response may not be great, and the first sign of a severe infection may be cognitive impairment. This is most often true in elders with borderline cognitive reserve or those who are already demented. The most common infections are pneumonia, urinary tract infection, and generalized sepsis. Thus, the evaluation of a sudden change of a frail elder's cognitive status should include a chest X ray, urinalysis, complete blood count, and, when indicated, blood culture. The same holds true in immunocompromised persons of all ages. In this group, which includes persons with acquired immunodeficiency syndrome (AIDS), lymphoma, or lymphocytic leukemia or those being treated with immunosuppressants, additional studies should include cerebrospinal fluid (CSF) examination and a computed tomographic (CT) scan of the head (with contrast) as part of a search for opportunistic infections.

Anoxia

Severe anemia, whether due to iron deficiency or blood loss, leads to impaired concentration, decreased effort, and consequent impairment of cognitive performance. Congestive heart failure may also lead to desaturation of arterial oxygen and relative brain anoxia. Cummings et al. (1980) cite a case of ventricular arrythmia worsening confusion in a man with a mild case of dementia. Chronic obstructive pulmonary diseases produce hypoxemia, hypercarbia, and acidosis. These patients are well-known to experience the form of delirium known as *sundowning* (i.e., worsening of sensorium and orientation in the evenings) and also manifest impaired neuropsychological performance (Prigatano et al. 1983). Improving oxygenation of blood improves cognitive function in these individuals (Krop et al. 1973). The cognitive impairment produced by these conditions is commonly superimposed on dementia produced by alcohol, AD, or VaD (Incalzi et al. 1993).

Vitamin Deficiencies

Thiamine (Vitamin B₁)

Wernicke's syndrome (polioencephalitis hemorrhagica superior) is characterized by sensorial impairment, apathy, and inattentiveness accompanied by nystagmus, abducens and conjugate gaze palsies, and ataxic gait. The symptoms are usually of abrupt onset and may occur singly or in various combinations. Prompt treatment with parenteral thiamine is indicated, with 100 mg qd given in divided doses until patients begin eating again, at which time they can take 100 mg qd po. There is usually prompt remission of the ophthalmoplegia and ataxia, but the majority of patients will continue to manifest deficits in memory and learning that are described as Korsakoff's syndrome (Victor 1993).

Korsakoff's syndrome (alcohol-persisting amnestic disorder) develops independently of Wernicke's syndrome in 75% of cases (Blansjaar et al. 1992), but Victor et al. (1971) found that 84% of Wernicke's syndrome survivors went on to manifest an amnestic syndrome. In this syndrome, immediate memory (as tested by digit span) is fairly well preserved, but short-term memory is devastated, and long-term memory is markedly impaired. A frequently reported aspect of Korsakoff's syndrome is confabulation—the tendency to invent memories. Confabulation is generally elicited by asking patients what they did and who they saw yesterday, and comparing the patient's account with that of a reliable witness. Psychological functions other than memory are affected in Korsakoff's syndrome. Executive cognitive functions, including abstract reasoning and the ability to change cognitive set are also impaired. With abstinence, some patients with Korsakoff's syndrome improve cognitively, with the recovery process taking as long as a year (Victor 1993). In both Wernicke's and Korsakoff's syndromes, there are lesions in the medial thalamic region, tegmentum of the pons, and cerebellar cortex. Victor (1993) attributes the memory disorder to the medial dorsal nuclei of the thalamus. Wernicke-Korsakoff pathology is found in 10%–15% of autopsied alcoholic persons, suggesting that thiamine should be prescribed routinely for these individuals (Victor 1993).

Intravenous glucose solution administered to a malnourished patient may precipitate a thiamine deficiency due to depleted reserves. Furthermore, administering thiamine may produce hypoglycemia in nutritionally deprived persons by stimulating the metabolism of glucose.

Cyanocobalamin (Vitamin B12)

Cyanocobalamin (vitamin B_{12}) deficiency affects the peripheral nerves, spinal cord, and brain. A megaloblastic anemia, it may be due to dietary lack or failure of absorption due to lack of intrinsic factor. The spinal cord lesions are termed *subacute combined degeneration* and affect the posterior and lateral columns. Symptoms usually begin with distal, symmetrical paresthesias in all limbs, followed by unsteadiness, stiffness, and weakness of the limbs. B_{12} deficiency may produce depression, psychotic states, and cognitive impairment. Because patients often receive folic acid in over-the-counter multivitamin preparations, the hematological findings characteristic of pernicious anemia may not be present and may be absent even without folate supplementation. Treatment involves a brief course of intramuscular injections of 1,000 µg of cyanocobalamin daily, followed by injections weekly and then monthly for the remainder of the patient's life.

Hector and Burton (1988) argue that their extensive literature review revealed little evidence of B_{12} deficiency associated with a full-blown dementia syndrome or that reversing B_{12} deficiency causes improvement in cognitive state. Unfortunately, those authors' criterion for dementia was a formal diagnosis of dementia rather than signs and symptoms of impaired cognition. Evidence of cognitive impairment was impressive in the studies they cited, but there was little evidence of improvement following B_{12} therapy. Of 1,457 cases of hypovitaminosis B_{12}, only one case showed cognitive improvement after replacement therapy. Thus, a subject's B_{12} level may not be a significant risk factor for dementia or for aggravating dementia symptoms in diseases such as Alzheimer's disease (Crystal et al. 1994). On the other hand, Gross et al. (1986) report two cases of B_{12} deficiency with abnormal Schilling tests in which there was cognitive improvement upon treatment. From a practical standpoint, a trial of weekly and then monthly parenteral B_{12} seems justified. There is little expense, no risk, and the possibility of gain.

Folic acid deficiency has also been reported as a cause of subacute combined degeneration (Pincus 1979), depression, and dementia (Strachan and Henderson 1967). Appropriate treatment is large oral doses of folic acid (Crellin et al. 1993).

Nicotinic Acid

The pellagrinous triad of dermatitis, diarrhea, and dementia due to nicotinic acid deficiency is now rare in this country, and it is limited to the alcoholic population in most developed countries. This disorder is characterized by a thickened, cracked rash in sun-exposed areas of the skin, occasionally accompanied by spastic leg weakness. It is difficult to ascertain how much of the symptom complex is due to nicotinic acid deficiency and how much is due to lack of other vitamins, such as pyridoxine. Pellagra is invariably associated with malnutrition; patients with this disorder require general nutritional measures in addition to specific vitamin supplementation.

Brain Disorders

Stroke (see also Vascular Dementia)

Single strokes have variable effects on cognition, depending on their size and location. Some strokes are essentially silent; many are highly symptomatic because of their interference with production or comprehension of speech, writing, or emotion. It is a reasonable assumption that all strokes involving the cerebral hemispheres will produce some degree of cognitive impairment due to interruption of association fibers or loss of specific cortical neurons. The mental impairment produced by stroke will ordinarily show partial resolution over time, with maximum resolution occurring after about 1 year.

Stroke raises a number of issues with regard to differential diagnosis. As mentioned in Chapter 1, dementia needs to be differentiated from expressive and receptive aphasia and from specific agnosias. In addition, depression is a frequent sequel of stroke. Its incidence is estimated conservatively at 25%–33% over a period of 2 years after a stroke (Robinson et al. 1984). Depression may occur immediately. If it does, it aggravates the apparent cognitive loss due to the stroke (Robinson et al. 1986). Depression due to left-hemisphere lesions may produce greater cognitive impairment than depression due to right-hemisphere lesions (Bolla-Wilson et al. 1989). Making the diagnosis of a poststroke depression is complicated by patients' communication problems (Ramasubbu and Kennedy 1994). Many are unable to report their mood or specifically deny depression. Examination may not reveal flattening of affective responses (Ross and Rush 1981). However, if observation and history indicate crying spells, lack of interest in the environment, irritability, uncooperativeness, loss of appetite, weight loss, and sleep disturbance with terminal insomnia, a trial of antidepressant medication (see Chapter 6) is indicated. Prompt, positive responses to such medication are frequently seen at low doses.

Trauma

An important cause of cognitive impairment in alcoholic persons and of suddenly worsened cognition in cognitively impaired elders is head trauma–induced subdural hematoma (Traynelis 1991). In these two groups, head trauma often results from an unremembered fall. In persons taking anticoagulant medication (including aspirin), the trauma may be trivial. Symptoms of increased intracranial pressure may be present. Localizing signs may or may not occur. A frequent sign is ipsilateral pupillary dilation caused by pressure of the herniating temporal lobe on the oculomotor nerve. Skull films may show shift of midline structures. CT scan shows hypodensity in the area of the hematoma, as does magnetic resonance imaging (MRI) (see Chapter 3, Figure 3–8), and an EEG shows reduced voltage over the hematoma and high-voltage slow waves on the opposite side (Adams and Victor 1989). A lumbar puncture may show xanthochromic fluid. Treatment of a subdural hematoma is neurosurgical evacuation of the clot after care has been taken to ascertain and correct any predilection to abnormal bleeding.

Concussive head injury may produce long-term impairment of concentration and recent memory, but it is not likely to produce a dementia syndrome. Concussion is accompanied by transient loss of consciousness and variable periods of retrograde and antegrade amnesia. Head injury with prolonged loss of consciousness (days to months) may be followed by a delirium and then a dementia syndrome or profound personality alteration (Capruso and Levin 1992).

HIV Infection

Infection with the human immunodeficiency virus type 1 (HIV-1) produces a dementia syndrome initially termed the *AIDS dementia complex* (Navia et al. 1986a, 1986b) and now designated HIV-1–associated cognitive/motor complex (American Academy of Neurology AIDS Task Force

1991). Two clinical categories are recognized: a more severe form known as HIV-1-associated dementia complex, and a less severe form known as HIV-1-associated minor cognitive/motor disorder. In the less severe disorder, despite demonstrable cognitive, motor, or behavioral abnormalities, only the most demanding activities of daily living are impaired.

HIV-1–Associated Dementia Complex

Associated dementia complex (ADC) is the most frequent neurological complication of HIV infection and in some individuals may be the earliest or the only clinical manifestation of HIV-1 infection. In the United States alone, an estimated 1 million persons are infected with HIV. Based on current rates of infection, 25–35 million cases are projected worldwide by the year 2000. Major high-risk groups for infection include bisexual/homosexual men, who constitute 70% of HIV cases, and intravenous drug abusers, who constitute 15%–20% of the total AIDS consort (Faulstich 1987). Early reports indicated that by 12 months after the first diagnosis of AIDS, 7% of patients were demented, increasing to 15% when the same patients were followed to death (McArthur et al. 1993). Untreated ADC may remain static or may fluctuate (American Academy of Neurology AIDS Task Force 1991). In a cohort of 536 neurologically symptomatic HIV-1-positive patients, those treated with ziduvodine (Retrovir) rarely developed ADC. Among the patients who developed ADC, survival was longer in the ziduvodine-treated patients (Portegies et al. 1993). The onset of HIV dementia is typically insidious; acute, abrupt onset usually occurs in the setting of systemic illness or secondary infection (Navia et al. 1986a). The earliest clinical features include subtle mood changes, inattentiveness, difficulty concentrating, distractibility, forgetfulness, and apathy. Patients often complain of being increasingly absent minded and mentally slow. Other early manifestations may include confusion, disorientation, malaise, lethargy, anhedonia, social withdrawal, diminished quality of work, and disinterest (Pajeau and Roman 1992). Motor symptoms such as clumsiness, deterioration in fine motor tasks, leg weakness, loss of balance, hyperreflexia, and sustention tremor may also be present (Simpson and Tagliati 1994). With disease progression, widespread cognitive impairment and psychomotor retardation dominate the clinical picture. Rarely, hallucinatory or delusional symptoms develop (Navia 1990).

The severity of clinical deterioration correlates generally with the severity of brain pathology. Some degree of cerebral atrophy is present in almost all demented HIV patients (Vago et al. 1990), with pathology found primarily in subcortical structures, particularly the basal ganglia and thalamus. Histological examination demonstrates diffuse pallor of the centrum semiovale with a mononuclear inflammatory response in the white matter and deep gray nuclei (Navia 1990). The presence of multinucleated giant cells and diffuse myelin pallor is specific for HIV dementia but is not seen in all clinically demented patients (Glass et al. 1993). The neuronal injury may be mediated by toxic substances produced by infected macrophages (Lipton and Gendelman 1995).

The neuropsychological deficits of HIV dementia include impaired attention and concentration, psychomotor slowing, diminished visuospatial performance, poor complex reaction time, memory disturbance, and personality/mood alterations such as apathy and irritability (see also Chapter 7). There is evidence for three distinct types of individuals seropositive for HIV-1: 1) a *subcortical* group, with depressed mood, psychomotor slowing, and forgetfulness; 2) a *cortical* group with verbal and visuospatial deficits, some psychomotor mood, and euthymia; and 3) a group without neuropsychological impairment (Van Gorp et al. 1993).

Neuroimaging techniques are valuable in the diagnosis and management of HIV patients (see also Chapter 3). CT and MRI show some degree of atrophy in almost all demented HIV patients. Ventricular enlargement, reflecting atrophy of the basal ganglia, is correlated with neuropsychological impairment (Aylward et al. 1993; Hestad et al. 1993). MRI typically reveals diffuse signal change in the subcortical white matter. Progressive multifocal leukoencephalopathy (PML) is the most common cause (Broderick et al. 1993; Olsen et al. 1988).

Functional imaging studies allow visualization of subclinical cerebral dysfunction at a time when CT or MRI may be normal (Rosci et al. 1992). Single photon emission computed tomography (SPECT) findings suggest a progression from subcortical asymmetry to cortical abnormality to more globally affected cerebral perfusion (Ajmani et al. 1991; Maini et al. 1990). Positron-emission tomography (PET) studies demonstrate relative hypermetabolism of the thalamus and basal ganglia in the early and middle stages of HIV infection. As dementia worsens, the temporal lobes become metabolically hypoactive (Van Gorp et al. 1992). Neuroimaging techniques are primarily helpful in ruling out opportunistic infections and focal lesions, although functional techniques now demonstrate disease progression as well as response to treatment (Brunetti et al. 1989).

The EEG often shows continuous or intermittent slowing in the anterior regions but may be normal in HIV dementia. Focal slowing or sharp wave activity is atypical and most often found with focal disease such as toxoplasmosis or lymphoma (Gabuzda et al. 1988). Lumbar puncture frequently reveals mononuclear pleocytosis, increased protein, and HIV p24 core protein. In the future, markers such as β-2-microglobulin may prove useful for staging disease severity and monitoring response to antiviral therapy (Brew et al. 1992).

Toxic encephalopathy may result from drugs used to treat AIDS. For example, alpha interferon has been associated with fatigue, drowsiness, disorientation, and withdrawal (McDonald et al. 1987).

Toxoplasmosis

The protozoan *Toxoplasma gondii* is an intracellular parasite that frequently produces CNS infections in AIDS patients (Bergen and Levy 1993; Pons et al. 1988). CT scan with contrast shows multiple-ring enhancing lesions in the deep white matter. MRI is highly sensitive to the lesions of toxoplasmosis (Rauch and Jinkins 1991) (see Chapter 3, Figure 3–13). Treatment with pyrimethamine and sulfadiazine supplemented by folinic acid is highly effective (Luft and Remington 1992).

Cryptococcosis

This fungal infection occurs primarily in chronically immunosuppressed individuals and presents as a subacute meningoencephalitis, with impaired cognitive function, cerebellar ataxia, or spastic paraparesis. Diagnosis is made by finding the organism in india ink preparations of CSF or by a positive latex agglutination test for the cryptococcal polysaccharide antigen (Kovacs et al. 1985). Treatment is the intravenous administration of amphotericin B. In AIDS patients, the relapse rate is high (Pons et al. 1988). Fluconazole is an alternative drug, particularly in patients with less severe disease.

Other nonviral infections include tuberculosis, infection with mycobacterium avium, candidiasis, aspergillosis, histoplasmosis, and coccidiodomycosis.

Progressive Multifocal Leukoencephalopathy

PML, which is caused by a papovavirus, also occurs in other states with impaired cell-mediated immunity, such as tuberculosis, sarcoidosis, lymphoproliferative disease, and neoplasms. It evolves subacutely with cognitive impairment as one of many symptoms, including multiple paralyses, cortical blindness, aphasia, ataxia, and dysarthria (von Einsiedel et al. 1993). CT shows subcortical areas of patchy attenuation. MRI findings are presented in Chapter 3, Figures 3–11 and 3–12. CSF is usually normal. Definitive diagnosis requires brain biopsy, which shows large multinucleated cells and particles that have been identified as a human polyoma virus (Padget et al. 1971). Cytosine arabinoside has been used to treat the disease. An occasional patient may have a transient clinical response, but the usual course is relentless deterioration of neurological function. Other opportunistic CNS viral infections include cytomegalovirus and herpes simplex virus. In addition, varicella-zoster encephalitis and Epstein-Barr virus encephalitis may occur (Simpson and Tagliati 1994).

Other Infections

Neurosyphilis may present insidiously as defects in memory, reasoning, deportment, and self-care. Small, irregular pupils probably occur more frequently than classic Argyll Robertson pupils. In addition, there may be dysarthria, myoclonic jerks, tremor, hyperreflexia, and Babinski signs. Polyradiculopathy and neuropathic pain are common (Scheck and Hook 1994). The diagnosis is made by examining CSF, which may show 200–300 cells/mm^3 (mostly lymphocytes), elevation of total protein up to 200 mg/dl, increased gamma globulin, and frequently a positive serological test. Treatment is intravenous aqueous penicillin G, 24 million units in divided doses for 14 days, followed by intramuscular benzathine penicillin G, 2.4 million units weekly for three doses (Centers for Disease Control 1989). CSF should be retested after 6 months. If all findings have reversed, no further treatment is indicated (Goldmeier and Hay 1993).

Permanent cognitive impairment occurs frequently after herpes simplex encephalitis and may manifest as an amnestic disorder or as a full-blown dementia. An EEG is usually abnormal, with focal epileptiform activity; a CT scan shows early lucent areas, with later breakdown in blood-brain barrier causing increased contrast enhancement. Early treatment (during the acute encephalitic stage) with acyclovir significantly reduces mortality and morbidity (Skoldenberg 1991).

Chronic meningitis may be associated with reversible cognitive impairment. Symptoms include headache, stiff neck, lethargy, and confusion. Chronic meningitis occurs in syphilis, tuberculosis, cryptococcosis, coccidioidomycosis, histoplasmosis, blastomycosis, and actinomycosis (Adams and Victor 1989). Lyme disease also causes chronic meningitis (Finkel and Halperin 1992).

Brain abscess usually presents as a focal brain process. In the past, it was often an extension of infection in the paranasal sinuses, middle ear, or mastoid. It is accompanied by rapidly developing signs of increased intracranial pressure and often by drowsiness, stupor, and inattentiveness that may obscure localizing signs. Fever and leukocytosis may not be present. CSF pressure is increased early, with a cell count ranging up to 300 white blood cells/mm^3, neutrophils accounting for 10%–80%. Protein content is mildly elevated, usually to less than 100 mg/dl. CT shows a low-density core and a contrast-enhanced capsule. Treatment is combined antimicrobial and surgical (Luby 1992).

Neoplasm

Brain neoplasms may be primary or metastatic and single or multiple. Neoplasm causes dementia by local tissue destruction or compression, compromise of blood supply, or obstructing outflow of CSF. Particularly when situated in the frontal lobes, slow-growing tumors such as meningiomas may produce prominent cognitive impairment without producing localizing signs (Sachs 1950). CT and MRI are the most useful diagnostic measures. Primary CNS lymphoma is the most common brain malignancy in AIDS patients, accounting for 5%–10% of CNS complications (So et al. 1988). The appearance on imaging can be nonspecific, and brain biopsy is often needed for diagnosis. Cytological examination of CSF may be helpful. Treatment is with antimetabolites and radiation.

Cerebral Vasculitis

Inflammatory disorders are characterized by the presence in the CNS of immune mediator substances such as antibodies and complement.

Systemic lupus erythematosus frequently involves the CNS (O'Connor and Musher 1966). Systemic manifestations of the disease (skin, joint, renal) are usually seen. CNS involvement tends to be strokelike with focal findings. An EEG may show focal or diffuse slowing. Imaging studies show areas of patchy destruction corresponding to the course of blood vessels. Inflammatory vessel changes are demonstrable on angiography. CSF protein may be increased; immunoglobulin G and IgG synthesis are increased. Treatment may involve the use of corticosteroids, cytotoxic agents, or plasmapheresis (Stahl et al. 1994).

There are occasional cases of a small-vessel giant-cell granulomatous arteritis confined to brain vessels. The presentation is similar to an encephalitis or low-grade meningitis.

Normal-Pressure Hydrocephalus

Hydrocephalus may result from blocked CSF flow within the ventricles (noncommunicating) or from a blockage to reabsorption outside the ventricular system (communicating). Noncommunicating hydrocephalus usually presents acutely or subacutely with signs of increased intracranial pressure; communicating hydrocephalus is associated with a triad of symptoms including slowly progressive dementia, gait disturbance, and urinary incontinence (Adams et al. 1965). This triad is designated normal-pressure hydrocephalus (NPH) because, on lumbar puncture, the opening pressure is frequently normal. The gait has been described as "magnetic" (i.e., the feet appear to be stuck to the floor) and is usually slow and shuffling, with small steps and a wide base (Friedland 1989).

NPH may follow subarachnoid hemorrhage, head trauma, and clinically evident meningitis, but the largest group is of unknown etiology. The diagnosis is made on the basis of the clinical triad, although incontinence tends to occur late (Vanneste 1994). CT shows minimal gyral atrophy and enlarged ventricles with periventricular lucency (see Chapter 3, Figure 3–5); MRI shows markedly increased periventricular signal. Cisternography is helpful in confirming the diagnosis. Drainage of 40–50 ml of CSF may predict clinical response to treatment (Sand et al. 1994), which consists of the placement of a ventriculoatrial or ventriculoperitoneal shunt. L. W. Thompson et al. (1989) found an overall cognitive improvement rate of 40%, with greater improvement in patients with known causes, short history, low CSF outflow, small sulci, and periventricular hypodensity on CT.

Multiple Sclerosis

Multiple sclerosis (MS) is the most common demyelinating disease. Beginning as early as puberty, MS has an intermittent course and is manifested by episodes of unilateral blindness (due to optic neuritis), diplopia, weakness, and sensory loss due to patchy demyelination of the CNS. It is accompanied frequently by impairment of cognitive function; the severity of impairment is usually related to the duration of the disease (Peyser et al. 1980). Laboratory aids to diagnosis include discrete areas of subcortical increased signal on T_2-weighted MRI (see Chapter 3, Figure 3–7) and the presence of mild mononuclear pleocytosis (less than 100 cells/mm^3) and oligoclonal banding in the CSF. Oligoclonal bands are present in 90% or more of MS cases and only rarely with other illnesses

(Schmidt and Neumann 1978). An additional helpful measure is the IgG synthesis rate. Multimodal evoked potentials give evidence of subcortical sensory pathway involvement (Sibley 1990). Acute episodes are treated with immunosuppressants.

Irreversible Dementias

A partial list of the irreversible dementias is shown in Table 4–3. The two primary entities discussed are AD and vascular dementia (VaD), both of which are largely associated with aging. Autopsy studies indicate that AD accounts for half of the cases of late-life dementia, vascular disease approximately 22%, and mixed AD and vascular disease approximately 14% (Wolfson and Katzman 1983). The next most common causes are intracranial neoplasm (5%) and Pick's disease (2%), with alcoholic dementia, Parkinson's dementia, and others each accounting for 1% or less. One study of community-dwelling elders suggests that AD may account for as many as 9 of 10 cases of dementia in persons 65 years of age and older (Evans et al. 1989). Recent advances in palliative drug therapy make a positive diagnosis of AD important (see Chapter 6).

Degenerative

It had been assumed throughout history that aging itself is the cause of cognitive decline in elderly persons. According to Folsom (1886), "Senile dementia is simply an excess of the natural mental weakness of old age . . . " (p. 174). That assumption was reaffirmed as recently as 1958, when Wechsler reported that "nearly all studies . . . have shown that most human abilities decline progressively after . . . ages 18 and 25" (p. 135). What was not attributable to normal aging was assigned to cerebrovascular arteriosclerosis and associated small strokes (Alvarez 1966). The former assumption was first challenged when Corsellis (1962) found a strong relationship between the severity of cerebral degenerative change and clinical diagnosis of patients who died in a psychiatric hospital. Of patients diagnosed as having organic mental disorder, 75% had moderate or severe cerebral degeneration, whereas only 25% of patients diagnosed with functional disorders showed comparable change in brain. Tomlinson et al. (1970) found soon afterward that half the brains of clinically demented elders bore the microscopic stigmata (neuritic plaques and neurofibrillary tangles) of a brain disease first described in a 51-year-old woman by alienist-pathologist Alois Alzheimer in 1907.

Alzheimer's Disease

AD is a disease of heterogeneous etiology that is characterized by the gradual erosion of intellectual function. It occurs primarily between the ages of 40 and 90, appearing on average at age 70 years in our clinic population but beginning at times by the end of the fourth decade of life (St. George-Hyslop et al. 1987). Disease onset is insidious; the average duration of symptoms prior to diagnosis in our clinic patients is 4 years. Estimates of the prevalence of AD in persons 65 years of age or older range from a high of 10.3% (Evans et al. 1989) to a low of 2.3% (Bachman et al. 1992). Prevalence increases with age, with estimates for persons 85 years of age or older ranging from 13% (Bachman et al. 1992) to 48% (Evans et al. 1989). The study reporting higher prevalence rates included mild cases but excluded institutionalized persons, whereas the study reporting lower prevalence included only moderate to severe cases of dementia but did include nursing home residents.

The age-specific prevalence for AD is higher in women than in men (Bachman et al. 1992), but women may be more often diagnosed than men for a host of reasons, including greater longevity.

Risk factors include advancing age, having an affected first-degree relative, Down's syndrome (trisomy 21), head injury (Mortimer et al. 1991), and inheritance of the E4 allele of apoliprotein E. Individuals with at least one first-degree relative with dementia may have a fourfold increase in risk for AD; those with two or more may have a 40 times greater than normal risk (Hofman et al. 1989). Identical twins, however, are not completely concordant for the disease (Kumar et al. 1991).

Nearly all Down's syndrome patients who reach the fifth decade of life show the microscopic brain stigmata of AD, and many have signifi-

---

Table 4–3. Irreversible dementias in adults

Degenerative	Infectious
Alzheimer's disease	Creutzfeldt-Jakob disease
Lewy body variant of Alzheimer's disease	Unknown
Pick's disease	Limbic encephalitis
Huntington's disease	Hereditary metabolic diseases
Progressive supranuclear palsy	Metachromatic leukodystrophy
Parkinson's disease	Adrenoleukodystrophy
Vascular	Adult polyglucosan disease
Vascular dementia	Ceroid lipofuscinosis
	Leigh's disease
	Gaucher's disease
	Niemann-Pick disease

cant cognitive decline (Wisniewski et al. 1985).The gene for amyloid precursor protein (APP) is reduplicated in Down's syndrome (Delebar et al. 1987), and the brains of persons with Down's syndrome show widespread cortical amyloid deposition (Hof et al. 1995), but the APP gene is not replicated in AD (Tanzi et al. 1991).

Severe head injury has been found to result within days in the deposition of amyloid plaques in brain (Roberts et al. 1991).

The most important risk factor in late-onset AD may be the inheritance of E4, a protein that binds to β-amyloid protein in neuritic plaques and spinal fluid. A single E4 allele is associated with a threefold increase of late-onset AD; homozygosity for E4 is associated with an eightfold increase (Corder et al. 1993).

The higher prevalence of the E4 allele in persons with late-onset AD might be accounted for in part by an increase in their survival time (Frisoni et al. 1995). There may be a synergistic effect between head injury and E4. Mayeux et al. (1995) found a 10-fold increased risk of AD in persons with both E4 and a history of head injury associated with loss of consciousness as compared with a twofold increase in persons with E4 alone. Possession of the E4 allele contributes to the deposition of brain amyloid in persons with Down's syndrome (Hyman et al. 1995) and increases the risk of mildly cognitively impaired elders developing AD (Petersen et al. 1995). Higher educational and occupational attainment may slow the clinical presentation of AD (Stern et al. 1994), but survival time after symptom onset may be shortened because more educated patients may be at a more advanced stage of disease when they present for avaluation (Stern et al. 1995).

Etiology of most AD cases is still unknown. Studies have thus far revealed seven separate point mutations in the APP gene on chromosome 21, each of which appears to account for the development of early-onset AD in a few families (APP is a normal constituent of cell membranes). Greater numbers of early-onset familial cases are linked to a location on chromosome 14 (Sherrington et al. 1995). Some families show linkage to chromosome 19, the chromosome containing the gene for apolipoprotein E, and still other familial cases are not linked to chromosome 21, 14, or 19 (Clark and Goate 1993). (Refer to Chapter 13 for further discussion of genetics.)

Other etiological theories include endogenous or exogenous toxins, autoimmunity, and transmissible agents. Many investigators (Baker et al. 1988; Blass et al. 1985; reviewed by Scott 1993) have suggested that generalized metabolic abnormalities may be present, citing findings in many tissues. Parker et al. (1995) have found deficiency in cytochrome c oxidase. Appel (1981) postulated the absence of a trophic factor, a hypothesis supported by the finding that cholinergic neurons in the nucleus basalis of Meynert are highly dependent on nerve growth factor (Perry 1990). Possible candidates for endogenous toxins include free radicals (C. D. Smith et al. 1991; M. A. Smith et al. 1995) and cortisol (Sapolsky 1992; Weiner et al. 1993). Aluminum was suggested as an exogenous toxin by Crapper et al. (1973) and Perl and Brody (1980), but it seems likely that accumulation of aluminum in brain is a result rather than a cause of the disease.

A possible inflammatory component is suggested by the presence in AD of antivascular antibodies in serum (Fillit et al. 1987) and evidence of immune-mediated damage to brain tissue (Rogers et al. 1992a, 1992b), as discussed in Chapter 13.

The demonstration of slow virus infections of the CNS (Gajdusek et al. 1966) raised the possibility that AD might be caused by a slow virus or other transmissible agent, such as the prion, which causes scrapie in sheep (Prusiner 1982). However, the pathology of AD resembles neither the pathology of the slow virus diseases nor the prion-related diseases, and the single report of AD transmission into laboratory animals has not been confirmed (Manuelidis et al. 1988).

The pathological microscopic stigmata of AD are neuritic plaques, neurofibrillary tangles, and granulovacuolar degeneration. Neuritic plaques are visible at low magnification (Figure 4–1). The plaques are 9–10 mm wide and consist of a central amyloid core surrounded by dystrophic and degenerating neuronal processes, reactive microglia, and phagocytes (Terry and Katzman 1983). Neurofibrillary tangles consisting of hyperphosphorylated tau protein occupy the cell bodies of medium and large neurons (Figure 4–2). Electron microscopy shows that they are masses of fibers made of paired helical filaments approximately 100 Å in width and crossing regularly at 800-Å intervals (Kidd 1963). Granulovacuolar degeneration consists of a small, dark, basophilic granule lying in a clear vacuole within the cytoplasm of hippocampal pyramidal cells (Terry and Katzman 1983).

Lewy bodies are found frequently in the cerebral cortex of patients with autopsy-confirmed AD. A hallmark of Parkinson's disease when found in the substantia nigra, these round, eosinophilic cytoplasmic inclusions have a diameter of 5–25 μm and are surrounded by a pale halo (see Figure 4–3).

The pathophysiology of AD includes amyloid infiltration of vascular walls (amyloid angiopathy). Its presence raises the question of whether amyloid is produced in the brain as a result of genetic influence, whether

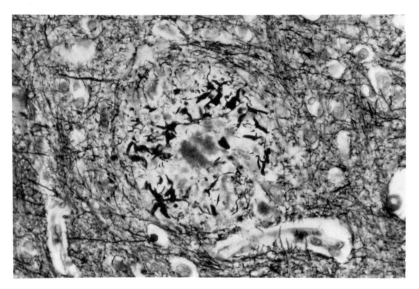

Figure 4-1.   Neuritic plaques (courtesy of Dr. Charles White).

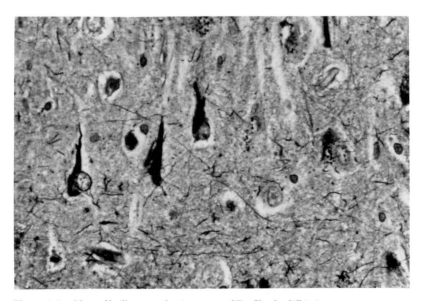

Figure 4–2.   Neurofibrillary tangles (courtesy of Dr. Charles White).

it is a product of the brain's reticuloendothelial system, or whether it leaks in through damaged blood vessels (Wisniewski 1983). Through immunohistochemical techniques, Joachim et al. (1989a) found a substance identical to brain amyloid in skin, subcutaneous tissue, and intestine, suggesting that the disease may be related in pathophysiology to systemic amyloidosis—a theory promulgated earlier by Glenner and Wong (1984).

Overproduction of amyloid has been suggested as a pathophysiological mechanism in AD. The gene for the β-amyloid of AD (Alzheimer precursor protein or APP gene) has been characterized and mapped to chromosome 21 (Goldgaber et al. 1987). β-Amyloid messenger ribonucleic acid (mRNA) is increased in the nucleus basalis, the site of pronounced cholinergic cell loss in AD (M. L. Cohen et al. 1988). The pathogenetic mechanism may be in the regulation of APP or in its catabolism (Selkoe 1993) or β-amyloid neurotoxicity in the mature CNS (Arispe et al. 1993; Yankner et al. 1990). Abnormal phosphorylation of the

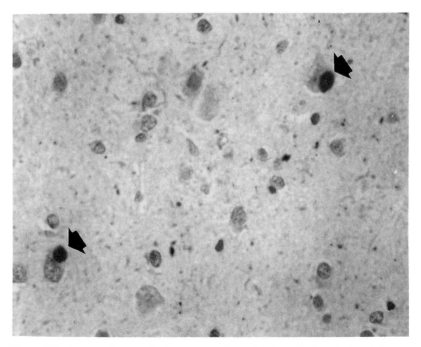

Figure 4–3.   Two small neocortical neurons, each containing a single cytoplasmic Lewy body (arrows) immunostained with an antibody to ubiquitin (magnification 125×; hematoxylin counterstain) (courtesy of Dr. Charles White).

normal cytoskeletal protein tau may be responsible for the formation of neurofibrillary tangles (Goedert 1993).

Numerous neurochemical abnormalities occur in AD brain tissue, presumably due to neuron loss. The first discovered was a marked decrease in cortical choline acetyltransferase (M. Davies and Maloney 1976). The reduced activity of this enzyme, which converts acetyl coenzyme A and choline to the neurotransmitter acetylcholine, suggested the possibility of a specific neurotransmitter deficit in AD, which is the basis for most present-day pharmacological interventions.

Loss of subcortical neurons occurs, including loss of cholinergic neurons of the nucleus basalis of Meynert, noradrenergic neurons of the locus coeruleus, and serotonergic neurons of the dorsal raphe nuclei, with an associated reduction of concentration of each transmitter in the cerebral cortex (German et al. 1987). Other neurotransmitters are affected and are discussed in Chapter 13.

The DSM-IV diagnosis of AD (dementia of the Alzheimer's type) has four basic requisites: 1) presence of dementia; 2) gradual onset with continuing cognitive decline; 3) exclusion of all other specific causes of dementia by history, physical examination, and laboratory tests; and 4) not occurring exclusively during the course of a delirium (American Psychiatric Association 1994). National Institute of Neurological and Communicative Disorders and Stroke—Alzheimer's Disease and Related Disorders Association (NINCDS-ADRDA) criteria for the clinical diagnosis of AD (McKhann et al. 1984), which are presented in Table 4–4, allow for the diagnosis of probable and possible AD. In a large autopsy series, the diagnosis of probable AD was confirmed in 92% of the subjects. Possible AD was pathologically diagnosed as AD in 87% of the subjects (Gearing et al. 1994).

The course of illness (see also Chapter 7) in AD starts most often in the seventh and eighth decades of life. Although DSM-IV divides AD into early-onset and late-onset forms, there is little evidence of important differences in the disease based on this distinction. Based on our experience with more than 400 cases of AD, the clinical presentation and course of the disease are diverse; but it most often begins as defects in memory, reasoning, and judgment. Among the frequent early signs are memory lapses common to all elders, such as forgetting where the house keys have been placed or where the car is parked in a shopping center. The disease occasionally presents as a delirium occurring when the person enters a strange environment or is hospitalized for medical treatment of an unrelated condition. Over variable periods, impairment of orientation occurs, and the ability to deal with abstract concepts and to

Table 4–4. NINCDS-ADRDA criteria for the clinical diagnosis of
Alzheimer's disease (AD)

Criteria for probable AD include:

1. Dementia established by clinical examination and documented by Mini-Mental State Exam, Blessed Dementia Scale, or similar examination, and confirmed by neuropsychological testing
2. Deficits in two or more areas of cognition
3. Progressive worsening of memory and other cognitive functions
4. No disturbance of consciousness
5. Onset between ages 40 and 90
6. Absence of systemic disorders or other brain diseases that in and of themselves could account for the progressive deficits in memory and cognition

The diagnosis of probable AD is supported by:

1. Progressive deterioration of specific cognitive functions such as language (aphasia), motor skills (apraxia), and perception (agnosia)
2. Impaired activities of daily living and altered patterns of behavior
3. Family history of similar disorders, particularly if confirmed neuropathologically
4. Normal lumbar puncture as evaluated by standard techniques
5. Normal pattern or nonspecific EEG changes, such as increased slow-wave activity
6. Evidence of cerebral atrophy on with progression documented by serial observation

Other clinical features consistent with probable AD after excluding other causes of dementia include:

1. Plateaus in the course of progression of the illness
2. Associated symptoms of depression; insomnia; incontinence; delusions; illusions; hallucinations; catastrophic verbal, emotional, or physical outbursts; sexual disorder; weight loss; and other neurologic abnormalities in some patients, especially with more advanced disease, and including motor signs such as increased muscle tone, myoclonus, or gait disorder
3. Seizures in advanced disease
4. CT normal for age

Features that make the diagnosis of probable AD uncertain or unlikely include:

1. Sudden, apoplectic onset
2. Focal neurologic findings such as hemiparesis, sensory loss, visual field deficits, and incoordination early in the course of the illness
3. Seizures or gait disturbances at the outset or very early in the course of the illness

Clinical diagnosis of possible AD:

1. May be made on the basis of the dementia syndrome; in the absence of other neurologic, psychiatric, or systemic disorders sufficient to cause dementia; and in the presence of variations in the onset, presentation, or clinical course
2. May be made in the presence of a second systemic or brain disorder sufficient to produce dementia, which is not considered to be the cause of the dementia
3. Should be used in research studies when a single, gradually progressive severe cognitive deficit is identified in the absence of other identifiable cause

Source. Used with permission from McKhann G, Drachman D, Folstein M, et al: "Clinical Diagnosis of Alzheimer's Disease: Report of the NINCDS-ADRDA Work Group Under the Auspices of the Department of Health and Human Services Task Force on Alzheimer's Disease." *Neurology* 34:939–944, 1984.

perform complex tasks is lost. Praxis difficulties may begin with dressing dyspraxias, such as inability to tie shoelaces or a necktie. Language becomes impaired, as manifested by difficulty in word finding and object naming, with resultant paraphasia. Constructional ability becomes impaired, rendering AD patients unable to copy simple diagrams or to draw a clock face (Sunderland et al. 1989). Patients also lose the ability to read and write. Prosopagnosia is common later in the disease, with patients frequently unable to identify loved ones or to recognize themselves in a mirror. Social judgment tends to be retained until late in the disease. Incontinence of bowel and bladder occur, and eventually AD patients become unable to walk or to perform other intentional acts, including self-feeding and eating. Death results from inanition, inability to maintain adequate pulmonary toilette, sepsis from urinary tract infection, or other intercurrent illnesses to which enfeebled elders are easy prey.

The duration of illness is variable, ranging from 4–10 years or more, depending on the patients' general health, the quality of nursing care available, and the vigor with which feeding and other life support measures are pursued in the later stages.

Neurological abnormalities often present in the middle or late stages of the disease. Cortical release signs including snout, suck, palmomental, and grasp reflexes appear. Myoclonic jerks occur often, as do mild extrapyramidal signs (Chen et al. 1991). Postural changes also occur, with turning en bloc a fairly frequent phenomenon, along with a lowering of the center of gravity that results in a bent-knee, shuffling gait. Contractures occur when patients become bedbound.

Psychiatric symptoms are common in AD (Burns et al. 1990a). Behavioral symptoms in early AD include passivity, agitation, low levels of interest, concentration, and energy (E. H. Rubin and Kinscherf 1989). Denial of memory deficit is common (Sevush and Leve 1993). Depressive symptoms are common, but full-blown major depression is rare (Weiner et al. 1991). Paranoid ideation is also common, and in one series it occurred in 31% of subjects (E. H. Rubin et al. 1988). The primary focus for these patients was on other people stealing objects from the home or of being the object of a foul plot. The delusion may develop that the spouse has a double or that the spouse is being impersonated. Visual hallucinations may occur in as many as 15% of patients and auditory hallucinations in 10% (E. H. Rubin et al. 1988). Hallucinations are no longer reported as language function disintegrates. Behavioral and psychiatric disturbances tend to increase as the disease progresses (J. K. Cooper et al. 1990; Swearer et al. 1988). Physical aggression is not rare (Deutsch et

al. 1991). It may be that much of the agitated behavior of severely demented patients is in response to ideas and perceptions they can no
longer communicate to others.

There are no laboratory findings specifically diagnostic of AD. Measurement of CSF-soluble amyloid β-protein precursor has been proposed as a confirmatory diagnostic measure; concentrations below 450
U/L suggest AD (Farlow et al. 1992), but low concentrations also occur
with Gerstman-Straussler Scheinker disease and hereditary cerebral
hemorrhage with amyloidosis (Van Nostrand et al. 1992). The discovery
by immunohistochemical techniques of β-amyloid in skin (Joachim et al.
1989a) raised the possibility of using skin biopsy to confirm the diagnosis
of AD, but this is not reliable (Heinonen et al. 1994). Sensitivity to the
mydriatric effects of dilute tropicamide (an acetylcholine receptor antagonist) was reported to differentiate between AD patients, normal individuals, and persons with other dementias (Scinto et al. 1994), but this
finding has been challenged (Treloar et al. 1995) and requires further investigation.

AD is detected early by signs of temporal and parietal lobe dysfunction, the triad of recent memory impairment, construction dyspraxia,
and dysnomia. Confirmation of diffuse cortical damage can be obtained
by neuropsychological testing (see Chapter 7). Signs of brain atrophy on
CT or MRI scans may be present early in the course of the disease. Frequent findings on both CT and MRI are shrinkage of the temporal lobes
with widening of the Sylvian fissures and hydrocephalus ex vacuo. On
MRI, the cortical ribbon is seen to narrow more than the white matter.
An EEG will usually show generalized slowing as the disease progresses.
SPECT regional cerebral blood flow studies performed with [133]Xe (Bonte
et al. 1986b) and ^{123}I-labeled iodoamphetamine (Jagust et al. 1987) and
other tracers show bilateral temporoparietal blood flow reduction. PET
with [^{15}O]- and fluorodeoxyglucose also shows reduction in temporoparietal blood flow, but other cortical regions have been found to be
involved. In a study of 32 AD patients (largely tissue confirmed), Haxby
et al. (1988) found that, in severe cases, premotor cortex involvement was
as severe as parietal. In a patient studied 16 months before death, PET
findings correlated well with microscopic findings of neuronal loss and
glial proliferation (McGeer et al. 1986).

There is no specific treatment for AD. Behavioral and emotional
complications are managed using psychological measures and drugs described in Chapters 5 and 6. Palliative drugs for cognitive deficit are
described in Chapter 6, experimental drugs in Chapter 15, and environmental measures are discussed in Chapter 7.

Lewy Body Variant of Alzheimer's Disease and Lewy Body Dementia

Patients with AD frequently develop parkinsonian symptoms. Some of these patients have both AD and Parkinson's disease. A small subset of these patients does not have pathological evidence of Parkinson's disease despite mild extrapyramidal symptoms during life. A larger group of these AD patients has the Lewy bodies and neuron loss in the substantia nigra characteristic of Parkinson's disease but also has Lewy bodies in the cortex (see Figure 4–3), where they are not usually found in Parkinson's disease. This Lewy body "variant" (LBV) of AD, which is present in nearly a third of autopsied clinically diagnosed AD patients (Hansen et al. 1990), is associated with the development of mild parkinsonian symptoms during the course of AD. These symptoms do not respond well to antiparkinsonian medications, and the patients often do not have tremor, although rigidity and gait disturbance are present. One group characterized LBV patients as having prominent hallucinations, paranoid ideation, unexplained falls, and loss of consciousness. Microscopically, the prevalence of neurofibrillary tangles was much less than in "pure" AD cases, but plaque counts were similar (McKeith et al. 1992). By contrast, Förstl et al. (1993) found extrapyramidal symptoms more common in LBV than AD, but there was no difference in hallucinations or in the overall course of the illness. All subjects had AD pathology but less severe than in age- and sex-matched AD patients. An important clinical characteristic of these patients is their sensitivity to the extrapyramidal effects of neuroleptics (McKeith et al. 1994).

In Lewy body dementia, there are Lewy bodies throughout the cortex without the pathology of AD. Much less common than either AD or LBV, we have seen one such case. This individual presented with two episodes of delirium that were several years apart. He slowly developed a dementia with extrapyramidal features.

Pick's Disease

Pick's disease is a form of cerebral degeneration involving both gray and white matter, with circumscribed areas of atrophy occurring predominantly in the frontal and temporal lobes. Histologically, there is a loss of neurons in the first three cortical layers. Remaining neurons are often swollen and contain silver-staining Pick bodies in the cytoplasm. In contrast to AD, there is no cholinergic deficit (Wood et al. 1983).

Pick's disease is not readily distinguishable from AD during the patient's life. There is often a "frontal" presentation (see Chapter 1), with apathy, abulia (slowing of thinking, speech, and activity), prancing gait, and prominent grasp and suck reflexes. Some patients giggle and appear silly. CT and MRI studies show areas of localized atrophy confined to the frontal and temporal lobes.

The etiology of this disease is unknown, although an autosomal dominant inheritance has been suggested (Heston et al. 1987). Its course is progressive and eventually leads to complete incapacity.

Huntington's Disease

Huntington's disease (HD) is a completely penetrant autosomal-dominant disorder. Its onset is usually between ages 35 and 45 years, but 25% of cases have onset of motor symptoms past the age of 50 years (Wojcieszek and Lang 1994). HD is characterized by loss of neurons in the caudate nucleus and the putamen of the thalamus. Various neurotransmitters are reduced in activity, including acetylcholine, γ-aminobutyric acid (GABA), substance P, cholecystokinin, and angiotensin-converting enzyme. The genetic abnormality is located on the short arm of chromosome 4 (Gusella et al. 1983). It consists of an excessive number of cytosine-adenine-guanine (CAG) trinucleotide repeats. With rare exceptions, persons destined to develop HD have 37–86 CAG repeats, in contrast to 11–34 repeats in normal individuals (Gusella et al. 1993). Thus, at-risk diagnosis is possible from DNA samples from individuals who have more than 38–40 repeats but is problematic for individuals with only 35–38 repeats.

Cognitive or affective disturbances are often the presenting symptoms. Typically, the dementia is frontal, with prominent behavioral problems and disruption of attention. Although choreiform movements are characteristic of the disease, it may present in the juvenile form as an akinetic-rigid disorder.

Physical signs include exaggerated deep tendon reflexes, cortical release signs, and signs of impersistence, such as inability to maintain tongue protrusion. Atrophy of the caudate nucleus is evident on both CT (see Chapter 3, Figure 3–4) and MRI scans, as is frontal atrophy. SPECT shows decreased frontal blood flow, and PET shows decreased basal ganglia metabolism.

HD is gradually progressive, eventually resulting in profound dementia and death. Choreic symptoms are treated with a dopamine blocker such as haloperidol in doses ranging from 2–10 mg qd, bearing in mind the possibility of inducing tardive dyskinesia. Baclofen, a GABA analogue, is also helpful as an antichoreic agent, as is low-dose bro-mocriptine.

Progressive Supranuclear Palsy

This disorder begins in late life and is characterized by difficulty in balance, falls, visual disturbances, slurred speech, dysphagia, and per-sonality change (Richardson et al. 1963). Dementia tends not to be pro-nounced. A characteristic triad of ophthalmoplegia, pseudobulbar palsy, and axial dystonia develops. First, downward gaze is impaired, then up-ward gaze, then voluntary gaze in all directions. If the eyes are fixed on a target and the head turned, full eye movement occurs, indicating the intactness of the motor nerves.

The etiology of this disease is unknown. Pathological findings in-clude loss of neurons, gliosis, and neurofibrillary tangles present in the surviving neurons in the midbrain, cerebellar peduncles, and subtha-lamic nucleus. Impairment proceeds to anarthria and total immobility.

Parkinson's Disease

Parkinson's disease exhibits resting tremors, rigidity resulting from in-creased tone in the axial musculature, and slowed, decreased motor ac-tivity. Gait is unstable, causing frequent falls. Facial expression generally decreases, rate of blinking diminishes, and arm swing diminishes during walking. The clinical syndrome is slowly progressive and appears to re-sult from loss of pigmented neurons in the pars compacta of the substan-tia nigra. Loss of these cells reduces dopaminergic input to the limbic system, forebrain, and the basal ganglia. Cells are lost in other pig-mented nuclei as well, including the locus coeruleus and the dorsal mo-tor nucleus of the vagus. Eosinophilic cytoplasmic inclusions called Lewy bodies are seen in surviving cells of the pigmented nuclei.

There is considerable pathological overlap between Parkinson's dis-ease and AD, with Joachim et al. (1988) reporting that 18% of their AD cases had sufficient neuronal loss and Lewy bodies in the substantia ni-gra to warrant a diagnosis of Parkinson's disease. Clinically, dementia occurs frequently in Parkinson's disease, with estimates ranging from 18% to 60% (Cummings 1985; Tison 1995).

Laboratory and neuroimaging studies are not helpful in the diagno-sis of Parkinson's disease. Treatment is with anticholinergics and dopa-mine agonists, but anticholinergic agents should be avoided in

Parkinson's disease patients with dementia because they are likely to increase confusion (De Smet et al. 1982).

Vascular

VaDs are the second most common dementia in elders in the United States, and VaD may complicate AD. VaD may result from multiple infarcts, strategically placed single infarcts, small-vessel disease, hypoperfusion, and brain hemorrhage. Dementia as a result of brain tissue infarction occurs in relation to the volume of tissue infarcted and to the location of the infarcts. Loss of approximately 100 ml of brain tissue produces severe cognitive impairment regardless of location (Tomlinson et al. 1970). Localized infarcts in the hippocampus, mammillary bodies, thalamus, or basal forebrain produce severe memory deficits (Scheinberg 1988). If small-vessel infarcts primarily involve white matter, the term *Binswanger's disease* is often used (Caplan and Schoene 1978; Román 1987). When brain tissue is reabsorbed following infarction, cavities develop. Figure 4–4 shows an MRI study of a man with a history of strokes, mild cognitive impairment, and sensory loss in both lower extremities. Multiple lacunes are present in the basal ganglia.

The following criteria have been proposed for the diagnosis of VaD (Román et al. 1993):

1. Dementia, defined by cognitive decline from a previously higher level of functioning with impairment of memory and two or more additional cognitive domains; established by clinical examination and confirmed by neuropsychological testing; severe enough to interfere with activities of daily living and not due to the physical effects of stroke alone.
2. Cerebrovascular disease (CVD), defined by focal neurological signs (with or without history of stroke) and evidence of relevant CVD by CT or MRI including multiple large-vessel infarcts, a single strategically placed infarct (angular gyrus, thalamus, basal forebrain, posterior cerebral artery, or anterior cerebral artery territories), and multiple basal ganglia and white matter lacunes or extensive periventricular white matter lesions.
3. A relationship between dementia and CVD as suggested by onset of dementia within 3 months following a recognized stroke; abrupt deterioration in cognitive function or fluctuating stepwise progression of cognitive defects.

VaD may exhibit predominantly cortical (aphasia, agnosia, apraxia, amnesia) or subcortical (slowness, depression, forgetfulness) signs but often presents with both. There may be pseudobulbar palsy and dysarthria. VaD is associated with hypertension, diabetes, and other evidence of cardiovascular disease, such as a history of myocardial infarction. There is often a history of transient ischemic attacks or frank stroke. VaD may progress in a stepwise fashion, with acute episodes of

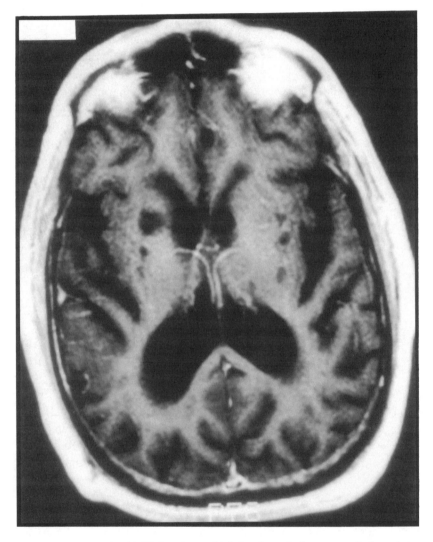

Figure 4–4. T_1-weighted MRI showing multiple basal ganglia lacunes, marked gyral atrophy and hydrocephalus ex vacuo (courtesy of Dr. Myron Weiner).

confusion accompanied by localizing or lateralizing neurological signs. Mental status examination may reveal a patchy pattern of deficit (see Chapter 1), but the deficit is often indistinguishable from AD. Depression and emotional lability are more characteristic of VaD than AD. There may be focal or generalized EEG slowing. When there are multiple infarcts, CT shows areas of lucency (Chapter 3, Figure 3–1), MRI shows areas of increased signal on TMv2-weighted images (Chapter 3, Figure 3–9), and SPECT indicates multiple areas of low flow that are wedge shaped when infarcts involve the cortex (see Chapter 3).

Treatment of VaD consists of prophylaxis, including control of hypertension and diabetes, and the use of aspirin and other drugs to reduce intravascular clotting (see Chapter 6). Anticoagulants are employed only when a definite cardiac embolic source has been identified or when repeated transient ischemic attacks occur in an individual with largely preserved function (Cummings 1987). Signs and symptoms of depression should be actively sought (see section on stroke in this chapter and also Chapter 1). In questionable cases, a trial of methylphenidate or low-dose antidepressant may be indicated, as suggested in Chapter 6.

Mixed Dementia

There are many cases in which the clinical picture has elements of both AD and VaD. There are cases in which the progress of the disease has been smooth, but unilateral hyperreflexia, dysarthria, unilateral facial palsy, or a unilateral Babinski sign is present along with CT or MRI evidence of an old infarct. In other cases, a smooth downward course is punctuated by one or more stepwise declines. Such cases—in which both diseases seem to be present but neither disease fully explains the clinical picture—are designated as mixed dementias.

Infectious

Subacute Spongiform Encephalopathy

Subacute spongiform encephalopathy (SSE, or Creutzfeldt-Jakob disease) is a rapidly progressive dementing disorder often accompanied by cerebellar ataxia and myoclonic jerks. The EEG frequently shows periodic complexes. Ordinarily a disease of older adults, death usually occurs within 6 months to a year. Sporadic cases are due to a transmissible agent (Gibbs et al. 1968) that is extremely small, resistant to chemical and physical agents, produces no inflammatory response, and lacks demonstrable nucleic acid or host protein (Lehrich 1985). The disease is diagnosed by detection of this prion protein in brain (Serban et al. 1990). The source of infection is not known in most cases. Known sources of transmission include corneal transplants, contaminated depth electrodes, and injections of human growth hormone from pooled cadaveric pituitary glands. In iatrogenic cases, the incubation period is 10 years or more (Gibbs et al. 1985).

Spongiform changes are present in the cerebral and cerebellar cortex. Heidenhain's variant of the disease affects the parietooccipital regions primarily.

The transmissible agent is of very low infectivity, but because of its transmissibility, precautions should be taken comparable to those taken with hepatitis B. Contact with body fluid requires that gloves be worn. Infected materials should be autoclaved at 132°C and 15 lb/in^2 for 1 hour or immersed in 1% sodium hydroxide for 1 hour.

Familial SSE and Gerstmann-Sträussler-Scheinker syndrome (GSS) are linked to the prion protein gene on chromosome 20 (Goldgaber at al. 1989). GSS has a course of about 5 years and is characterized by cerebellar ataxia and dementia. A GSS-associated mutation of the prion protein may produce a neurodegenerative disorder in transfected mice (Hsiao et al. 1990).

Unknown

Limbic Encephalitis

Limbic encephalitis is a progressive dementia, often preceded or accompanied by agitation, depression, and behavioral disturbances. It is associated with systemic neoplasms, including oat-cell lung carcinoma, and with carcinoma of the ovary, breast, uterus, and stomach (Massachusetts General Hospital 1985). Autopsy reveals an inflammatory reaction confined largely to the temporal lobes, including hippocampus and amygdala (Brierley et al. 1960).

CSF may show mild lymphocytosis. An EEG may be normal or abnormal. A CT scan may reveal no abnormality, whereas MRI shows medial temporal lobe enhancement. Treatment of the related malignancy does not reverse the course of the illness.

Adult Forms of Hereditary Metabolic Diseases

Hereditary metabolic diseases that manifest in adults include metachromatic leukodystrophy, adrenoleukodystrophy, and adult polyglucosan body disease.

Metachromatic leukodystrophy is caused by lack of the enzyme aryl sulfatase. It is transmitted as an autosomal recessive, usually manifesting in the first decade of life. There is widespread degeneration of myelinated fibers in the central and peripheral nervous system, leading to combined upper and lower motor neuron signs. Adults may become demented, but they also lose deep tendon reflexes and have upturned toes. Cases are reported to occur as late as 62 years of age (Bosch and Hart 1978). Diagnosis is by sural nerve biopsy demonstrating the metachromatic material (3'-sulfogalacto-cerebroside).

Adult polyglucosan body disease may develop in late adulthood, with upper and lower motor neuron involvement, marked sensory loss, neurogenic bladder, and dementia. In this disease, there is massive accumulation of polyglucosan bodies throughout the central and peripheral nervous system. Diagnosis is made by sural nerve biopsy demonstrating polyglucosan inclusions (Lafora bodies) in processes of nerve cells and in astrocytes (Gray et al. 1988) (see Chapter 1).

Adrenoleukodystrophy (also termed *adrenomyeloneuropathy*) generally presents with spastic paraparesis and peripheral neuropathy (Menza et al. 1988) but occasionally causes dementia. It is a peroxisomal disorder that results in the systemic accumulation of very long chain fatty acids, with concentrations highest in the adrenal cortex and CNS. Although transmitted as an X-linked recessive, it is occasionally symptomatic in women. The diagnosis is made by demonstrating elevated C26/C22 fatty acids in serum and tissue assay (Moser et al. 1985).

According to Adams and Victor (1989), adult cases of the following disorders have also been observed or reported. Ceroid lipofuscinosis (Kufs' disease form of lipid storage disease) may begin in adolescence or early adulthood, with personality changes, myoclonus, and seizures. Later, cerebellar ataxia spasticity and rigidity of limbs and dementia develop. Patients may survive Leigh's disease in a helpless state for many years. Adolescents have been found with Gaucher's disease or Neimann-Pick disease. Other diseases not mentioned earlier that can manifest past the age of 50 are Hallervorden-Spatz syndrome and choreoacanthocytosis (Civil et al. 1993).

Summary

This chapter deals with the most common causes of the dementia syndrome. Although treatable dementias are far less common than irreversible dementias, they occur sufficiently often that all dementia syndromes warrant a search for either a reversible etiology or a reversible component. Accurate diagnosis of the irreversible dementias is important as a basis for family counseling and for identifying patients who may respond temporarily to palliative therapies or who can participate in studies that may lead to cure.

CHAPTER 5

Psychological and
Behavioral Management

Myron F. Weiner, M.D.
Linda Teri, Ph.D
Brent T. Williams, B.A., M.S.

Emotional and behavioral problems are thought to affect 70%–90% of patients with Alzheimer's disease (AD) (Reisberg et al. 1987; Teri et al. 1992) and are highly prevalent in other dementing illnesses. Such problems seriously impair quality of life for patient and caregivers alike (Drinka et al. 1987; Haley et al. 1987; Swearer et al. 1988). Many of the emotional and behavioral consequences of dementia can be managed by psychological or behavioral means (Baltes and Zerbe 1976; Teri 1985; Wragg and Jeste 1988), either alone or in conjunction with medications. Certain principles apply to the psychological and behavioral management of persons with dementia, but the most efficacious interventions are based on understanding the individual patient's disease, the patient as a person, and the social and interpersonal context in which he or she lives. The interventions described are not applied directly to patients in a one-to-one relationship and then applied by patients in their day-to-day living, as they would be in the course of formal psychotherapy. Although all but the most deteriorated dementia patients are capable of some learning, impaired brain function materially reduces the likelihood of dementia patients generalizing from one situation to another. Thus, clinicians address themselves largely to caregivers, who carry out clinicians' suggestions in their everyday contact with patients.

In this chapter, we describe the physiological and psychological factors that determine the most helpful type of psychological or behavioral intervention for dementia patients and provide a set of general principles governing such interventions. We also discuss specific behavioral interventions for dealing with depressed mood and disruptive behaviors. Nursing issue behaviors are discussed in Chapter 11, and environmental factors that contribute to and ameliorate dementia-related behaviors are described in Chapter 12.

Physiological Factors

The physiological factors that dictate the types of intervention to be employed include the amount of brain function compromised (severity of brain damage), the predominant function(s) lost or impaired, and whether the impairment of function is static, reversible, or progressive.

Severity of Brain Damage

In cerebrovascular disease, a relationship has been shown between the amount of cerebral tissue infarcted and the appearance of dementia (Tomlinson et al. 1970), although the amount of tissue lost does not always parallel loss of function. In AD, there is a relationship between cortical synapse loss and the severity of dementia (Terry et al. 1991), but the loss of brain volume as determined by sulcal widening and gyral atrophy on computed tomographic (CT) or magnetic resonance imaging (MRI) is not a useful index.

The cerebral cortex and its association pathways enable the formulation and understanding of symbolic communication. The greater the neuronal damage or loss, the greater the impairment of comprehension and reasoning, and the greater the difficulty in symbolic communication to and by brain-damaged persons. For the purpose of discussion, it is useful to "stage" cognitive impairment. A convenient hypothetical staging for the purpose of patient management follows Piaget's (1954) description of cognitive maturation in children.

1. Sensory motor.   In this stage, what cannot be experienced by the senses does not exist. The child is unable to maintain a mental image of a person or an object and experiences an intense affective storm when the nurturing person or object disappears from view at a time the child is experiencing physical tension such as hunger or thirst. Adults functioning at this level frequently "shadow" their caregivers. This can be seen as an attempt to physically maintain the "object constancy" that they are unable to maintain cognitively. At times, they will accept a substitute caregiver, but many times, they will not. Such individuals may find a soft, fuzzy toy animal or even a blanket a source of comfort.

2. Preoperational. Preoperational children can remember objects and actions and grieve when important persons or objects are lost from view, but they have learned that matter is conserved and will search for what has been lost. Thus, the brain-damaged person, whose possessions now seem unfamiliar, may engage in extensive rummaging in search of unnamed objects that appear to be lost. Wanting to "go home" also seems related to this level of function. Not recognizing present surroundings but remembering having felt comfortable elsewhere, the patient longs to "go home."

3. Concrete operations. At the stage of concrete operations, children can change their thinking when evidence is presented that their view is incorrect. Children at this stage can imagine what an object looks like from another physical point of view or imagine how others might react in a given situation.

Many dementia patients have difficulty with depth perception, possibly related to difficulty sorting the significant from the insignificant aspects of their sensory input. A change in the texture or color of floor covering suggests a change in the level of the floor, and patients may attempt to step up or down. Having made this mistake several times, patients can learn that there is no change in level. Dementia patients who hallucinate can sometimes learn that their perceptions are false and can describe them as hallucinations.

4. Formal operations. In this stage, which Piaget states only 30% of adults achieve, children become able to transcend reality and imagine what could be. It allows the generation of hypotheses that can be tested by observation and experimentation.

Persons who have achieved the stage of formal operations in their development often maintain the ability to use their imagination early in the course of a dementing illness. They imagine what it will be like when they can no longer reason or remember. Many have written moving accounts of anticipating loss of their personhood (Cohen and Eisdorfer 1986). The following was written by a man with a cognitive disorder:

Old Man on the Curb
Who is he, who sits there at twilight,

head bowed, with feet in the gutter?
—that old man on the curb?
As the universe and its throbbing
activity of mankind, its
dreams, its threats
Demand more, more, more.
The old man on the curb stares
only at the darkening pavement.
"ITS NIGHT AND COLD, OLD MAN;
BETTER GO HOME BEFORE ITS ON YOU."
Then he lifted his eyes, void of
hope or expression,
"Night and home, you say—
night and home?"

RL

Parkland Hospital

11-24-75   3 A.M.

Although still oriented to time and place, the writer was losing both his identity and his ability to connect thoughts. Progressively dementing persons still functioning at the level of formal operations can understand the need for a joint bank account, for making a will, and for assigning power of attorney.

Often, however, the dementing process has reduced cognitive functioning to the preoperational stage by the time it is formally detected. In such cases, the dementia patient may be unable to understand the need for changes, such as relinquishing the checkbook and the steering wheel, nor is the person able to learn from mistakes. It is often necessary, at this stage, to employ subterfuge to avoid the adult equivalent of a temper tantrum. For example, when a woman with dementia who was accustomed to paying household bills realized that they were probably due, her husband said that he did not want to bother her and mailed them in her stead and offered to let her see what he had done. When poor judgment and memory impair driving at this stage of thinking, the husband can tell his wife that the car is being repaired, that the keys have been misplaced, or that their daughter has borrowed it.

When functioning at the preoperational level, many persons are fearful in the absence of their spouse and are not consoled when told that the spouse will return soon, because they cannot remember the reassurance. Shadowing of spouses, as indicated above, also substitutes for the patient's inability to hold the spouse in memory and anticipate his or her return.

The Piagetian stages do not exactly parallel the development of dementia. Young children are able to remember and thus learn, whereas much of the behavior seen in dementia results from an admixture of retained and lost ability to understand various means of communication, including spoken and written language, signs, and symbols.

Placing a DO NOT ENTER sign on a door may deter the entry of a person mildly affected with dementia who maintains the ability to read and to understand that the sign indicates a prohibition. Telling a person about to enter an off-limits area "No!" and accompanying the "no" with appropriate gestures may be a deterrent as long as emotional speech and symbolic gestures can be comprehended. A person profoundly affected with dementia who can no longer read or understand verbal communication may respond to a physical cue to stop or may be distracted into some other activity. When even that level of reaction to the external environment is gone, physical means must be found to prevent such behavior; this may consist of making door opening a two-stage procedure requiring the throwing of a bolt and the turning of a knob, or it may involve substituting a thumb latch for a doorknob. At worst, physical restraint may be temporarily necessary.

A common incitement to agitation is when caregivers use modes of communication that patients can no longer understand. Caregivers then become angry with patients' seeming obstinacy, followed by the patients reacting in self-defense. Thus, effective communication with dementia patients, based on knowledge of their impairment, is a good prophylactic for agitated behaviors.

Predominant Function(s) Lost or Impaired

Piagetian or other staging models based on cognitive or psychomotor development are useful conceptual tools for patient management but are not useful for staging dementing illness, because dementing illness may not progress along the same lines as healthy maturation. Tissue destruction may be confined to one area of the brain or may not be symmetrical, even when the pathology is diffuse and bilateral. AD or Pick's disease may present with predominant left- or right-hemisphere symptoms. The most complex functions may not be those first affected, and the functions damaged may have been developed to different levels before they were compromised. Well-socialized AD patients, for example, may preserve their ability to act appropriately in social situations until they become severely impaired. DSM-IV (American Psychiatric Association 1994) and other recent classification schemes take these factors into account by describing a group of disorders instead of the unitary organic mental syndrome presented in DSM-I (American Psychiatric Association 1952).

Careful evaluation of patients will reveal the extent to which aspects of cognitive functioning are impaired, including understanding of spoken language, written language, affective communication, memory, spatial orientation, orientation to self, judgment, and so on. Orientation to self serves as an example. When a patient is well oriented to self, calling her "Mrs. Smith" helps preserve her dignity as an adult. When orientation to self is impaired, she may no longer remember her married name. Thus, addressing her by her first name at this stage is better than using her married name.

Another type of loss that occurs in dementing illness is loss of executive or regulatory functioning, the ability to concentrate or focus attention, the ability to distinguish the important aspect of a task or a situation from an unimportant one, the ability to prioritize, the ability to perform mental or physical activities in proper sequence, and the ability to modulate behavior based on social cues. Many dementia patients are stimulus bound. They react to stimuli without regard to context. They open drawers or doors because they have knobs whose function is to open them. They put on two pairs of underwear because there are two pairs of underwear in the drawer. Recognizing deficits in regulatory function and constructing the environment and personal demands on dementia patients to match their level of function reduce frustration for both patients and caregivers. For example, knobs can be removed from drawers to prevent rummaging. Door knobs can be concealed to prevent inappropriate entering and exiting, or a special set of drawers can be provided to enable rummaging as a time-filling activity.

Reversibility and Progression

Dealing with a person with a reversible dementia differs from dealing with a person who has a static or a progressive dementia. When there is reasonable expectation that certain functions will return, patients can be challenged to use those functions. A person who is reversibly demented can be encouraged to remember the day of the week or the month of the year. When confronted with a problem such as counting change, such a person can be encouraged to attempt to do it correctly. The presumption in this instance is that challenge will stimulate attention and help the individual improve function through concentration and practice. Similarly, in the months following a stroke, it is useful to challenge patients to function to the limit of their abilities so that they can employ maximally the functions that have been preserved and can learn to compensate for functions that have been damaged or lost.

When dementia is fixed, as is often the case 1–2 years after head injury or stroke, it is no longer useful to challenge the patient. The patient's limits will have been established by this point. If there is some question, they can be formally assessed through history taking, mental status examination, and neuropsychological testing. Patients are then helped to find the optimal environmental circumstances in which to operate. Many persons can live independently; others require supervision. Some persons who require supervision will require assistance in dressing and grooming. Others will be able to manage those functions on their own but will become lost if unescorted. The principle to be observed in the management of fixed dementia is to encourage patients to function autonomously but not so close to maximal function that they continually experience or anticipate failure. For each patient, a "comfort zone" can usually be established. Many patients will rail against their limitations and experience disappointment that they are no longer the person they once were. In general, this is dealt with by praising them for the level of function that they are able to achieve and involving them in distracting activities that are experienced as pleasant diversions or seen as worthwhile pursuits. Some dementia patients do well with distracting activities such as simple games or taking walks. Others are more concerned with the value of their activities. They can be occupied in helping perform household tasks that they can manage well, or they can be employed in sheltered workshops. When dementia patients seem unwilling to make an effort because of discouragement, they should be evaluated for depression.

The management of a progressive dementia begins with the principle of accepting patients at their present level of function. After having established their level of function by history and appropriate clinical means, including caregiver questionnaires (Baum et al. 1993), caregivers are encouraged to support, not challenge patients. It is common for dementia patients to turn to accompanying loved ones for the answer to questions they cannot manage. In the clinical setting, we discourage this so that an adequate evaluation can be performed. We advise to the contrary in the caregiving situation. We advise caregivers to observe a second principle: filling in for the functions lost by persons with progressive dementia. To deal with memory problems, we ask caregivers to do the remembering or to supply sufficient cues so that the dementia patient can remember. Medication taking illustrates this principle. Patients who are mildly affected can be reminded to take their medications by laying out the medications for the day with reminders of the times they are to be taken. Compliance is assessed by counting the pills at the end of the day. When it is obvious that compliance cannot be maintained by reminding, it becomes the caregiver's job to actually administer the medication at the appropriate time in the appropriate dose. The strategy of filling in avoids painful confrontation of dementing persons with their fading abilities.

Another strategy in dealing with progressive dementia is finding a person with whom the dementia patient has rapport and designating certain aspects of care to that person. That person is frequently a housekeeper or a sitter from whom the dementia patient can accept both nurturance and limits. Usually, such a person is affectionate, has a sense of humor, and has the ability to be set limits without being punitive. Positive bonding may occur in these cases through prolonged acquaintance or may occur almost instantaneously as a special kind of rapport. This type of caregiver often serves as a bridge between family members and dementia patients who have difficulty tolerating role reversal with adult children and who thus can save face with the family by depending on the professional caregiver instead of their children. Although it would seem as if the dynamism of "face" operates at a higher level of abstraction than might be possible in dementia, it appears to weigh heavily in the behavior of many brain-damaged persons. For example, an elderly woman with dementia who was unable to manage her financial affairs relied on her accountant to do so. She insisted, however, that he account to her for the checks he wrote, despite the fact that she did not understand what expenses she was covering.

Psychological Factors

The psychological factors important in patient management are 1) coping ability (ego strength) in relation to demands of conscience, ego ideal, and biological/psychological drives; 2) predominant coping mechanisms; and 3) predominant defense mechanisms.

Personality Structure

Persons with dementia respond in different ways to their brain damage depending on their psychological makeup. Those with punitive conscience or with high performance standards have a difficult time maintaining their self-esteem. It is important for these persons, when mildly demented, to find activities that they view as productive. This may require some rudimentary cognitive reframing, such as suggesting to a patient that helping to prepare meals, cleaning up the kitchen, or doing the laundry is in fact productive. With more demented persons, for whom autonomy and individuality remain an issue, it may be better to assign simple, repetitive tasks, such as drying dishes or taking out the trash, so that they can perform independently. Others seem more comfortable operating in tandem with another person on whom they can lean cognitively and psychologically.

Some persons with dementia pose problems because they become overly aggressive or inappropriately sexual as cortical inhibition diminishes. In many cases, aggression arises out of misunderstanding the behavior of caregivers, seeing them as hiding possessions instead of helpfully placing them where they can be found later. Inappropriate sexual display is frequently a consequence of having the urge to urinate or being interrupted during toileting and forgetting to cover up. With irritable dementia patients, efforts are made to reduce the number and frequency of stimuli, such as keeping patients in quiet areas devoid of objects that can be thrown or damaged. Aggressive confrontations are also avoided, with caregivers stepping out of the way when violence is threatened instead of demanding that dementia patients control themselves. Sexual display is managed in the same way. Without a confrontation, clothing is arranged to cover the sexual parts. If masturbation occurs, patients can be steered into a place where others do not have to watch. Special care may need to be taken that caregivers are not sexually stimulating to dementia patients. The issue of continued sexual activity with spouse or lover is discussed in Chapter 8.

Predominant Coping Mechanisms

Normal coping mechanisms are described in Chapter 2 and summarized in Table 2–1. Enabling patients to use their most intact or most needed mechanisms serves to heighten self-esteem and to reinforce a sense of personal integrity. The needs to make decisions, to employ one's own will, and to assume responsibility remain strong in many dementia patients, often leading to conflict between them and their caregivers. The best general management principle is to allow decision making, exercise of will, and assumption of responsibility to the extent of the patient's capability. Dressing is a good example. As dementia becomes more severe, patients have increasing difficulty choosing clothing. In a mild dementia, this may cause only minor hesitation. In a more severe dementia, inappropriate clothing may be chosen for both the weather conditions and the events of the day. In the former case, nothing need be done. In the latter case, caregivers can lay out two sets of appropriate clothing and allow a choice. Mastery can be exercised in less complex tasks. Many persons who can no longer function at complex jobs or pastimes can still perform many household tasks well. Keeping the yard neatly trimmed and adequately watered in summer and free of leaves in the winter can provide both needed activity and a needed sense of mastery.

Many persons who are aware of their cognitive deficits hold the hope that they will improve or at least remain static. If the dementia is deemed reversible or if the person's functioning appears to be worsened by emotional factors such as anxiety or depression, hope of improvement can be reinforced. Where the dementia appears irreversible and psychological and environmental factors do not seem to be reducing performance, the most reasonable attitude is to offer hope that the patient's condition will not progress or that it will progress slowly. Hope is also maintained by seeing patients at 6-month intervals. Patients who are self-aware appreciate being reevaluated to validate their own perception of the course of their illness or the extent of their cognitive dysfunction. Maintaining patients' hope also involves maintaining caregivers' hope. To that end, they are allotted time alone with the clinician to share their observations at the time of diagnosis and at reevaluations and to share their feelings. Patients are helped to be reasonable in their expectations of themselves and of the person in their care and to recognize that their feelings of anger and frustration are common and appropriate.

Some patients and caregivers can regard their cognitive impairment with humor. In our clinic, we often poke fun at our own difficulty with memory, pointing to the various memory cues that we employ. For example, Polaroid photographs are taken of each patient and the accompanying caregiver so that the staff will recognize patient and caregiver on return visits. The extensive records we keep are evidence that memory difficulties are common and that the person with dementia is not so different from others. Altruism can also play a role in maintaining morale. Many patients seen by our clinic value the opportunity to be involved as research subjects. It gives meaning to their lives and enables them to give to others, not only as passive subjects for study and experimentation but also as active teachers about dementia.

Defense Mechanisms

The most common defense mechanisms, as pointed out in Chapter 2, are denial and projection. Apparent denial may be a function of brain tissue loss but may also be psychological in origin. Projection is a common means to avoid awareness of defects in memory and orientation. Patients frequently blame caregivers for stealing or may hide their possessions to keep them from being stolen, thus worsening the problem when they cannot remember where objects are hidden. Whatever defense mechanism is employed, it generally should not be challenged. Patients who deny their inability to drive are usually not confronted. They are told that the car is in the shop, that the keys have been lost, or that it has been borrowed. They may be told that the doctor does not want them to drive because of his or her concern over memory function, that they are being treated for memory dysfunction, and that when they improve, they will be allowed to drive again. In this way, caregivers avoid the primary responsibility of saying no and place the decision beyond their control, a ploy that partially diverts the patient's anger from the caregiver. Another way to deal with the driving issue is to arrange a driving test with the state department of motor vehicle safety, allowing its examiners to be the judges.

Acting out of impulses may be related to diminished cortical inhibition and occurs often in crowded dementia units in nursing homes. Dementia patients in nursing homes often strike out at others who get in their way or who appear to be invading their territory. Because such aggression is usually justified in patients' minds, it does little good to reason with them. Instead, it is best to remove the patient or the aggravating stimulus from the scene and to distract the patient into some other activity. Lecturing about the evils of violence does no good because the lecture will not be remembered, and the chastising tone sets caregiver and patient in opposition. Repeated violence in response to trivial environmental stimuli may require relative isolation of certain patients or placement in a simplified environment with few stimuli. When objects are consistently broken, it may be necessary to remove all breakable objects from patients' rooms and from their path if they cannot be constantly supervised. Some extremely aggressive or episodically violent nursing home residents will require psychiatric hospitalization for the management of their behavior.

General Principles

The general principles of managing dementia patients summarized in Table 5–1 lay the groundwork for the A-B-C approach described later in this chapter. The principles take into account dementia patients' impairment of new learning. Some patients with early progressive or mild fixed dementias retain an ability to learn from verbally presented or written information. Later, they learn by imitation and physical guidance. Means to compensate are found for areas of function in which there is irreversible loss.

Correcting Sensory Impairment

Every person with an apparent dementia requires an assessment of vision and hearing. An adequate screening eye examination includes evaluation of distant and near vision and funduscopic examination. An adequate screening hearing evaluation includes assessing the ability to understand whispered speech and direct inspection of the auditory canals and ear drums. The patient's hearing evaluation is important for the caregivers as well, many of whom attribute the patient's lack of comprehension to hearing impairment rather than cognitive dysfunction. Caregivers can consequently focus their efforts on the modality of communication rather than sheer volume. Correction of presbyopia with magnifying lenses and improvement of hearing by removal of impacted cerumen are simple measures that can improve the ability of dementia patients to understand their environment. It has been our experience that the introduction of electronic hearing aids is not useful for hearing-impaired dementia patients. The process of inserting and tuning them is too difficult to master, and they are often lost or thrown away. Mildly

Table 5–1.   General principles of managing dementia patients

Correcting sensory impairment	Reinforcement
Nonconfrontation	Reducing choices
Finding optimal level of autonomy	Optimal stimulation
Simplification	
Structuring	Avoiding new learning
Multiple cuing	Determining and using overlearned skills
Repetition	Minimizing anxiety
Guiding and demonstration	Distraction

impaired persons accustomed to hearing aids may profit from having them adjusted if they are still able to manipulate them.

Even with maximal correction, many persons still have significantly compromised vision and hearing. For that reason, it is useful to speak and interact at a closer distance than would ordinarily be interpersonally appropriate and to face dementia patients when addressing them. A hand on the shoulder while addressing these persons also serves to reinforce their attention. In addition to having frequent physical contact when interacting, the use of gestures or other nonverbal communication often facilitates communication.

Nonconfrontation

The principle of nonconfrontation is important in dealing with persons who are unaware of their deficits or who need to deny them. A nonconfrontational approach requires caregivers to note the abilities and disabilities of dementia patients and to then matter-of-factly help fill in or compensate for those disabilities. A story is told of a woman with a mild case of dementia who was reluctant to attend a family gathering for fear she would be embarrassed by not remembering names. Her daughter cheerfully told her not to worry, she would help. She did so by greeting everyone by name. Her mother then repeated the name and continued the conversation.

Caregivers often attempt to teach skills that have been lost or to encourage dementia patients to use their memory in the hope that those functions will be stimulated and return. Such attempts may be useful after an acute insult such as a stroke or when a delirium is clearing. Otherwise, these well-intentioned attempts ignore the destruction of the physical substrate of skills and memories and frequently result in a cyclic pattern of caregiver frustration and patient agitation. Caregivers are also frustrated when dementia patients ask the same questions repeatedly. To the limit of caregivers' patience, questions can be answered succinctly, and a distracting activity or line of conversation can be introduced. Family members are often concerned that dementia patients will become too dependent on others thinking for them and will fail to do what they are actually able to do. It can be gently suggested that the issue is not whether their loved one is dependent on them but on the quality of that dependence. Those who are sure that they have someone to depend on are often more secure in doing what they can for themselves. Those who sense their caregivers abandoning them to their own meager cognitive resources are more likely to become emotionally determined burdens.

Many dangers can be avoided without making an issue of them. The gas or electric supply to a stove can be turned off. Weapons such as guns can be removed from the house. Poisons can be removed from places where they might be confused with foods. Excuses can be made for the nonworking condition of the stove; weapons can be "borrowed." These nonconfrontational subterfuges help to maintain the patients' sense of autonomy without reminding them of the painful facts of their disabilities.

Optimal Autonomy

To a greater or lesser extent, all persons value their ability to govern themselves and their environment. The task in dealing with dementia patients is helping them to find and operate at the level of autonomy most consistent with their personal needs and coping ability. Much of the distress suffered by these individuals and their caregivers results from tension over this issue. The most common problem is that the patients' ability to regulate their own behavior and environment is not commensurate with their psychological need for autonomy. Indeed, part of the normal need for autonomy is exaggerated by a need to demonstrate that nothing is really wrong. More compromised persons with dementia demonstrate their autonomy by negativism. Although they do not know exactly what they want, they know what they do not want, for example, conforming to the caregiver's schedule for taking a bath.

Another autonomy-related issue is "space." Territory becomes important to persons whose living space has become greatly encroached on, as in nursing homes in which residents' private living space is reduced to one room or half a room. Many persons become very upset when other residents enter their room or a roommate crosses into "their" half of the room; after all, neither resident selected the other to share living space. In these situations, the right of the person intruded on needs to be defended, and the simplest way to do so is to divert the offending person. Attempting to explain that the intruder meant no harm is often beyond the ken of the nursing home resident with dementia. The staff needs to serve as protectors in this instance, even if the reaction is out of proportion to the realistic danger posed by the intruder.

Simplification

Simplification refers to reducing the number and complexity of environmental demands (Mace and Rabins 1991) and introducing tasks in simple steps rather than as a set of serial or contingent ("if this happens, then do such-and-such") instructions. Many patients with dementia are able to remain at home and can answer the telephone if the caller wishes to communicate directly with them. On the other hand, they are not able to take telephone messages for others when alone because they forget the content of the messages or forget to write them down. The life of a dementia patient who is left alone at home during the day can be simplified by turning off the telephone ringer and turning on an answering machine to take messages. In this way, the patient can still make outgoing calls, but there will be no arguments over untransmitted messages for other members of the family and no signing up with telephone solicitors for unwanted magazine subscriptions, and so on. When asked to do chores, serial instructions, such as "Sweep the kitchen floor and then take out the trash," are to be avoided. Instead, it is preferable to say, "Sweep the kitchen floor, please," while handing a broom to the person as an extra cue. Contingent instructions are to be avoided as well. Instead of, "Look to see whether the water on the stove is boiling, and if it is, turn the heat down," the better instruction is, "Tell me if the water on the stove is boiling." If the water is found to be boiling, a second instruction can be given to turn the heat down.

Simplification is especially useful with persons who have difficulty dressing and undressing. For men, beltless trousers are the most convenient clothing. For women, house dresses are the simplest clothing. On the other hand, it is better not to argue with the dementia patient whose identity demands wearing a girdle or panty hose.

Structuring

All persons attempt to organize their activities and environment to suit their abilities and personal needs. Dementia patients are limited in their ability to provide structure for themselves, and structuring daily activities and the environment often becomes the responsibility of caregivers. Some dementia patients require little structure and seem very comfortable without any planned or organized activity. They may sit for hours reading and rereading the same magazine or watching the same videotape. Persons who require activity are in greater need of structure because they are frequently unable to organize their own activities. Such persons may need a day-care program or at least a structured daily routine. Providing structure often reduces the tension and restlessness of being unable to channel energy in a consistent direction without guidance.

Closely related to a need for structure is a need for environmental constancy or predictability. Most adults are faced with an everchanging environment. Jobs demand change. Children grow up. Parents grow old. All of these changes require adaptation. Persons with dementia are markedly limited in their adaptive ability and therefore require sameness to function comfortably. Sameness means having meals at roughly the same time each day, going to bed at roughly the same time each evening, managing personal hygiene at the same times each day, and going for walks or engaging in other activities at the same times daily. Each day has an orderly progression with which patients with mild-to-moderate dementia can become familiar. There is not the challenge of having to understand different activities or having to modify the overall daily schedule. Whereas persons mildly affected with dementia may enjoy a varied weekend schedule, those with more severe dementia seem to do better with the same routine every day of the week.

Multiple Cuing

Multiple cuing refers to using several different types of cuing to initiate a suggested action. Cuing to sweep the floor, for example, can be done by giving the verbal instruction and pantomiming sweeping the floor or actually picking up a broom and demonstrating briefly. The capacity to understand nonverbal cues and to imitate are maintained longer than the capacity to understand verbal communication; therefore, nonverbal cues are useful augmenting devices.

Repetition

Repetition is necessary because of attentional deficit and slowness of information processing. If attempting to engage a person with dementia in a new activity, such as going for a walk, the person's attention must be first engaged, usually by calling out his or her name. If the response is uncertain or not apparent, the person's name is repeated until attention is secured. The verbal repetition may be underscored by an additional cue of placing a hand on the person's arm and entering the field of vision. In keeping with the principle of simplification, it may be wisest to begin with the suggestion of standing up, reinforcing that suggestion with a hand under the elbow or a gesture indicating rising: "Let's stand up," followed with reinforcers such as, "Good!" and, "There, you're up," and then, "Let's go for a walk." Lesser amounts of repetition are necessary when comprehension is greater, but it is better to be overly repetitive than to further aggravate confusion.

Guiding and Demonstration

Accompanying commands and suggestions by pantomiming movements or direct physical guidance reinforces the communication and serves as a reminder of how things are done. Guiding a hand when urging patients to draw or to paint helps to overcome their difficulty with initiating an activity and helps establish a new activity set. In initiating a singing session, the leader names a song, starts the music, begins to sing, and then asks patients to join in. Having established that they are singing, patients can be asked to name and sing their favorite songs with others reinforcing their singing.

Reinforcement

Reinforcement may help to shape behavior in cognitively impaired persons who cannot foresee or understand the long-term consequences of their actions. To shape behavior effectively, the reinforcing stimulus must immediately follow the behavior to be reinforced or extinguished. In the case of a rapidly progressing dementing illness, reinforcement is of little use. However, in a slowly progressive or a fixed dementia, it has been reported to be useful in controlling and regulating some behaviors (Wisner and Green 1986). Toileting behaviors can be reinforced (Hussian and Davis 1985). Urinary incontinence usually begins as an occasional incident, often causing great embarrassment. Patients are helped to avoid repetitions of this behavior by reminding them to go to the bathroom or taking them to the bathroom at fixed intervals during the day (Pinkston and Linsk 1984). Times are marked on a piece of paper and checked off by the caregiver until the caregiver has the routine down. Each time patients succeed in urinating when they are taken to the bathroom, they are praised.

Eating behavior can be reinforced by having dementia patients eat in the company of others in designated eating areas at designated eating places (see also Chapter 11).

Reducing Choices

As long as individuals maintain a sense of selfhood, being able to make choices concerning themselves is important as confirmation of intactness and of having worth and dignity. Advanced cognitive impairment makes choosing difficult; it is no longer possible to easily weigh the relative value of multiple alternatives. It is not possible to hold them in memory long enough to compare and contrast them or to assign them relative weights. The use of choices in relation to dress was illustrated earlier. Patients are not asked what they would like to wear but are instead given a choice of two ensembles and asked which they prefer. It may not be possible to give a choice of when or what to eat in an institutional setting, but it is possible to give patients a choice of what they would like to have first: meat or vegetables, milk or salad. By offering limited choices, individual dignity is maintained without creating intellectual chaos for dementia patients or environmental chaos for their caregivers.

Optimal Stimulation

The need for stimulation varies greatly depending on many factors, including cognitive intactness, alertness, emotional state, and physical state. The amount of stimulation received also influences each person's behavior. Minimizing stimulation leads to sleep. Moderate amounts of stimulation awaken and may arouse interest and attention. Intense stimulation may cause overload with emotional distress, retreat, or aggression. Generally speaking, the more severe the dementia, the fewer stimuli that can be integrated; the more advanced the dementia, the simpler the stimulation must be. For example, it may not be possible for dementia patients to tolerate being in a room with a TV or radio blaring while they are trying to play cards. Attempts should be made to determine what is an optimal level of stimulation for each person at various times of the day. Often, relatively complex situations can be tolerated in the morning but not in the afternoon, when many persons are fatigued. The early evening may provide insufficient orienting cues, contributing to *sundowning* (increasing confusion as sensory cues wane in the evenings) in some patients. For such patients, stimulating activities may be offered in the mornings, afternoons may involve quiet TV watching, and in the evenings, brief walks or social interaction.

Avoiding New Learning

Although total impairment of new learning ability is not usual in dementia patients, the best assumption is that, if an activity requires learning new principles, such as bidding conventions in bridge, it is more likely to be frustrating than entertaining. If a newly introduced card game is based on already-learned principles, such as matching suits or arranging cards by face value, dementia patients are more likely to grasp them. Sometimes a demand for new learning cannot be avoided; for instance, parents may move into the home of their adult children. However, their bedroom can be fitted out with their own furnishings, and the hallway can be decorated with pictures from their former home that are arranged as they previously were in relation to the bathroom.

Reality orientation, a frequent institutional psychosocial approach to caring for dementia patients, attempts to bring dementia patients into contact with their present-day reality, including date, day, time of day, and geographical location (Taulbee and Folsom 1966). This type of program has been practiced as a 24-hour system in which the staff provides orientation and reality cues at every contact with patients. The method has also been developed as formal didactic classes meeting 30 minutes per day. Vigorous reorientation is appropriate in delirium. Delirious persons tend to be calmed by developing a sense of where they are in time and space. Dementia, as noted previously, may preclude learning material that needs to be memorized, and when such material is constantly represented, it leaves dementia patients frustrated and painfully reminded of their deficits (Dietch et al. 1989). Therefore, vigorous attempts at reality orientation seem inappropriate in the progressive dementias. Responding to patients' requests for orienting information is quite another story. Such requests should be answered succinctly and matter-of-factly, recognizing that the information may not be retained and that the same questions may be asked again.

Determining and Using Overlearned Skills

Memories and skills that are well imprinted often remain. For example, an accountant who was no longer able to do simple mathematical operations was still able to umpire softball games. Many musicians continue to play their instruments. These overlearned behaviors can be used to advantage and are established by taking a history of both occupational and avocational pursuits. Families are then encouraged to facilitate the use of these talents and abilities. Making a scrapbook from old family photographs is a good pastime and leaves patients on familiar ground. Cooking may no longer be feasible, but setting and clearing the table may still be possible. The process of planting seeds and weeding a garden is usually well understood. A list of potential activities for patients is limited only by the imagination and ingenuity of the caregivers and the time and energy available to supervise and participate in these activities.

Minimizing Anxiety

Cognitively impaired persons often become anxious when they cannot adequately comprehend their environment. The additional load of anxiety can trigger suspiciousness, transient delusion formation, or frank delirium. For this reason, attempts are made to minimize patients' anxiety. This is accomplished by many of the means already discussed: keeping the environment simple, providing a structured routine, reducing choices, avoiding new learning, and so on. In addition, it is also useful to reduce anticipation, whether it is of positive or negative events. Discussing plans for a trip months in advance gives time for anticipatory fears to develop. Mentioning a visit to the doctor a week in advance is likely to stimulate incessant questions as to why the trip is necessary. Because dementia patients lack the ability to rehearse or plan effectively, they are relatively helpless to manage their normal anticipatory anxiety. This is dealt with most effectively by not burdening dementia patients with information about the future and keeping them focused on the present day.

Distraction

Distraction is the most useful means for dealing with the mounting frustration of trying to master a task that is cognitively out of reach. It is also useful in helping to manage anger, anxiety, or lowered mood. Thus, a woman struggling angrily to master her checkbook can be distracted by calling her attention to the weather or a photograph of a favorite grandchild. The anger having been interrupted, it is then possible to suggest that she put aside the checkbook for a while and return to it another time. Later, when calm, she can be asked to allow the caregiver to help her. The dynamic is similar to that in dealing with a small child experiencing intense emotion: the emotion propagates itself and becomes less and less controllable. Suggesting that agitated dementia patients calm down is frequently asking for something beyond their voluntary control and intensifies their agitation as they struggle vainly to assert self-control. Instead, caregivers find means to help patients calm down.

Depression

Depression is a treatable condition that may be confused with dementia; however, many patients have depression concurrent with dementia. Caregivers often equate the loss of interest and initiative that occurs in dementia with depression. Patients who express persistent feelings of worthlessness or guilt or thoughts of death or suicide, or who become appear apathetic or withdrawn should be evaluated for depression. Antidepressant medication is useful for major depression, but behavior measures are useful in both major depression and more transient, less severe lowering of mood (Teri, in press; Teri and Gallagher-Thompson 1991). Many dementia patients become demoralized and have a sense of lowered worth because of their decreased ability to work and to deal with the problems of daily living. It is therefore useful to engage persons capable of focusing their energy in simple repetitive projects with which they are familiar, at which they can succeed, and for which they can be praised. Raking the leaves in the fall, and turning and weeding a garden in the spring are good examples. Walking the dog is another activity that is both energy and time consuming. Demoralized persons in nursing homes can be engaged in simple occupational therapy activities such as making lanyards, belts, and ceramic ashtrays and in recreational activities such as sing-alongs and shuffleboard. These activities also serve to distract from self-directed thinking.

Behavioral interventions in depression are based on breaking up a self-reinforcing cycle in which decreased positive person-environment interactions and increased aversive interactions increase depressed mood. Also, depressed persons do little that is pleasant, and the less they do, the worse they feel. Using the A-B-C model described above, strategies are devised to deal with events that lead or reinforce depressed mood. In addition, patient and caregiver work from a Pleasant Events Schedule (Teri and Logsdon 1991) to increase activities that the patient enjoys presently or enjoyed in the past. A comparison of depressed AD patients on a waiting list with AD patients in a 9-week behavioral treatment program showed no change for the persons on the waiting list and significant decreases in depressive symptoms in the treated group (Teri 1994). For pleasant events to achieve the desired effect, they should be enjoyable, easily achievable, accessible, and reinforced. They must be introduced slowly and in small steps and be consonant with the patient's current cognitive and functional ability. Caregivers need to gently motivate patients to be involved in activities and to be flexible in their approach. If patients do not enjoy the activities in which caregivers are attempting to enlist them, other activities should be sought.

A corollary to increasing pleasant events for depressed dementia patients is decreasing unpleasant events. Activities that are too demanding are unpleasant and likely to reinforce a sense of demoralization.

There can be reinforcing consequences to depressive symptoms, as with any other symptoms. Consequences may be special privileges, such as not having to wait in the nursing home cafeteria line or receiving special attention from the nursing staff. In those instances, it may be necessary to advise the staff to "get tough" and to chide patients for not doing all they can for themselves. This type of chiding, when dosed properly, tends to arouse defiance and helps patients to mobilize their remaining resources. Maintaining a mildly critical attitude such as "I know you can really push a shuffleboard puck harder than that, Mr. Smith!" often stimulates greater effort—the implied message being that the patient is really capable but choosing not to use those capabilities.

Delirium

The principle of optimal stimulation is most important in the psychological management of delirium. Both too little and too much stimulation may aggravate delirium. Maintaining orienting stimuli by keeping window blinds open during the day and a light on at night is important, but televisions that cannot be seen well by visually impaired patients may overburden them and worsen agitation. Having familiar objects such as photographs, blankets, or pillows can be helpful in reducing confusion, as can the presence of a caregiver who is friendly and reassuring. It is useful to attempt orientation of patients with a mild underlying dementia to place, year, month, and day of the week. For those with more severe dementia, attempts at orientation add a further cognitive burden and compound confusion. Caregivers need to frequently identify themselves to patients with delirium and to communicate their presence through physical contact. Soft chest and extremity restraints may be necessary to keep patients in hospital beds or to keep them from dislodging or pulling out intravenous lines, endotracheal tubes, catheters, and so on. When possible, verbal restraint by a caregiver is preferable to mechanical restraint. When sundowning occurs, it may indicate a need for more environmental structure, such as evening activities.

Anxiety

The psychological management of anxiety is similar to that of discouragement. Patients who can be engaged in activities often find temporary relief through distraction. Both anxiety and depression interfere with cognition and often result in patients repeatedly asking the same question, in part for information and in part as a form of clinging. Attempts to cut question asking short or writing down the answers to questions are generally of no avail, because the need for reassurance and comforting usually generates further questioning. Unlike the anxious person who is cognitively intact, it is not possible to put off the anxious person with dementia. Allowing these anxious persons to "shadow" caregivers is frequently helpful, providing a concrete response to the implicit request, "Do not desert me." This proximity is very tiring for caregivers, who may then need more frequent relief. Repetitive questions should be answered briefly. Then, with emotional arousal to augment learning, patients can be told firmly, and sometimes with a hint of anger, "That's enough for now" and be taken for a walk or seated in front of the television set, with the caregiver remaining in full view.

Anxiety is frequently aggravated by caregivers attempting to interrupt clinging behavior by threatening desertion, by insisting that patients already know the answers to the questions they are asking, or by pushing patients to perform activities that are beyond their cognitive or emotional resources. Caregivers can be instructed to look for early signs of frustration and examine the underlying causes of past anxious episodes. In addition, it is important to reduce possible reinforcement by praising and paying attention to patients during nonanxious times to reinforce patients' behavior when they are behaving well. Patients who become anxious during social activities can be allowed to withdraw to more solitary activities. Those who become anxious when deprived of social contact can be kept in contact with others. Caregivers often come to discount the communications of chronically anxious patients and may thereby ignore needs that could be met, thus escalating anxiety over abandonment. It is therefore important that attention be paid by caregivers each time they are approached so that no important message (e.g., "I have wet myself, I am too embarrassed to say so, and I'm too impaired to know what to do") is overlooked.

Disruptive Behaviors

The term *disruptive behaviors* has been used to categorize a variety of behaviors that are problems for patients, family, and professional caregivers. Disruptive behaviors include agitation, verbal and physical aggression, and catastrophic reactions and have been studied most extensively by Cohen-Mansfield (Cohen-Mansfield and Billig 1986). Physically aggressive behaviors occur in 25%–50% of community-dwelling dementia patients and even more frequently in nursing home patients (A. H. Mann et al. 1984; Nilsson et al. 1988; Ryden 1988). The antecedent for many disruptive behaviors is lack of appropriate stimulation, which may mean either increasing or reducing the frequency and nature of the stimulation patients receive. When they are engaging in appropriate, nonagitated behaviors, such patients should receive additional praise. All too often, a kind touch or word is the consequence of agitated behaviors and may be a reinforcer. Identifying triggers for agitation can be used to prevent these behaviors. If that is not possible, distraction, altering the environment, or removing patients from situations in which they become agitated can alter the behavior as well.

Examination of catastrophic reactions will often reveal a chain of events that initiate and maintain them. They include too many or too complicated physical and emotional demands, too many questions, noise, criticism, and fatigue. Many times, dementia patients impose these demands on themselves, as in the case of a woman who insisted on coming to our clinic alone. She arrived several hours early for a 1 P.M. appointment. The staff explained to her that she had arrived early and attempted to keep her occupied. She stayed fairly calm until lunchtime, when the staff left. Then, responding to her own hunger and her frustration over waiting, she exploded and stormed out.

Wandering

Many dementia patients seek to "go home" because they no longer recognize their own homes. Others seem to roam purposelessly from place to place where they reside, exiting when they have the opportunity but having no obvious goal in mind. The latter group are the wanderers. Wandering is not in itself dangerous unless patients are able to leave safe environments, and wandering behavior generally does not need to be interrupted. When wanderers are relatively intact cognitively, they can be engaged in activities as a substitute for wandering, including simple games and chores. Wandering behavior usually responds well to redirection, even in advanced dementia. Unfortunately, wandering behavior may occur when caregivers are not present or are asleep, necessitating mechanical restraint from wandering, such as double-locking exits from the home and locking doors of areas into which patients should not wander.

Wandering is a major issue, especially in nursing homes. The principal means of dealing with patients who wander into other patients' rooms or out the door is to have an adequate number of staff members to provide supervision and electronically controlled exits. Wandering behavior may be interrupted in more cognitively intact persons by calling out to them and distracting them by verbal means. Patients who are beyond verbal restraint can be distracted by physically interrupting their course of action and gently redirecting them. Much wandering is due to patients' inability to find their own rooms. Means for minimizing wandering are discussed in Chapters 11 and 12.

Sleep-Wake Disturbances

The principles of sleep hygiene are discussed in Chapter 6. The most important principle is to provide a structured routine that maintains daytime physical and mental activity. The best way to do this is through establishing a daily routine that is constantly reinforced and does not involve asking patients' permission or stimulating their interest; for example, "It's 10 o'clock and time to walk the dog," or "It's nearly noon and time for you to help me make lunch." Patients who are not ambulatory can be helped out of bed and into chairs and stimulated by engaging them in brief conversation or by turning on a television.

Suspiciousness and Delusion Formation

Patients' suspiciousness and delusional thinking must be attended to be certain that they do not endanger themselves or others should they attempt to attack or defend themselves against imagined persecutors. Often, such delusions will be verbalized when patients are placed in situations they cannot master cognitively. The principle of nonconfrontation is the most important in dealing with suspiciousness and delusion formation. Instead, effort is made to determine under what circumstances suspicion and delusion formation are increased and to find means to avoid those situations.

Common causes of suspicion are changes in daily routine and the presence of strangers. The common accusations, "Someone has entered my room," or "Someone has changed my room," can be managed by asking, "Do you want to see if anything is missing?" Such accusations usually arise when a patient cannot remember what the room looks like; the accusations are often worsened if objects in the room are rearranged in well-meaning efforts to tidy up or to place them more conveniently.

Suspicious patients frequently hide certain of their belongings and later complain that they are missing. It is the caregivers' responsibility to note favorite hiding places so that objects can be more easily retrieved. An outburst of delusional accusations following a social outing or a trip to the grocery store may indicate that the trip was too long, the setting was too stimulating, there was too much activity going on, or the pace was too fast. All of these elements can be modified. However, it may be necessary to temporarily suspend such trips. Minimizing anxiety is another important means of reducing suspiciousness and delusion formation. For that reason, it is best not to inform suspicious dementia patients of plans for a visit to the doctor or a trip to the grocery store until immediately beforehand. That reduces the period of time during which tension can develop.

Prosopagnosia contributes to delusion formation, such as Capgras's syndrome, in which a patient develops the delusion that spouse, children, or other important persons have been replaced with evil look-alikes (Hayman and Abrams 1977). In this situation, it is best if the spouse or caregiver dresses nearly the same way each day as much as possible, wearing the same jewelry, the same perfume, using the same color lipstick, and so on. A matter-of-fact assertion that "I am your wife, Mary" is all that is useful in response to an accusation of being a double or an impostor. More vigorous assertions and offering various types of proof tend only to increase puzzlement as to why a person would go so far to impersonate a spouse.

Hallucinations

Hallucinations are common in dementia, but their form and content should be ascertained, because this information may suggest a treatable disorder. For example, tactile hallucinations accompanied by frightening visual hallucinations may point to a drug-induced delirium in dementia patients. Auditory hallucinations commanding patients to kill themselves may be part of a treatable major depression. Visual hallucinations are the most common in dementia (see Charles Bonnet syndrome in Chapter 2). A frequent complaint is that children, little adults, or strange creatures are entering the house, but they are often dealt with casually or humorously by the patient. Frightening hallucinations will usually require medications to dampen patients' emotional reactions, but they can also be dealt with by optimizing perceptual cues and encouraging patients to stay physically close to their caregivers. Hallucinations and delusions in elders with dementia are often concretizations of their wishes and fear—and a principal fear, as noted previously, is that of abandonment. The fear is best alleviated by having caregivers be visible and constant. As is the case with the previously cited disturbances, distraction is often the best course of action in mitigating the distress of hallucinations. Also, the patient's environment may be changed. If the patient insists that there is a strange or threatening person in the mirror, the mirror can be covered up or removed. The environment should be checked for noises that might be misinterpreted and for lighting that may glare or cast shadows. Frightening hallucinations often subside in well-lighted areas where other persons are present.

Apathy and Withdrawal

Loss of interest in formerly valued activities and withdrawal from social situations are noted frequently by families of dementia patients. Early in the course of a progressive dementia, efforts can be made to maintain involvement in these activities and in unstructured socialization. It is important for caregivers to develop realistic expectations with regard to the patient's abilities. If frustration and discouragement arise due to the patient's realization of the loss of former abilities, caregivers can intervene and provide the needed assistance and structure, praising the skills that remain. Later, apathy and withdrawal can be dealt with by engaging patients in structured activities. Often caregivers attempt to place themselves in the patient's position and express difficulty in understanding how such activities could be rewarding. Although apathy and withdrawal can be successfully addressed, it is important that caregivers understand the stimulus limitations that cognitive impairment places on their loved ones.

Apathy and withdrawal are common behaviors in nursing homes. They are often defensive responses to abandonment and to living among strangers. Rather than reach out to staff who may be transient and roommates who remind them of their own condition, patients may keep to themselves and withdraw from emotional involvement with others. Caregivers need to determine the risk-benefit ratio of pushing patients to be more active and more involved with other persons. If a patient's apathy is the product of extensive frontal lobe damage, attempts to activate that patient are not likely to be worth the caregiver effort involved. If apathy is part of a reversible depression, increased activity is part of the treatment. When apathy is a temporary reaction to a new environment, patients can be stimulated gradually to be more active. Patients who become overtly paranoid or violent when stimulated to interact are best allowed the protective mechanism of withdrawal from stimuli that they cannot manage.

In drawing apathetic or withdrawn dementia patients into activities, it is best to start by allowing them to be spectators or passive participants, engaging them gradually. In the home environment, nonchallenging activities such as watching TV or taking short walks may be a good way to start. In institutional settings, attending group meals or sing-alongs is relatively unchallenging.

Driving

This section deals with an issue for caregivers and persons with dementia that defies easy classification. From the standpoint of the dementia patient, driving a car is related to both autonomy and identity. Freedom for many persons is the ability to drive where and when they want. For many persons, driving also symbolizes adulthood and competence, especially for the many individuals for whom driving was part of their livelihood. It is obviously best for the public at large to curtail patients' driving before an accident occurs. Dementia patients seldom have difficulty with the mechanics of driving. They can start the car, shift gears, turn it, put on the brakes, and turn off the ignition. Their loss of executive function and their orientation and visuospatial problems lead to driving in the wrong lane, inattention to traffic lights and warning signs, inappropriate responses in emergency situations, misjudging distances, and getting lost (van Zomeren et al. 1987). To date, no accurate means have been found to distinguish between dementia patients who are able to drive and those who are not. In a small study of 12 very mild (Clinical Dementia Rating [CDR] = 0.5) and 13 mild (CDR = 1.0) AD cases, L. Hunt et al. (1993) found that all of the very mild and 62% of the mild AD patients "passed" a 1-hour test of driving under light traffic conditions. Gouvier et al. (1989) found that the digit-symbol section of the Wechsler Adult Intelligence Scale (WAIS; Wechsler 1981) correlated well with driving ability. A simple and useful test of dementia patients' driving ability is to ask caregivers whether they are comfortable driving with the patient. The best test, of course, is assessment of skills through an actual driving examination.

It is best, as far as patients' self-esteem is concerned, to allow persons for whom driving is an issue of autonomy or identity to drive as long as possible. Observation may be all that is necessary in mild dementia, when orientation is relatively intact, when attention to traffic signs and signals is not greatly impaired, and when the driving is done in familiar areas. A spouse or another caregiver may ask to go along "just to get out of the house." More advanced dementia will require supervision of driving, with caregivers making active suggestions as to when to come to a stop or to make a turn. If suggestions are resisted or if driving creates too much tension in the caregiver, it needs to be suspended in ways suggested earlier.

Memory Training and Retraining

It has been well demonstrated that cognitively intact persons can greatly increase their ability to memorize lists of related and unrelated words through the technique of associating visual images with the words to be remembered (Patten 1972). Many studies have been done on memory retraining in persons who have the memory deficits of normal aging and in persons who are brain damaged (Lewinsohn et al. 1977; Patten 1972; Poon 1985). The memory deficits that accompany normal aging include greater difficulty encoding in secondary memory and difficulty with retrieval from secondary memory. Primary memory (immediate recall, as tested by digit span) and tertiary memory are relatively unaffected. The greatest decrements in secondary memory occur when the memory task requires some organization of the material, as in paired-associate learning or list learning. In terms of day-to-day functioning, this means that normal elders require more repetitions to remember new information and that, once learned, such information requires more cues to recall. Most studies show that using a mnemonic improves the paired-associate and list-learning performances of elderly subjects. In addition, age differences can be reduced through techniques of organizing new learning, practicing, and then adapting the pace of new learning to the individual (Poon 1985).

Not all normal elders profit from mnemonic training; furthermore, they tend not to maintain the techniques they have learned unless reminded (Schaffer and Poon 1982). "Internal" memory aids, such as organization and visual imagery, are seldom used by either young or old persons in everyday situations. "External" memory aids, such as making notes, keeping a diary, or tying a string on a finger, are employed most of the time. Yesavage et al. (1988) found that elders' scores on the WAIS vocabulary subscale increased with treatment combining mnemonics with verbal elaboration techniques and that elders' scores on a measure of anxiety were reduced in response to a treatment combining relaxation training with mnemonics. In the first group, subjects associated names to parts of a face as the mnemonic technique. The elaboration technique involved subjects making a judgment about the images they produced: pleasant or unpleasant, silly or logical. Subjects were trained for 2 weeks and tested immediately afterward. There was no long-term follow-up.

Persons with static mild organic deficits due to acute episodes such as stroke, head trauma, or central nervous system infection appear to profit from memory training. Their ability to identify frequently seen faces and often-visited places can be improved significantly (Wilson 1987). They also can be helped to recognize the need to pace themselves slowly, to stay with what is familiar, and to use external reminders. Such training is also helpful in combating discouragement and depression. It would not be reasonable to expect that psychological measures could overcome the effects of a progressive disorder; but if it were possible to arrest the course of a progressive dementia, memory retraining might be useful.

Formal Psychotherapy

To our knowledge, there are no controlled outcome studies of formal psychotherapy in dementia patients. Those who are cognitively handicapped (i.e., low IQ or educationally deprived) or who have mild static cognitive impairment can be treated individually (Weiner and Crowder 1986) or in groups (Weiner 1988), with techniques such as paradoxical intervention, task assignment, promoting identification, reinforcement, education, and advice. These techniques are part of a general style or level of psychotherapy characterized as repressive psychotherapy and are well described elsewhere (Weiner 1986). Thompson et al. (1989) have proposed the use of cognitive-behavior therapy for depressed early AD patients, but only anecdotal reports of positive outcome are available.

Early anecdotal reports of formal psychotherapy with dementia patients give insufficient information about the patients treated and do not suggest significant gains (e.g., Linden 1953; Manaster 1972). It is possible, however, that individual or group psychotherapy for early dementia patients might help reduce anxiety and depression and provide emotional support. It would be expected that these patients would respond best to techniques that do not involve reflective self-observation or the acquisition of large amounts of new information. They can learn to attempt only one task at a time and to make lists to augment memory function. They can accept advice, such as avoiding jobs that involve new learning, and can learn the names of persons to help them negotiate the various agencies with which they interact. In groups, they can be praised for their warmth, openness, and sound advice to others. In our experience, persons with dementias often seek out and enjoy interactions in which they are treated with warmth and respect. The most successful caregivers are those who throw their arms around the patients and say, "I love you."

Activity Therapies

Activity therapies differ from psychotherapies in that their emphasis is on activity instead of self-observation and verbally mediated learning. Patients' attention is drawn away from themselves and toward the accomplishment of pleasurable or useful tasks. Distracting dementia patients from dwelling on themselves and directing their attention to tasks they can accomplish and enjoy is probably more useful than formal psychotherapy. In fact, much of what dementia patients probably gain in psychotherapy groups is just such temporary distraction from themselves. Activity or recreational therapies can readily employ the general principles elaborated earlier in this chapter. They avoid confronting patients with their disability, allow the level of autonomy best tolerated by the patient, simplify activities to the point that they can be mastered, provide adequate structure, and so forth. Patients use overlearned skills, such as singing songs or performing familiar repetitive activities. As a result of feeling valued and competent, the patients' morale and self-esteem are maintained. Detailed descriptions of activity therapies are presented by Burnside (1984).

Medically Ill
Dementia Patients

The behavioral suggestions for the management of dementia patients at home or in the nursing home also apply to the management of medically ill dementia patients. An individual with dementia who is calm at home is more likely to remain calm in a hospital setting if accompanied by a familiar person who can serve as an intermediary and as a source of emotional support and orientation. After determining the need for hospital treatment, the physician asks the family whether they can arrange for family members to be with the patient during the daylight hours and evenings, explaining that this is the best way to prevent delirium and to ensure the highest quality of medical care. Professional sitters can be arranged for if family members are not available. The least desirable alternatives are for confused persons to be sedated or restrained. It is helpful to explain to family or professional sitters what procedures are being carried out, what they entail, and why they are being undertaken. Dementia patients do not usually tolerate long explanations well; on the other hand, they can comprehend the gist of a procedure. Thus, an MRI scan becomes a brain X ray, and a lumbar puncture becomes a spinal fluid test or a little "stick" to draw fluid from the back. Because of attention, concentration, and memory difficulties, dementia patients cannot be expected to carry out instructions such as being asked to lie flat for several hours following a lumbar puncture. Such instruction must be given to the nurse or the sitter. Because these patients frequently cannot develop a rational understanding of a medical procedure or adequately suppress their emotional reactions, they should not be subjected to prolonged or frightening procedures without the presence of a calming person or the use of a calming medication. For example, we prefer MRI to CT as the routine imaging procedure of choice in the assessment of dementia. In some instances, MRI is unsuccessful because of patients' poor ability to tolerate this frightening, incomprehensible new environment. In these situations, we employ CT as our imaging procedure and sedate our patients with 0.5–1.0 mg of lorazepam im 20 minutes before the procedure, as indicated in the sections on the management of agitation and delirium in Chapter 6.

Delirium is a common complication of hospitalization and may be related to the medical condition under treatment, to prescribed medications, or to being in an unfamiliar environment. It is dealt with behaviorally and medically as indicated earlier in this chapter and in Chapter 6.

Compliance with posthospital medical treatment is a substantial problem for dementia patients who live alone. There are numerous reminder strategies that can be used, including posting checklists on the refrigerator or labeling various kinds of pill containers specifying when, where, and how medications are to be taken. However, there is no adequate substitute for direct supervision. Compliance is best ensured by prescribing medication that can be taken once a day and by having a family member or neighbor check daily or several times a week to be certain the medication is taken.

The ABCs of Behavior Management

The general principles elaborated in the previous sections can be used to help deal with the emotional, behavioral, ideational, and perceptual disturbances that are common in dementia patients, with an ABC approach to analyze the specifics of the problem under consideration. *A* refers to the antecedents of *B*, the behavior. Did anything or anyone trigger the behavior? What was happening before the behavior started? *C* refers to the consequences of the behavior. What happened as a result of the behavior? What was the caregiver's response? Although many behaviors appear to arise de novo, this is seldom the case. By carefully examining the ABCs of behavior, factors that trigger and maintain the behavior can be identified and modified.

When multiple behaviors must be dealt with, it is useful to begin with one behavior at a time and to restrict its definition to observable phenomena. In addition to ascertaining precisely what the patient does and what the caregiver does, it is also important to know how often the behavior occurs, when it happens, where it happens, and with whom it happens. Interventions are developed with the following characteristics:

- They address an antecedent or a reinforcing consequence of the behavior.
- They have objective, realistic, clearly defined goals and identified steps to meet these goals.
- The steps to goal attainment are objective, realistic, and clearly defined. They are small, simple, straightforward, easily achievable steps to the larger goal.
- Each step is constantly reevaluated. Problems may resolve quickly, but they more often require time, creativity, and flexibility. It is necessary to continually modify and adapt solutions to patients' current level of cognitive and functional impairment and behavioral disturbance.

The A-B-C approach is illustrated by the following case:

Mrs. B., a woman with AD, tended to act up in church when taken by her daughter. The mother's acting up consisted of talking loudly during the church service (the behavior). On reflection, the daughter recalled that her mother tended to be more vocal after interacting with her friends (the antecedent) before the service began and that her friends seemed to enjoy her obstreperousness. The daughter dealt with the situation by arriving exactly on time for services, thereby avoiding the stimulating interaction of her mother with her friends until after services were over.

For shaping the behavior of more severely demented persons, McGovern and Koss (1995) suggest that foods and drinks (the consequence) may be more effective than attention or praise.

Summary

The psychological and behavioral management of persons with dementia is based on a global assessment of these individuals and their surroundings. Changes in caregiver attitudes and behavior and environmental changes can precipitate maladaptive, alienating, or dangerous patient behaviors. When dementia patients who have been easily manageable become restless and agitated, it is important to look for antecedent sources of stress and for consequences of restlessness and agitation in addition to examining the patients directly. An understanding of patients' cognitive, emotional, interpersonal, and environmental assets and liabilities enables clinicians to decide how to construct an interpersonal environment that maintains patients at the best level of function for them as individuals. Dementia patients are often able to participate in such decisions. Many will raise the question of their own ability to drive or to live independently and will respond to direct suggestion. Others will require environmental manipulations to ensure that they do not endanger themselves or others.

Persons with static dementia, such as a dementia that follows a head injury, can be challenged to develop their remaining resources. Progressively dementing persons are constantly losing ground and therefore best dealt with by accommodating their deficits. Autonomy and self-care are promoted when they are not too demanding of these individuals and their caregivers. In other instances, initiative may be discouraged and dependence fostered. In all cases, but especially in the progressive dementing diseases, what is best for patients changes in relation to the progress of their illness and the demands of their interpersonal environment. Ultimately, patients with progressive dementing illnesses may deteriorate beyond the reach of formal language. Communication then becomes nonverbal, conveying to these persons through touch and tone of voice what one would want to convey to a preverbal infant: gentleness, affection, and a consistent soothing response to evidence of discomfort. Unlike infants, persons with profound dementia are unable to learn that their environment is consistent, and they often do not learn to soothe themselves when caregivers are temporarily unavailable. Thus, caregivers are often unrewarded for their efforts and come to feel frustrated when their charges do not appear to respond to their ministrations. For this and other reasons, caregivers themselves require the various kinds of support described in Chapter 8.

CHAPTER 6

Pharmacological Management and Treatment of Dementia and Secondary Symptoms

Myron F. Weiner, M.D.
Lon S. Schneider, M.D.
Kevin F. Gray, M.D.
Robert G. Stern, M.D.

Drugs are used to manage dementia-related symptoms and behaviors and to ameliorate cognitive deficit. The former drugs are designated as psychotropics, the latter as nootropics or cognitive enhancers. In this chapter, we discuss the general principles of drug administration to frail adults and elders, certain specifics with regard to the dementing disorders, and the types of symptoms and behaviors dealt with by psychopharmacological means.

General Principles

The rational use of drugs to manage dementia-related symptoms and to ameliorate cognitive deficit requires an accurate diagnosis of the dementia-causing condition and knowledge of patients' medical history and current medical status and of the medications currently prescribed or self-administered. In some instances, addressing the cognitive and behavioral symptomatology must await adequate diagnosis and treatment of a medical condition such as heart failure, pneumonia, or hypothyroidism. The medical, social, and psychological histories are important because they give clues to the factors precipitating the presenting symptoms, such as a change of environment, as indicated in the following example:

175

The daughter-in-law of Mrs. A., an elderly woman who was enrolled in a nootropic drug study, called in an alarmed manner stating that Mrs. A. initially had a good response to the drug, but had suddenly worsened. When asked to describe what had happened, she told the physician that Mrs. A. had been living with her and her husband for about a month. They had gone to the apartment where Mrs. A. had formerly resided to pack up more of her possessions. While there, Mrs. A. suddenly became so confused that she no longer recognized her son. They took her back to their home, where she sat on her bed crying out for her own mother. The physician reassured the daughter-in-law that the mother had experienced a catastrophic response to the emotional stimulus of giving up her apartment and her former lifestyle and that with a good night's rest, she would probably settle down. The daughter-in-law called the next morning to say that indeed all was well again.

A list of medical conditions that may manifest as dementia is presented in Chapter 4. Having ruled out or ameliorated the medical conditions that may precipitate or aggravate the symptoms of dementia, physicians next review patients' medications for drugs that may dull sensorium, produce delirium, or increase agitation. In some cases, the indicated pharmacological intervention is reducing the dosage or eliminating the use of a cognition-impairing medication the patient is currently taking, such as the beta-blockers propranolol and methyldopa, or benzodiazepine tranquilizers or hypnotics. Learoyd (1972) found that, of 236 persons over age 65 years who had been hospitalized for behavioral disturbances, 16% had disorders directly attributable to the effects of psychotropic drugs.

Certain classes of drugs are to be avoided or employed in minimal dosages, depending on the type of dementia underlying the patient's symptomatology. The cholinergic deficit in Alzheimer's disease (AD) makes AD patients highly susceptible to further impairment of sensorium by drugs with strong anticholinergic properties. Thus, the use for sedation of antihistamines such as diphenhydramine is probably contraindicated, as is the strongly anticholinergic antidepressant amitriptyline for either its sedative or antidepressant effect. Indeed, elders in general are sensitive to medications with anticholinergic actions, including many psychotropic, gastrointestinal, and other medications.

Age-Related Considerations

In treating elders with dementia, special consideration must be given to certain age-related phenomena. They include changes in absorption, distribution, protein binding, hepatic metabolism, renal excretion, receptor sensitivity, and neurotransmitters.

The absorption of psychotropic drugs administered by mouth is relatively unaffected by age (Salzman 1987). It is possible, however, that the concomitant use of anticholinergic drugs might reduce the rate of absorption by reducing gastrointestinal mobility and that the use of antacids and calcium might delay absorption of psychotropic drugs by decreasing their ionization.

In the aging process, lean muscle mass and body water decrease while total body fat tends to increase (Fryer 1962), despite a tendency toward overall weight loss in late old age. Thus, the majority of psychotropic drugs, which are lipophilic, will be more widely distributed through the body, whereas lithium carbonate will be less widely distributed because of reduced body water content (Chapron et al. 1982). Because serum albumin may be lowered by more than 15% in the elderly (Bender et al. 1975), less protein binding occurs and more free drug is available to receptor sites.

The efficiency of the liver in detoxifying and eliminating drugs decreases with age (Vestal and Wood 1980), due in part to decreased cardiac output with diminution of hepatic blood flow. As a result, the first-pass effect (the rapid elimination of the first dose of a drug by the liver) may be considerably reduced. Therapeutic levels of psychotropic drugs may be reached more rapidly in elders than in younger persons. Drugs with multiple metabolites will have inordinately long half-lives—in the case of diazepam, 89 hours at age 80 years, in contrast to 24 hours at age 20 years (Klotz et al. 1975). Renal function also diminishes with age (D. F. Davies and Shock 1950). Lithium carbonate dosage must therefore be reduced by about 30% (Hewick and Newbury 1976). Renal excretion of drugs may be further compromised by sodium-depleting diuretics, nonsteroidal anti-inflammatory drugs, and drugs such as propranolol that reduce glomerular filtration (Abernethy 1992). Decreased brain levels of dopamine (D. S. Robinson et al. 1972) and acetylcholine (Perry et al. 1977) make elders relatively more susceptible to the side effects of dopamine blockers and anticholinergic agents that cross the blood-brain barrier.

Psychotropic Drugs

Psychotropic drugs are employed to treat the behavioral effects of the dementing process, emotionally based responses to the dementing illness, or inability to adequately understand and cope with the environment. These responses include the following:

- Depression
- Delirium
- Anxiety and restlessness
- Agitation and aggression
- Sleep-wake disturbance
- Suspiciousness and delusion formation
- Hallucinations
- Apathy and withdrawal
- Inappropriate sexuality

In addition to their dementia and its direct and indirect effects on psychological function, patients may have a preexisting mental illness such as schizophrenia, manic-depressive illness, or major depression, or they may develop mania or depression after having become cognitively impaired. Although the fundamental psychopharmacological treatment of these illnesses is not different in a dementia-affected population than in a nondementia-affected population, dementia and physical frailty impose additional considerations in determining choice of medication, dose, and treatment regimen.

Depression

Depression is a frequent concomitant of dementia. A preexisting depressive illness may also continue to manifest in dementia patients. Early dementia may lead to depression when the individual, no longer able to live up to his or her standards of mental functioning, experiences self-criticism and lowering of self-esteem. In addition, the relative norepinephrine deficiency that accompanies aging may create a biological predisposition or further aggravate a long-standing tendency. In most cases of depression as an emotional reaction to dementia, sad thoughts and self-criticism are self-limited. They can be diminished by distracting dementia patients from thinking about their limitations by drawing them into overlearned pleasurable activities (Teri and Gallagher-Thompson 1991). Major depression can mimic dementia in terms of slowed thinking, speech, and movement, as well as loss of interest in the environment (Weiner and Fitzpatrick 1987).

Antidepressants are effective in treating depression in cognitively impaired persons (Greenwald et al. 1989; Reynolds et al. 1987). The indication for antidepressant medication in dementia patients is the presence of signs and symptoms characteristic of major depression, although less severe mood disturbances may also respond to treatment. Depression may be accompanied by psychotic features. Common delusions include that patients are being persecuted for past misdeeds, that they are about to be prosecuted or executed, or that the world has been destroyed. A foul body odor may be hallucinated. Somatic delusions also occur, in which patients imagine themselves to be riddled with cancer or filled with feces. If profound anorexia, refusal to eat, or suicidal ideation are prominent, patients should be hospitalized, either in a closely supervised general medical unit accustomed to managing depressed patients or in a psychiatric unit. Hospitalization can prevent death from dehydration, malnutrition, drug effects, or suicide. Cognitively impaired elderly depressed patients have been found to require longer periods of inpatient treatment and more often require high-potency neuroleptics than do noncognitively impaired elderly depressed patients (LaRue et al. 1986).

Electroconvulsive Therapy

Electroconvulsive therapy (ECT) is the treatment of choice for psychotically or melancholically depressed persons, especially if there has been rapid weight loss, sleeplessness, and profound suicidal or homicidal ideation or a suicide attempt (Karlinsky and Shulman 1984). In Greenwald et al.'s (1989) study of 10 demented/depressed patients, half required ECT to achieve remission. Psychotically depressed dementia patients who are unwilling to undergo ECT or for whom ECT is contraindicated should be started first on a neuroleptic, with dosage based on state of health, physical strength, adequacy of hydration, and cardiovascular status. Physically frail persons are generally treated with small doses of high-potency neuroleptics, such as 0.5–2.0 mg qd of haloperidol administered bid po, or 2–20 mg qd of trifluoperazine po bid. High-potency neuroleptics are employed because they are not cardiotoxic, have little anticholinergic activity, and produce little orthostatic hypotension. Neuroleptics prescribed by the authors are listed in Table 6–1, along with their antipsychotic equivalence to chlorpromazine, the reference drug for the neuroleptic class. Neuroleptic side effects are listed in Table 6–2. Many medications are available to treat depression. Table 6–3 shows the dosage and therapeutic blood levels of certain antidepressant drugs; Table 6–4 shows their side effects. Because antidepressants are roughly equivalent in therapeutic effect, choice of antidepressant is based more on the desired or undesired side effects. An adequate trial of antidepressant medication is 4 weeks (at therapeutic blood levels for tricyclics). Some depressed patients (especially outpatients) may take more than 7 weeks to respond (Georgotas et al. 1987b). Should one drug fail, the patient may be changed to another drug of the same or another class. A washout period of 7–10 days is desirable between antidepressant medications, and 10–14 days is safest when making the transition between selective serotonin reuptake inhibitors (SSRIs) and monoamine oxidase inhibitors (MAOIs) or vice versa. The transition from fluoxetine to an MAOI may require even longer because of fluoxetine's prolonged half-life. Because of their benign side-effect

Table 6–1. Dosage of selected neuroleptic drugs

Generic name	Trade name	Smallest tablet (mg)	Liquid	Adult dosage (mg/day)	Geriatric dosage (mg/day)	Equiv.[a]
Chlorpromazine	Thorazine	10	10 mg/5 ml	200–400	10–300	100
Thioridazine	Mellaril	10, 15	25 mg/5 ml	200–400	10–300	95
Trifluoperazine	Stelazine	1	10 mg/ml	10–20	4–20	5
Thiothixene	Navane	1	5 mg/ml	10–20	4–20	5
Haloperidol	Haldol	0.5[b]	2 mg/ml	4–8	0.25–6	2
Risperidone	Risperdal	1[b]	–	2–6	1–2	?

[a]Equivalent in antipsychotic effect to 100 mg chlorpromazine.
[b]Scored tablet.

Table 6–2. Neuroleptic side effects

Generic name	Class	Sedation	Hypotension	Extra-pyramidal symptoms	Anticholinergic effects
Chlorpromazine	Phenothiazine (aliphatic)	++++	++++	++	++++
Thioridazine	Phenothiazine (piperidine)	++++	++++	+	++++
Trifluoperazine	Phenothiazine (piperazine)	+	++	+++	++
Thiothixene	Thioxanthine (piperazine)	++	++	+++	++
Haloperidol	Butyrophenone	+	+	++++	—
Risperidone	Benzicoxazole	++	++	+	+

profile, their low toxicity, and positive case reports (Burke et al. 1994), SSRIs are the first-line drugs for treatment of depression in dementia patients, despite the absence of confirmation studies in this population.

Table 6–3. Dosage and therapeutic range of selected antidepressants

Generic name	Trade name	Initial dosage	Adult dosage	Geriatric dosage*	Thera-peutic range
Fluoxetine	Prozac	20	20–80	10–20	?
Sertraline	Zoloft	50	50	25–50	?
Paroxetine	Paxil	20	20–40	10–20	?
Imipramine	Tofranil SK-Pramine	25–50	50–300	20–100	150–200 ng/ml
Desipramine	Norpramin Pertofrane	25	75–200	25–75	50–150 ng/ml
Nortriptyline**	Pamelor	25	50–150	25–100	50–100 ng/ml
Phenelzine	Nardil	15	30–60	15–60	?
Tranylcypromine	Parnate	10	20–30	5–15	?

*mg/day.
**Available as liquid.

Table 6–4. Antidepressant side effects at therapeutic dosages

Generic name	Class	Sedation	Hypo-tension	Anti-cholinergic Effects	Cardio-toxicity
Fluoxetine	SSRI	—	—	—	—
Sertraline	SSRI	—	—	—	—
Paroxetine	SSRI	—	—	—	—
Imipramine	Tertiary amine	+++	+++	+++	+++
Desipramine	Secondary amine	+	+	+	+
Nortriptyline	Secondary amine	+	+	+	+
Trazodone	Cyclic (other)	++	++	+	—
Phenelzine	MAOI	+	+++	—	—
Tranylcypromine	MAOI	—	++	—	—

SSRI = selective serotonin reuptake inhibitor; MAOI = monoamine oxidase inhibitor.

Selective Serotonin Reuptake Inhibitors

Fluoxetine, sertraline, and paroxetine are highly selective SSRIs. They are virtually devoid of anticholinergic, antihistaminic, or antiadrenergic side effects, but paroxetine is mildly anticholinergic. All have long half-lives. Fluoxetine and its active metabolite norfluoxetine have a total half-life of up to 12 days; sertraline and its active metabolite have a total half-life of as long as 4 days, and paroxetine, with no active metabolite, has one as long as 24 hours. All three drugs are dosed once a day. They are administered in the morning because of their tendency to stimulate. SSRI lethality in overdose is low. All three medications may produce nausea, anxiety, restlessness, and sleep loss. Fluoxetine may produce hyponatremia by inducing inappropriate secretion of antidiuretic hormone (Hwang and Magraw 1989). SSRIs should not be taken in combination with MAOIs or tryptophan (Sternbach 1988). The serotonergic state resulting from such combinations ranges from simple agitation to hyperthermia, muscular rigidity, delirium, coma, and death.

In frail or elderly dementia patients, fluoxetine is initiated at 10 mg qd, sertraline at 25 mg qd, and paroxetine at 10 mg qd, with weekly titration upward as indicated and tolerated (see Table 6–3). If fluoxetine is too stimulating dosed once a day, it may be dosed qod. Withdrawal symptoms, including agitation, sleepiness, vivid dreams, and hypomania, have all been reported with paroxetine.

Cyclic and Heterocyclic Antidepressants

Cyclic Antidepressants

The cyclic antidepressants include the tricyclic tertiary amine group such as amitriptyline, imipramine, and doxepin; their secondary amine active metabolites, including desipramine and nortriptyline; and those with atypical or heterocyclic structures such as maprotiline and amoxapine. These drugs are more toxic in physically ill persons and elders because of decreased protein binding, slowed demethylation in the liver, and reduced hepatic and renal clearance. The diminished first-pass effect renders patients susceptible to the toxic effects of both the primary drugs and their active metabolites. Imipramine and nortriptyline produce moderate norepinephrine and serotonin blockade, whereas desipramine strongly blocks norepinephrine reuptake. Elders are more liable to the therapeutic and toxic effects of these drugs because of decreases in norepinephrine, serotonin, and acetylcholine.

Secondary amines are the preferable tricyclics in elderly or physically ill patients; they have fewer side effects and are less sedating. Although desipramine, the demethylated metabolite of imipramine, is the least anticholinergic of the tricyclic antidepressants (TCAs), it produces anticholinergic side effects. TCAs as a group cause postural hypotension in some patients, and may cause agitation (Salzman and van der Kolk 1984). Nortriptyline, the demethylated metabolite of amitriptyline, is low in anticholinergic and sedative side effects compared with the tertiary amines (Gerson et al. 1988). Even in frail elders, plasma levels correlate well with dosage. In a group of such patients with an average age of 84 years, a dose averaging 80 mg qd was required to produce a plasma level of 100 ng/ml (Katz et al. 1989). In a study of 21 elderly depressed patients with heart disease, there was no effect on ejection fraction and minimal orthostatic hypotension (Roose et al. 1986). Kumar et al. (1987) found significant orthostatic hypotension, no significant electrocardiogram (ECG) changes, and plasma levels and elimination half-life similar to young adults. First-degree atrioventricular (AV) block and right bundle branch block have been reported during nortriptyline treatment (Schneider et al. 1988).

Amoxapine, a dibenzazepine tricyclic, is metabolized to 7-hydroxy-amoxapine, a dopamine antagonist documented to cause tardive dyskinesia (Jenike 1985).

Administration and Dosage

If a TCA is to be administered, a careful check must be made of cardiac status and blood pressure. An ECG and standing and sitting blood pressure should be obtained. Because of a strong correlation between antidepressant effect and plasma concentration of certain TCAs (see Table 6–3), an attempt is made to reach a plasma level of 150–200 ng/ml in healthy adults. There is no improvement or worsening above that concentration. Nortriptyline has a therapeutic window at 50–150 ng/ml documented largely in inpatients with major depression. The lower therapeutic blood level range for elderly patients has not been established; elders may have clinical responses at low doses. The best starting dose for elders is 10–25 mg hs. (TCAs can be given once a day because of their long half-lives.) Amitriptyline, imipramine, and doxepin are strongly sedating and may produce morning grogginess. Thus, it is best to administer them no later than 9 P.M. Nortriptyline and desipramine may stimulate and thus may best be given as a single morning dose. If there are no significant side effects, dosage can be increased 10–25 mg every 2–4 days to a maximum of 50–150 mg qd, except for nortriptyline (25–100 mg qd).

Side Effects

The common side effects of TCAs are sedation, orthostatic hypotension, cardiac toxicity, and anticholinergic toxicity. All of these side effects are most common with the tertiary amine group (see Table 6–4), which should probably not be used in elders with dementia and other frail individuals (Cassem 1982; Gerson et al. 1988). Orthostatic hypotension often leads to falls in frail patients. Slowing of conduction in the His-Purkinje system of the heart necessitates careful monitoring in patients with bundle branch disease, heart block, cardiac arrhythmias, congestive heart failure, or past history of myocardial infarction. Bifascicular block, 2:1 AV block, and left bundle branch block are important predictors of orthostatic hypotension with tricyclic use (Roose et al. 1986). TCAs have quinidine-like effects and should be used with caution in patients taking quinidine or procainamide.

Anticholinergic side effects include dry mouth, constipation, urinary retention, precipitation or aggravation of narrow-angle glaucoma, impairment of memory, and delirium. Dry mouth may result in candidiasis or parotitis or may lead to excessive water intake and hyponatremia. It can be reduced by the use of sugarless candies or gum. Constipation can be reduced by using stool softeners. Impairment of cognition is best dealt with by changing to a less anticholinergic medication.

Anticholinergic delirium.   Anticholinergic delirium is first treated by discontinuing the offending medication. Although anticholinergic delirium is reversible by physostigmine (Weiner and Davis 1986), the potential toxic effects of cholinergic excess require that physostigmine be used in well-supervised medical environments. If the agitated dementia patient is strong and healthy, 0.015–0.030 mg/kg (approximately 0.5–2 mg) of physostigmine can be slowly administered intravenously over 10 minutes after first recording pupil size, pulse, temperature, and bowel sounds. A syringe containing 1 mg of atropine should be available in case overtreatment results in a physostigmine-induced cholinergic state of bradycardia, asystole, meiosis, increased secretions, abdominal cramping, and urinary frequency or urgency. Approximately 0.5 mg of atropine intravenously will be required to reverse the effects of every 1.0 mg of physostigmine administered.

The slow intravenous administration of 0.5–2 mg of physostigmine can also be used to diagnose anticholinergic delirium. An anticholinergic delirium is suggested if the patient becomes more alert and less confused while the physostigmine is being administered. Despite the usefulness of physostigmine, it is less dangerous to treat an agitated delirium in frail or ill persons with a high-potency neuroleptic. Low-potency neuroleptics are to be avoided because of their anticholinergic effects.

Heterocyclic Antidepressants

Trazodone, a triazolopyridine, is very specific for the serotonergic system and has little effect on dopamine, norepinephrine, histamine, and cholinergic systems. It has a low cardiovascular risk profile, low toxicity with overdose, absence of anticholinergic effects, and minimal effects on cognition (Gerner 1987). Trazodone is highly sedative and produces occasional orthostatic hypotension, probably related to α-adrenergic blockade. The rare effect of priapism may be avoided by warning male patients in advance and discontinuing the drug should it occur (Hayes and Kristoff 1986). Because of its 4- to 6-hour half-life, it requires tid dosing.

Should other classes of antidepressants prove too toxic for an individual patient or be ineffective after an adequate period at an adequate blood level, the next group of drugs to be tried are the MAOIs.

Monoamine Oxidase Inhibitors

The enzyme monoamine oxidase (MAO), which degrades the transmitters norepinephrine, serotonin, and dopamine, increases with increasing age (Robinson 1975). This class of drugs presumably acts by inhibiting MAO, thereby increasing the availability of norepinephrine and serotonin. The most common side effect of these drugs is orthostatic hypotension. Less common are stimulation, dry mouth, and weight gain. Because MAOIs interfere with their metabolism, pressor amines and sympathomimetic drugs may not be used during MAO treatment. The pressor amine tyramine in foods must also be avoided by eliminating from the diet aged cheeses, yeast extract, caviar, sausage, herring, beef and chicken liver, and large amounts of avocado, chocolate, caffeine, and Chianti. MAOIs may have significant adverse interaction with SSRIs and should not be administered with them.

The two commonly used drugs in this class are phenelzine and tranylcypromine. In elders, phenelzine is prescribed in an initial dose of 7.5 mg (½ tablet), raising the dose every 3–4 days to a maximum of 15–60 mg qd in divided doses. Tranylcypromine, which appears to have greater stimulating effect, is started in elders at 2.5–5 mg (½–¼ tablet) qd and increased to 5–15 mg qd in divided doses.

Stimulants

The use of stimulants such as D-amphetamine, methylphenidate, or magnesium pemoline in depressed dementia patients is controversial (Chiarello and Cole 1987). Because of their risk of abuse and because they can agitate, induce, or exaggerate paranoid thinking; increase blood pressure and heart rate; interact adversely with antihypertensives (Crook 1979); and aggravate depressive symptoms when withdrawn, stimulants are not employed as primary treatments for depression. Their main use in elders is in short-term treatment of withdrawn depression, in medically ill patients with significant cardiovascular disease (Satel and Nelson 1989), and with withdrawn apathetic behavior in dementia patients that cannot be differentiated clearly from depression (Kaplitz 1975) (see section on apathy and withdrawal in this chapter).

Delirium

The best treatment for delirium is treatment of the underlying medical disorder, which may be pneumonia, congestive heart failure, a urinary tract infection, or other causes. Environmental and interpersonal measures are the first to be instituted in dealing with the cognitive and affective consequences of delirium. Patients should be kept in well-lighted rooms so that they are not confused by shadows or vague outlines. If possible, the room should have a window so that the person can be oriented to day and night. Staff should constantly reintroduce themselves, briefly describe their role ("I am your nurse") and mention the place and the day ("This is the Sunnyside Nursing Home; today is Wednesday"). If possible, familiar people (with whom the delirious person has a positive relationship) and objects (e.g., photographs of loved ones, a pillow, a comforter, a stuffed animal) should be in the room. Mechanical restraint is to be avoided in favor of distracting the delirious person from pulling out nasogastric tubing, indwelling catheters, and so on. Delirium that occurs quietly and without agitation requires no psychotropic medication. The following is an example of the development and resolution of a typical delirium:

> A 66-year-old man was admitted to the hospital in 1984 for shortness of breath and chest pain probably due to coronary artery disease. He was kept under observation and given nitroglycerin as needed for pain. On the third hospital day, he became disoriented to time and place and mistook the intern for his nephew. The psychiatric consultant found him alert but agitated. The patient reported that he was scared of being in the "'factory' and wanted to speak to his 'nephew'" the intern. He thought the year was 1979 and had markedly impaired recall and short-term memory. He was treated with orienting and supportive measures, and by the 7th day of hospitalization, his disorientation and confusion had cleared sufficiently that he was able to be discharged to his own care with the supervision of a visiting nurse. A computed tomography (CT) scan performed during his hospitalization showed hydrocephalus ex vacuo and marked cortical atrophy.

Psychotropic drugs are used when delirious persons become difficult to manage—refusing to remain at needed bed rest, pulling out catheters and intravenous tubes, or attacking staff members and family. Neuroleptic medications are the treatment of choice except in withdrawal deliria. When agitation is mild, these medications should be given orally. When there is danger to life, medication should be administered parenterally, because peak blood levels can be achieved in 30 minutes instead of the 4–6 hours required for medication administered orally (Settle 1984). A relatively safe drug to use in an agitated delirium is haloperidol, which may be administered intravenously or intramuscularly if needed. An adequate oral, intravenous, or intramuscular dose for an agitated, physically frail person ranges from 0.5 to 2 mg. A physically strong person may require a larger dosage. As soon as delirious patients calm down (usually within 24 hours), the neuroleptic medication may be administered orally at twice the total daily dose of the parenterally administered drug, given in divided doses. Thus, if 10 mg iv haloperidol were required the first day, 20 mg would be administered as 5 mg qid or 10 mg bid. Typically, 3–4 days of a gradually lowered dose of neuroleptic medication are required. The chief complication of this technique of rapid neuroleptization is acute dystonia—dramatic, painful tonic contraction of neck, tongue, and mouth muscles. Oculogyric crisis may occur, as may contraction of large muscle groups. Acute dystonia is treated by the intravenous administration of diphenhydramine 25 mg or benztropine maleate 2 mg iv (Baldessarini 1977), followed by discontinuance of the offending drug. It is wise to follow the intravenous use of these medications with 1–2 mg of benztropine maleate bid for several days, because neuroleptics are long acting.

In the case of severe agitated delirium, and when it is essential to achieve sedation (e.g., for patients struggling against physical restraints), haloperidol may be combined with lorazepam in a ratio ranging from 3:1 to 5:1 and administered intravenously in the same syringe.

If the patient's delirium is due to withdrawal from minor tranquilizers, barbiturates, or glutethimide, pentobarbital may be used in 200- to 400-mg doses every 4–6 hours sufficient to cause nystagmus, slurred speech, drowsiness, and/or mild ataxia within an hour after drug administration. When an adequate 24-hour dose is established, it is maintained for several days and then reduced by approximately one-tenth of the total dose (but not more than 100 mg) per day. Barbiturates are used in preference to benzodiazepines because it is essential to use a drug that is substantially cross-tolerant with the drug being withdrawn.

The beginning stage of delirium tremens, usually manifested by diaphoresis and tremulousness, can be treated using benzodiazepines with a long half-life, such as 10–25 mg of chlordiazepoxide po qid or 2–10 mg diazepam po q 4 h as needed. An intravenous dose of 5–10 mg of diazepam may be used for severe agitation, followed by 5 mg iv every 5 minutes until the patient is calm. An oral dose of 5–10 mg of diazepam every 1–4 hours may then be administered (Beresford et al. 1984). Diazepam should not be administered intramuscularly because it is poorly and irregularly absorbed. Patients with alcohol dependence, alcohol withdrawal, or delirium tremens also require treatment with 100 mg qd of thiamine orally or parenterally, especially if intravenous dextrose solutions are employed. Inadequate stores of thiamine to metabolize a sugar load can produce an acute, potentially lethal case of Wernicke's syndrome (Adams and Victor 1989). Too-rapid hydration with lowering of serum sodium to less than 130 mEq/L can produce central pontine myelinolysis (Adams et al. 1959).

As pointed out in Chapter 1, delirium is often superimposed on a preexisting dementia syndrome. Dementia patients are easily made delirious by mild metabolic or toxic insults and, as indicated in Chapter 4, by psychotropic medications including antipsychotics. Furthermore, preexisting dementia is a strong predictor of postoperative delirium. Delirium superimposed on dementia may respond to very small doses of haloperidol (0.25–1 mg po or iv). In elders, intravenous administration is preferable to intramuscular administration to avoid tissue damage. As indicated above (see Anticholinergic delirium), physostigmine may be used to reverse anticholinergic delirium.

Anxiety and Restlessness

Many dementia patients experience anxiety and restlessness. Mild anxiety and restlessness are dealt with by the behavioral and environmental means suggested in Chapter 5, after having made certain that these symptoms are not the result of medications such as bronchodilators, sympathomimetics, or antipsychotics.

Minor Tranquilizers

Minor tranquilizers of the benzodiazepine class (Table 6–5) are drugs of choice for the treatment of anxiety disorders in cognitively intact patients. Benzodiazepines are metabolized either by conjugation or oxidation (Shader and Greenblatt 1977). Benzodiazepine oxidation by hepatic microsomal enzymes is inhibited by cimetidine, erythromycin, fluoxetine, isoniazid, and omeprazole (Wengel et al. 1992). Sedative effects are antagonized by theophylline, increased by acute alcohol ingestion, and reduced by chronic alcohol use. Because hepatic oxidation may be impaired in elders, benzodiazepines metabolized by conjugation, such as oxazepam, lorazepam, and temazepam, are preferred (Salzman 1992).

The side effects of benzodiazepines are sedation, memory impairment, and muscular uncoordination leading to dysarthria and ataxia. Withdrawal symptoms occur frequently, especially with triazolam and alprazolam. Therefore, if benzodiazepine withdrawal is undertaken, it should be done slowly to prevent severe withdrawal symptoms, including gastrointestinal upset, tremor, agitation, and (occasionally, after abrupt cessation of high doses) seizures (Salzman 1987). There do not seem to be important age differences in benzodiazepine withdrawal.

Table 6–5.   Dosage of selected benzodiazepine tranquilizers

Generic name	Trade name	Adult dosage*	Geriatric dosage*	Frequency of dosage in adults	Frequency of dosage in elders
Chlordiaze-poxide	Librium	20–40	20–40	tid	bid
Diazepam	Valium	10–20	2–20	tid	qd/qod
Oxazepam	Serax	45–60	15–60	tid	tid
Lorazepam	Ativan	2–4	0.5–4	tid	bid/tid

*mg/day

A study contrasting withdrawal (reduction of dose by 25% per week) in elderly chronic benzodiazepine users and in young adults showed somewhat lower symptomatology in the older group (Schweizer et al. 1989).

Persons taking high therapeutic ranges doses of benzodiazepines for long periods perform poorly on neuropsychological tasks involving visuospatial ability and sustained attention (Golombok et al. 1988). In elders, cognitive impairment may develop insidiously, becoming evident only after years of treatment (Larson et al. 1987).

Self-reported anxiety may accompany or be aggravated by mild to moderate dementia. There have been few controlled studies of benzodiazepines in dementia patients. In a comparison with oxazepam, chlordiazepoxide, and placebo, oxazepam (with 76% of patients improved) was superior to chlordiazepoxide (23% improved) and placebo (7% improved), but half of the chlordiazepoxide group were oversedated, ataxic, or dizzy (Chesrow et al. 1965). Diazepam improved daytime restlessness in dementia patients, but 85% appeared oversedated (DeLamos et al. 1965). Because of its long half-life, clonazepam may be useful in tapering alprazolam discontinuation or when alprazolam is ineffective for panic symptoms.

Because they may cloud sensorium, impair memory, and produce ataxia, benzodiazepines should generally be avoided in dementia patients. In addition, there is concern that they may produce a disinhibition syndrome of rage or agitation. On the other hand, many mildly to moderately cognitively impaired patients have been taking such medications for years, and discontinuing the medication results in further increases in agitation that are not well relieved with other classes of drugs. In such instances, the wisest course of action is to determine the smallest dose of benzodiazepine needed to control the patient's restlessness and to maintain the patient on that dose. It is not possible to determine whether one is treating the patient's anxiety, preventing withdrawal symptoms, or dealing with family members' inability to cope in these instances, as indicated in the following case:

> Mrs. G., a 75-year-old woman, was referred for evaluation of her irritability and forgetfulness. She had been well from the emotional standpoint until 12 years earlier, when she began to suffer gastrointestinal complaints including "nervous stomach," diarrhea, and anorexia. A prescription of 5 mg of diazepam tid was taken from that time forward. Following a hysterectomy at age 73 years, Mrs. G. became increasingly irritable, forgetful, and repetitious. After a severe quarrel with her husband 6 months earlier, she was hospitalized for 21 days in

a psychiatric unit. She received a single ECT during that admission, following which she became extremely confused. She continued to take diazepam in addition to 25 mg of amitriptyline hs after discharge.

On examination, Mrs. G. was cognitively impaired and mildly to moderately depressed. She reported both appetite and weight loss. The examiner thought that both of her medications might be contributing to her cognitive impairment and asked that they be gradually withdrawn. Attempts to withdraw the diazepam resulted in Mrs. G. experiencing escalating agitation and making demands for her "nerve medicine" that exceeded her husband's ability to set limits. An attempt was made to resolve the situation by changing the dose of diazepam to 2.5 mg bid by giving her half a tablet at a time. Difficulty with sleep was dealt with by using imipramine 25 mg in place of amitriptyline. Her husband was unable to limit her intake of medication, and it was eventually necessary to place her in a nursing home as her confusion increased with her advancing dementia. At that time, it was possible to slowly discontinue her medications.

Agitation and Violence

Behaviors such as agitation and violence occur in a substantial minority of dementia patients. Nondirected violent or aggressive behavior occurs more commonly than specific, directed violence. As noted in Chapter 5, verbal and physical violence are often precipitated by interpersonal events (such as unpleasant confrontations) or misperceptions due to patients' cognitive impairment. There have been a few randomized placebo-controlled pharmacotherapeutic studies of agitation and aggression in dementia patients. Some have been reviewed previously (Schneider and Sobin 1994; Schneider et al. 1990). The information presented in the following paragraphs is taken largely from controlled studies, case reports, and expert physician evaluations. Drugs used include neuroleptics, lithium, anticonvulsants, β-adrenergic blockers, and serotonergic agents.

Neuroleptics

Neuroleptics are the drugs of choice for agitated, restless behavior that is not a consequence of major depression, an abstinence syndrome, a neuroleptic, or a serotonergic state. They are consistently more effective than benzodiazepines (Schneider and Sobin 1994). Given in a single daily dose at bedtime, neuroleptics provide some degree of sedation or sleep induction and reduce daytime agitation. Higher-potency neuroleptics are useful for persons sensitive to the anticholinergic effects, sedation, or postural hypotension produced by these medications. Low-potency neuroleptics can be used if more sedation is needed or if patients are susceptible to the extrapyramidal side effects of the high-potency neuroleptics. The dosage ranges and side-effect profiles for a representative group of these drugs are shown in Tables 6–1 and 6–2. Plasma levels are not helpful in determining dosage, which is established by striking a balance between calming effects and side effects. These medications are effective by mouth, and, with the exception of thioridazine and molindone, they can be administered parenterally. Parenteral administration of chlorpromazine is generally undesirable because of its irritating properties and hypotensive effects. When severe agitation occurs, neuroleptics may be given intramuscularly in approximately half the recommended adult or geriatric dose. Haloperidol may be administered intravenously at the intramuscular dose. Haloperidol and thioridazine are among the few medications that have been demonstrated to be effective for agitation and other symptomatic behaviors in dementia patients in randomized trials. As noted above, the neuroleptics are somewhat more effective than benzodiazepines (Schneider and Sobin 1994).

Molindone and loxapine are useful neuroleptics but their half-lives are considerably shorter than other neuroleptics. Both are moderate in sedative, extrapyramidal, and anticholinergic effects. They may be initiated at 5–10 mg tid, with increases in daily dose of 10–25 mg every 3–4 days to a maximum of 225 mg qd.

Clozapine, a dibenzodiazepine derivative, may be used when other neuroleptics fail to control symptoms or have dangerous or disabling side effects. Clozapine does not cause acute dystonia, parkinsonism, akathisia, or tardive dyskinesia. On the other hand, the drug often causes sialorrhea, somnolence, and, occasionally, irreversible agranulocytosis and death from sepsis (Alvir et al. 1993). It has also been reported to cause severe orthostatic hypotension accompanied by cardiovascular and respiratory collapse and cardiac arrest. Low-dose clozapine has been found effective, in doses generally lower than 75 mg qd, in controlling agitation in dementia patients (Oberholzer et al. 1992). Clozapine can also be used to treat psychotic symptoms in Parkinson's disease patients (J. H. Friedman and Lannon 1989). Dosing should begin with 12.5 mg qd, increasing as needed and tolerated to bid or tid dosing. Monitoring of total white cell and neutrophil counts are needed weekly for the first 6 months, then biweekly, with discontinuance of the drug if white count falls below 3,500/mm^3 or neutrophil count falls below 1,500/mm^3 (Gerson 1993).

Risperidone, a neuroleptic that produces only moderate D_2 receptor blockade, may also be effective in treating psychotic symptoms and agitation in dementia patients. In doses below 5 mg qd, it is not as potent at causing extrapyramidal effects. The manufacturer (Janssen Pharmaceutica, personal communication, April 14, 1994) recommends an initial dose of 0.5 mg bid in elderly or debilitated patients with severe renal or hepatic impairment or for whom hypotension would pose a risk. Dosage increases above 1.5 mg bid should be made at no less than 1-week intervals. Doses above 6 mg qd were not found to be more effective than lower doses.

Toxic Effects

Most neuroleptic drugs have a wide margin of safety. Except for clozapine, there is little danger of death from deliberate or accidental overdose unless combined with other drugs. On the other hand, they have a variety of toxic long- and short-term effects. For the low-potency neuroleptics, the prominent short-term toxic effects are anticholinergic, sedative, and hypotensive. For the higher-potency neuroleptics, the prominent short-term toxic effects are dystonias, parkinsonian symptoms, and akathisia (an involuntary restless pacing). Dystonias are treated acutely as described previously. Parkinsonian symptoms are best treated by lowering the dosage of the neuroleptic drug. If that is insufficient, the antiparkinsonian drug amantadine may be administered in a dose ranging from 100 to 300 mg qd. It is used in preference to drugs such as benztropine, diphenhydramine, and trihexyphenidyl in elders. It has been shown in healthy elders that amantadine does not impair memory (it appears to act by enhancing the action of dopamine), as opposed to drugs such as trihexphenidyl that do impair memory, possibly because of their strong anticholinergic effects (McEvoy et al. 1987). It has also been shown in healthy volunteers that benztropine impairs memory more than amantadine (Gelenberg et al. 1989). Akathisia responds best to lowering the dose of neuroleptic and may respond to doses of propranolol as low as 30–80 mg qd (Lipinski et al. 1984).

Neuroleptic malignant syndrome. An extremely important toxic effect of neuroleptics is neuroleptic malignant syndrome (Caroff 1980). This life-threatening complication occurs in approximately 0.9% of patients exposed to neuroleptics (Keck et al. 1987) and is characterized by muscular rigidity, akinesia, fever, diaphoresis, and increased pulse and blood pressure. It may progress rapidly to coma (Pearlman 1986). Laboratory findings include elevated white blood cell count, elevated liver enzymes, markedly elevated creatinine phosphokinase (up to 20,000 U/dl), and myoglobin in plasma due to muscle tissue breakdown. The latter may result in acute renal shutdown. Symptoms evolve over 24–72 hours and are frequently related to an injection of a long-acting neuroleptic such as fluphenazine decanoate. Treatment is withdrawal of the neuroleptic agent, intravenous fluids, and body-cooling measures. Because the syndrome presumably arises from intense dopaminergic blockade, the treatment of choice is to counteract dopaminergic blockade and to achieve muscle relaxation (Granato et al. 1983). The dopamine agonist bromocriptine is administered 5 mg q 4 h (po or nasogastric tube). Muscle relaxation is achieved by using the skeletal muscle relaxant dantrolene 4–8 mg/kg qd po in four divided doses. It may also be administered intravenously beginning with 1 mg/kg to a maximum cumulative dose of 10 mg/kg.

Tardive dyskinesia syndromes.   The tardive dyskinesia (TD) syndromes consist of involuntary movements appearing after a minimum of 3 months of neuroleptic treatment and for which alternate etiologies of dyskinesia have been excluded (Chouinard et al. 1979). Their principal determinants are prolonged neuroleptic exposure and advancing age, but a primary psychiatric diagnosis of mood disorder and the presence of brain injury may also be predisposing factors (Marsden et al. 1972). Persons who have received neuroleptic medication for more than a year are estimated to develop TD at a rate of 3% per year. TD syndromes may be reversible or irreversible and are frequently unmasked by antiparkinsonian medication.

Five principal TD syndromes have been identified (R. G. Davis and Cummings 1988): classic tardive dyskinesia, tardive dystonia, tardive akathisia, tardive Gilles de la Tourette syndrome, and tardive complex (simultaneous presence of three or more movement disorders). Classic TD consists of ticlike or choreiform movements, usually beginning with the tongue, facial, and neck muscles and involving arms and hands. Chewing movements of the mouth and sudden protrusions of the tongue are commonly seen. These movements are worsened by physical activity and emotional distress but disappear during sleep. Early facial dyskinesias are difficult to differentiate from the chewing movements that occur in elders who have not been exposed to neuroleptics (Varga et al. 1982). Tardive dystonias may display as wry neck, truncal muscle spasm, blepharospasm, oromandibular dystonia, or laryngospasm; tardive Tourette's syndrome exhibits as involuntary coprolalia, palilalia, or echolalia.

These syndromes are probably due to increased numbers of postsynaptic dopamine receptors that appear in response to chronic dopaminergic blockade. For that reason, they often appear when neuroleptic dosage is reduced. Although no safe and effective treatment is available (American Psychiatric Association 1992), discontinuing the causative medication may result in reduction of symptoms after a period of months. When the medication cannot be safely discontinued, a small increase in dosage may ameliorate symptoms by increasing the dopaminergic blockade. Despite the fact that anticholinergics may unmask some cases of TD, Gardos et al. (1986) found that antiparkinsonian drugs were helpful in cases of TD with symptoms such as drooling, akathisia, and tremor. They also found benzodiazepines frequently useful but did not have success with lecithin, baclofen, propranolol, or levodopa (L-dopa). There have been several trials of vitamin E with inconclusive results (Feltner and Hertzman 1992).

Unlike the treatment of schizophrenia, in which chronic neuroleptic treatment may be required, the need for neuroleptics in dementing illness is usually time limited. Thus, periodic attempts should be made to slowly withdraw neuroleptics in these patients. We do not employ chronic neuroleptic treatment to manage infrequent episodes of agitation. We attempt to treat patients with neuroleptics in sufficiently small doses that they do not produce extrapyramidal symptoms and thus rarely use antiparkinsonian agents. We tend to augment neuroleptics with trazodone rather than increasing dosage to the point of producing extrapyramidal symptoms. Patients who require chronic neuroleptics should be assessed approximately every 3 months for evidence of TD by using the Abnormal Involuntary Movement Scale (AIMS) (Guy 1976; see Appendix 11) and by making serial comparisons. If symptoms appear, a decision can be made about medication reduction or treatment as indicated above.

Lithium Carbonate

Lithium carbonate is specifically indicated as a prophylactic agent in the management of bipolar disorder. Bipolar disorder may present de novo in dementia patients or may be a continuation of a preexisting illness. Manic behavior frequently includes agitation and restlessness and may progress to combativeness and physical exhaustion. Hypomania may occur without depression in dementia patients (Joyce and Levy 1989). The accompanying ideation is usually grandiose, with inflated notions of importance and a sense of enormous personal power. Mood is generally euphoric but many manic patients are quite irritable and paranoid ideation is common. Lithium carbonate appears to dampen mood swings in this illness; the mechanism of action is unknown. In acute manic attacks, it should be combined with a neuroleptic.

Lithium has also been used to control violent behavior in many different populations, including epileptic patients with interictal aggression (Gershon 1968), brain-damaged children (Annell 1969), brain-damaged prisoners (Tupin et al. 1973), and demented elders (Salzman 1988). The single systematic study of 10 elderly dementia patients showed no effect of low-dose lithium after 4 weeks (Holton and George 1985). K. H. Williams and Goldstein (1979) treated 10 brain-damaged patients with lithium carbonate 1,200 mg qd in divided doses and found reduced agitation and pacing in 8 patients, not including the single AD patient in the group. Response times ranged from 2 to 6 weeks. Others have reported less success (Randels et al. 1984).

The starting dose of lithium in healthy adults is 300 mg tid, with an ultimate total daily dose in the range of 900–1,800 mg qd. Therapeutic serum level in acute mania is 0.8–1.5 mEq/L; maintenance level is 0.6–1.2 mEq/L (Jefferson et al. 1986). Elders and persons with impaired renal function should be started at doses of 75–300 mg qd. The 75-mg dose can be achieved using concentrate; 150-mg doses can be obtained by breaking 300-mg tablets in half. Effective plasma levels in elders are approximately half those for healthy adults. Red blood cell lithium levels rise before plasma levels and may be a better indicator of impending toxicity (Foster 1992).

Toxic Effects

Toxic lithium effects include mental confusion, nausea, vomiting, diarrhea, tremor, goiter, polyuria, and flattened or inverted T-waves on ECG. Additional effects of lithium in elderly patients include induction or exacerbation of extrapyramidal symptoms, ataxia, cardiac sinus node dysfunction, and a Creutzfeldt-Jakob–like syndrome (J. M. Smith and Kocen 1988). In contrast to lipid-soluble neuroleptic drugs, lithium is water soluble. Lithium levels tend to be higher in elders because of decreased total body water and decreased renal function. Therefore, it is advisable before undertaking lithium treatment to obtain a baseline ECG, thyroid function studies, serum creatinine (if not a creatinine clearance test), urinalysis, and urine osmolality. Lithium levels may be raised by increased pituitary antidiuretic hormone secretion in patients who are receiving concomitant neuroleptics. The development of lethargy may be due to relative overdosage of lithium or to lithium-induced hypothyroidism. If lithium-induced tremor becomes disabling, small doses of propranolol are useful, as is substitution of carbamazepine for lithium.

Because of the relatively low efficacy of lithium and its frequent toxic effects, the use of lithium in dementing illness is not encouraged.

Anticonvulsants

The anticonvulsant drug carbamazepine has been found useful in the treatment of manic-depressive illness (Ballenger and Post 1975). It can be combined with lithium to reduce rapid cycling and may be substituted for lithium in elders with conditions such as congestive heart failure and hypertension that require treatment with high-dose diuretics (Salzman 1988). It may also be substituted for lithium in patients with markedly reduced renal clearance and may be used in combination with lithium to protect against lithium-induced diuresis (Vieweg et al. 1987). Based on its effect in decreasing aggression in patients with functional psychotic disorders, Jenike (1985) proposed the use of carbamazepine for violent dementia patients who were without evidence of affective disorder.

The beginning dose is one-half tablet (100 mg) once a day, taken at mealtime. Dosage may be increased by 100 mg qd in divided doses with meals to a maximum of 1,200 mg qd (300–800 mg qd in elders). The recommended plasma level is in the range of 8–12 µg/ml (4–8 µg/ml in elders).

Carbamazepine side effects include nausea, vomiting, drowsiness, dizziness, and blurred vision. Hepatotoxicity and bone marrow suppression are occasional complications. It is imperative that a complete blood count and liver function tests be obtained before beginning this drug. Such tests should be repeated at 3- to 6-month intervals. Carbamazepine also acts as an antidiuretic agent and may thereby lower serum sodium. This action can be protected against by lowering the dose through the concomitant use of lithium (Vieweg et al. 1987).

Valproic acid has been reported useful in alleviating manic-delirious episodes accompanying multiple sclerosis and systemic lupus erythematosus (Kahn et al. 1988). The drug has side effects that include peripheral edema, rash, blood dyscrasias, and hepatotoxicity and requires periodic clinical monitoring. It also interacts with other anticonvulsants and, when used concomitantly with phenobarbital or phenytoin, requires careful monitoring of those drugs. The recommended initial dose is 15 mg/kg per day (approximately 250 mg), increasing by 250 mg qd to 250 mg tid or 50–100 µq/ml. Mazure et al. (1992) found valproate effective in two brain-damaged elderly patients with severe agitation. Mellow et al. (1993) reported efficacy in three of four dementia patients with severe behavioral disturbance.

Beta-Adrenerglc Blockers

Case reports support the use of propranolol in managing aggression in demented elders (Jenike 1983; Petrie and Ban 1981) and in younger brain-damaged patients who are unresponsive to neuroleptics (Mansheim 1981; Yudofsky et al. 1981). Greendyke et al. (1984) found propranolol reduced assaultive behavior and agitation in seven of eight patients with organic mental disorders. Hypotension and bradycardia were the most frequent side effects. Surprisingly, the effects of this drug are not immediate; 2–4 weeks are required. Effective doses range from 60 to 800 mg qd (Hales et al. 1990). At any dosage, the use of propranolol requires monitoring of pulse, blood pressure, and (in frail elders) creatinine level to ensure the adequacy of renal blood flow. The drug is contraindicated if there is a history of asthma or if bronchopulmonary disease is present.

Pindolol is a beta-blocker with partial intrinsic sympathomimetic activity. It was found effective in controlling agitation and assaultiveness in a double-blind, placebo-controlled crossover study of 11 "worst cases" of organically based agitation and assaultiveness gathered from several Veterans Affairs hospitals. Most diagnoses were brain disorder due to alcohol and trauma. Significant therapeutic effects were achieved without sedation and with no bradycardia or hypotension. The optimal dose was 40–60 mg qd, with no benefit apparent from higher doses (Greendyke and Kanter 1986). Metoprolol was used successfully at 200–300 mg qd in two brain-damaged persons who had developed sedation and depression on propranolol (Mattes 1985).

Serotonin Agonists

Cell loss in AD often occurs in the dorsal raphe nucleus of the brain stem, the site of serotonergic innervation of the forebrain (Yamamoto and Hirano 1985). As a result, brain serotonin metabolites are reduced 30%–40% in AD (Gottfries et al. 1983). Low blood levels of serotonin metabolites have been reported in aggressive children (Greenberg and Coleman 1976) and adults (Brown et al. 1979). Adverse reactions tended to occur when such persons were treated with drugs that further lowered serotonin metabolite concentration in blood (amitriptyline, diphenhydramine, reserpine, and high-dose trifluoperazine and chlorpromazine). Calming occurred with drugs that increased serotonin metabolites (thioridazine, mesoridazine, primidone, methsuximide, and lithium carbonate) (Greenberg and Coleman 1976).

Trazodone

Trazodone, an antidepressant that blocks serotonin reuptake, has been used alone or in combination with the serotonin precursor tryptophan. In a literature review, Schneider and Sobin (1994) found 23 cases of agitated dementia patients treated with trazodone. Dosages ranged from 150 to 500 mg qd. Of the 23 cases, at least 9 (39%) improved. Response time ranged from 2 to 4 weeks. The drug was discontinued in only one case, and that was due to edema. An open study (Houlihan et al. 1994) of trazodone in 22 behaviorally disturbed dementia patients on a geropsychiatric inpatient service showed moderate to marked improvement in 82%. Patients were dosed at 172 ± 107 mg qd for an average of 20 days. At the time of discharge, trazodone dosage ranged from 25 to 500 mg qd. Two patients became delirious, but no other side effects were noted. In the authors' experience, sedation can be a significant side effect. A multicenter randomized trial comparing trazodone and haloperidol is under way, sponsored by the National Institute of Aging.

Buspirone

A serotonin-1A agonist, buspirone, which is generally employed as an anxiolytic, has been reported as effective in two case reports of severe agitation in demented elders, one with AD (Colenda 1988) and the other with MID (Tiller et al. 1988). In a small open study of the drug in demented, agitated elders (primarily residents of a long-term care facility), 6 of 16 patients were rated as much improved or very much improved (Herrmann and Eryavec 1993). An attempt was made to give each patient at least a 1-month trial. Dosage ranged from 10 to 15 mg tid. One patient, who was concomitantly receiving loxitane, suffered a dystonic reaction. Another became much more agitated, necessitating withdrawal of the drug after 4 days.

Sleep-Wake Disturbance

The management of daytime sleepiness begins with reducing sedating drugs to the smallest possible dose. The most likely culprits are antianxiety drugs, neuroleptics, muscle relaxants, and analgesics. The next step is maximizing out-of-bed time and finding a means, if possible, to keep patients physically active or at least cognitively in touch with the environment. Stimulants such as coffee, tea, and cola drinks can be used in the mornings and afternoons but not after the evening meal. The use of other stimulants is discussed in the section on management of apathy and withdrawal.

Nighttime sleeplessness is best combated by keeping patients active during the day and postponing bedtime until after 9 P.M. Generally speaking, it is best to have the patients keep the same bedtime every day of the week. Once depression, sleep apnea, and other medical causes of insomnia have been ruled out, small doses of various medications may be prescribed. Small doses of antidepressant medications may be used as sleep aids. These are not habit forming, tolerance does not develop, and withdrawal symptoms do not occur. The medications employed most commonly are 0.5–1 mg of haloperidol, 2 mg of trifluoperazine, 50–100 mg of trazodone, 10–25 mg of thioridazine, 10–25 mg of imipramine, and 10–40 mg of doxepin. The latter three medications have relatively strong anticholinergic properties, but these are useful at night for delaying bladder emptying, and the latter two medications potentiate the effect of analgesics for those persons whose sleep is disturbed by arthritis or other pain. The benzodiazepine hypnotics temazepam and triazolam may also be prescribed. Temazepam is administered in doses of 15–30 mg per hour before bedtime because of its slow absorption. Triazolam is administered in doses of 0.125–0.25 mg. Flurazepam has a half-life of more than 24 hours in healthy adults and 100–200 hours in elders and thus seems contraindicated in elders, dementia patients, or physically debilitated persons because of its potential for accumulation and clouding of sensorium. Other short-acting benzodiazepines such as oxazepam may also be used in 10- to 15-mg doses for nighttime sedation. However, these should be administered 1 hour before bedtime because of slow absorption. Barbiturates are contraindicated because they cloud sensorium, produce respiratory depression, and patients rapidly develop tolerance. Antihistamines may be relatively contraindicated in Alzheimer's disease because of their potential for causing anticholinergic delirium and in debilitated patients because of mucosal drying. Zolpidem, which is a rapid-acting nonbenzodiazepine hypnotic, has been proposed for use in elderly patients at a recommended dose of 5 mg. However, tolerance, withdrawal symptoms, and amnestic episodes occur, as with benzodiazepines (Ayd 1994).

Suspiciousness and Delusion Formation

Blaming others for not being able to find familiar objects is a common occurrence in dementia. Angry questions such as, "Where did you put my hair brush?" or "Why did you take the money from my dresser?" are common. Some dementias are engrafted on a suspicious, blaming premorbid personality. Dementia patients may develop general suspiciousness or may fix their suspicion on one person, usually a caregiver. On rare occasions, delusions of persecution develop, but they are seldom organized into a complex plot, as occurs in paranoid disorder or paranoid schizophrenia. After having ruled out aggravation of sensorial impairment by drugs or the development of a major depressive episode, the drugs of choice are the antipsychotic medications in the doses suggested in Table 6–1. Should increased confusion follow use of these drugs, an anticholinergic delirium should be suspected and the drug withheld or the dose lowered. Benzodiazepines are not generally useful in the management of suspicion and delusion formation unless they result from barbiturate or benzodiazepine withdrawal.

In most cases, suspiciousness and delusion formation do not abate completely with the use of drugs, but their interference with patient management and with the patient's daily living needs is usually reduced. For example, patients who formerly refused to eat because they feared poisoning may afterward refuse to eat only certain foods or only in certain circumstances.

Hallucinations

Many brain-damaged persons experience hallucinations. These hallucinations are usually visual but may be auditory, tactile, gustatory, or olfactory, depending in part on the damaged area of the brain and whether the damaged area becomes an irritable focus. Typical hallucinations of dementia were described previously. The presence of hallucinations per se is not an indication for psychotropic drugs. To the extent that dementia patients can regard hallucinations with humor or do not react to them (e.g., trying to catch an imagined intruder), no drug treatment is required. The development of hallucinations demands an investigation of etiology, which may include delirium due to prescribed or unprescribed drugs; infectious, metabolic, or toxic factors; severe depression; or a new environment. Hallucinations may also indicate the development of an irritable brain focus.

The primary treatment of hallucinations (usually visual but sometimes tactile) due to delirium consists of treating the underlying condition. The use of drugs in delirium was discussed previously. Auditory hallucinations commanding a severely depressed person to commit suicide are best treated by ECT. Less threatening auditory hallucinations may remit with the use of a combined antipsychotic-antidepressant drug regimen. Hallucinations in other nondelirious dementia patients that are not due to an irritable focus are often not greatly ameliorated by psychotropic drugs. If patients become greatly disturbed by their hallucinations, antipsychotic drugs may be useful in less-than-full antipsychotic doses for reducing emotional distress.

Apathy and Withdrawal

After having ruled out major depression, stroke, the exacerbation of a chronic illness or the occurrence of an acute illness, various kinds of stimulation can be used to combat apathy and withdrawal. The first is social stimulation, as was discussed previously.

The psychostimulants dextroamphetamine and methylphenidate have been used successfully to treat apathy and anergy developing in the course of a physical illness (Woods et al. 1986). Several reports have appeared on the treatment of AIDS dementia complex (ADC) with both drugs (Fernandez et al. 1988a, 1988b). These patients responded promptly, whether symptoms of depression were due to affective disorder or ADC. Significant side effects, other than an uncovering or worsening of existing dyskinesias, were not found. Appetite stimulation was observed in lower dose ranges. Psychostimulants should be avoided in patients with a history of seizures, and special care must be taken in patients with a history of manic-depressive illness and in the face of congestive heart failure or significant hypertension.

Based on experience with three very old dementia patients (ages 81, 86, and 95 years), methylphenidate has been proposed as a first-line approach in very old, long-institutionalized dementia patients who become apathetic and stop eating (Maletta and Winegarden 1993). In the three patients treated, response times ranged from 2 to 10 days, with optimal response to 10 mg po on arising and at noon. No adverse effects occurred. One patient was successfully tapered off the medication after 9 months; another after 2 years. The third was still on the medication after 16 months at the time of the report. It was not possible to determine whether these patients were depressed, because they lacked the ability to convey their mood state.

Methylphenidate is preferable to dextroamphetamine because it produces minimal appetite suppression and has a half-life of 2–6 hours, in contrast to 18 hours for dextroamphetamine. It is initiated at 5- to 10-mg increases in total daily dose every 2 or 3 days. The average response range in ADC is 30–45 mg daily; as much as 120 mg qd has been required. Methylphenidate in very old patients (age 80+ years) may be effective in dosages as small as 1.25 mg qd (Gurian and Rosowsky 1993).

Oral pemoline has been suggested as a potential third-line drug in ADC, conferring the advantage of once-away dosing (Goodkin 1988).

Inappropriate Sexuality

A number of case reports indicate that the antiandrogen medroxyprogesterone is effective in reducing sexual drive and sexually aggressive acts in both cognitively intact and brain damaged men, including AD patients (Cooper 1988). With daily or weekly dosing, side effects are minimal and include blood pressure elevation and pedal edema. We found in two cases that doses of 150–200 mg of medroxyprogesterone acetate im every other week eliminated hypersexual behavior within a month (Weiner et al. 1992). One was a long-standing pedophile whose behavior was aggravated by a brain injury; the other was an AD patient. The pedophile died within 6 months. The AD patient's treatment was discontinued after 6 months, with no return of aggressive hypersexual behavior but with a continued tendency to touch women who sat next to him.

We employed medroxyprogesterone to reduce nonsexual aggression in dementia patients on several occasions but found it ineffective at 200 mg im every other week.

Nootropic Drugs

The term *nootropic* was coined by Giurgea (1972), who combined the Greek *noos* (mind) with *tropein* (toward) to designate psychoactive drugs that selectively improve efficiency of learning and protect against the effects of hypoxia or electroconvulsive shock on learning. Other terms such as *cognitive enhancers* and *cerebroactive drugs* have been proposed to designate the broad class of drugs that appear to improve cognitive function by putative mechanisms ranging from facilitation of cerebral blood flow to enhancement of neuronal metabolism (Spagnoli and Tognoni 1983).

In this section, the discussion concerns drugs or substances currently available by prescription or as food substances in the United States or other countries for enhancing cognition. Promising and experimental drugs or substances are discussed in Chapter 11. None of the drugs discussed has had more than modest effects when administered to large groups of patients, despite individual reports of marked improvement. No differences have yet been found between responders and nonresponders. There are other important flaws in many older drug studies. They are often uncontrolled. Many investigators did not differentiate between types of dementia. Ratings were frequently the unsystematized subjective reports of patients and their families. Even in the best of studies, it is not possible to be certain of patients' diagnoses without postmortem confirmation. There is a clear need for antemortem markers for the various dementing diseases to enable physicians to provide effective drug treatment. It must also be recognized that enhancement of cognition is only a palliative treatment in dementia due to progressive brain disease.

Vasodilators

In theory, vasodilators might be useful in cases of cerebrovascular insufficiency, but there is no evidence for their efficacy. Studies with the vasodilator acetazolamide have shown that blood flow actually diminishes in ischemic areas after drug administration because it reduces perfusion pressure throughout the brain and results in a "steal" of blood from areas of high resistance (Bonte et al. 1986a; P. Cook and James 1981). Nevertheless, putative cerebrovascular dilators are widely used. The prototypical drug is the alkaloid papaverine, which is also used to treat peripheral vascular disease. It acts by reducing smooth muscle spasm. Side effects include nausea, abdominal distress, anorexia, constipation, diarrhea, general malaise, and drowsiness.

Blood Viscosity Reducers and Antiplatelet Drugs

This class of drugs would seem a logical means to slow or arrest the progress of vascular dementia (VaD). Prevention of sludging and platelet aggregation should prevent the formation of clots on arterial atherosclerotic plaques and possibly help maintain arteriolar patency.

Aspirin is the most widely used drug of this class. In low doses, aspirin inhibits the enzyme cyclooxygenase, which is responsible for the synthesis by platelets of thromboxane, a substance that promotes platelet aggregation and causes vasodilating properties of prostacyclin (Amano and Meyer 1978). Aspirin's effectiveness in preventing transient ischemic attacks and reducing thrombotic strokes and myocardial infarction is well known (Aspirin Myocardial Infarction Study Research Group 1980; W. S. Fields et al. 1987; Swedish Cooperative Study Group 1987). In a randomized study of 70 VaD patients (325 mg aspirin qd versus no treatment), Meyer et al. (1989) demonstrated actual improvement in the cognitive state of the aspirin-treated patients over the first 2 years of a 3-year follow-up period, whereas the control group deteriorated slightly. Studies of cerebral blood flow with ^{133}Xe showed improvement in the aspirin-treated group and deterioration in the no-treatment group over the same period.

Ticlopidine hydrochloride is a platelet antiaggregant that inhibits the adenosine diphosphate pathway of platelet aggregation. It does not inhibit the cyclooxygenase pathway, or block the production of thromboxane by platelets or the production of prostacyclin by endothelial cells (Hass et al. 1989). When compared with placebo in 1,072 subjects with completed strokes, ticlopidine (250 mg bid) reduced the rate of stroke or stroke death by 33.5% over 3 years (Gent et al. 1989). Compared with aspirin at a dose of 325 mg qid, 250 mg bid ticlopidine reduced the rate of strokes in more than 3,000 persons with prior cerebrovascular symptoms (transient ischemic attacks, amaurosis fugax, mild stroke), 21% more than did aspirin, and was equally effective in men and women (Hass et al. 1989). The chief side effects of ticlopidine are diarrhea and skin rash. An uncommon but important side effect is severe reversible neutropenia, which occurs within the first 3 months of treatment.

Pentoxyphilline is a xanthine derivative reported to reduce blood viscosity by increasing fibrinolytic activity, inhibiting platelet aggregation, and increasing the flexibility of red blood cells (Spagnoli and Tognoni 1983). Its effectiveness in VaD was shown in early double-blind studies (Harwart 1979), but a more recent review suggests lack of efficacy in stroke prevention (Fitzgerald 1987); it is dosed at 400 mg tid. Nausea, dizziness, and abdominal discomfort are the principal side effects.

Metabolic Enhancers

The three ergoloid mesylates—dihydroergocornine mesylate, dihydroergocristine mesylate, and dihydroergocryptine (in equal proportions by weight)—comprise Hydergine, the most widely used of the nootropic drugs. In use for nearly 50 years, Hydergine was thought originally to be a vasodilator. It does appear to correct EEG alterations in models of impaired brain function and in vivo appears to be a central nervous system dopamine and serotonin agonist (Loew and Weil 1982). It is thought to be useful in treating both AD and VaD. There are a number of major reviews of Hydergine studies (C. P. Hughes et al. 1976; Loew and Weil 1982). McDonald (1979) found that Hydergine significantly improved 13 of 32 symptoms in at least 50% of six or more double-blind studies. The specific effects after 12 weeks were increased alertness, recent memory, self-care, cooperation, sociability, and appetite, with decreased confusion, emotional lability, anxiety and/or fears, dizziness, fatigue, and bothersomeness. The most recent large study reported no effectiveness of the drug in AD (Thompson et al. 1990), and a meta-analysis of 47 double-blind, placebo-controlled randomized clinical trials suggested only a modest overall clinical effect, somewhat stronger for VaD and little efficacy for AD. A dose-response relationship suggested greater efficacy with doses higher than currently approved (Schneider and Olin 1994). Conventional dosage is 1 mg tid. In our experience, doses up to 9 mg qd are well tolerated; an adequate trial is 3–6 months. Side effects are uncommon and include nausea and agitation. Because of its mild stimulant effect, Hydergine is probably contraindicated in patients with known seizures. Its use was associated with new onset of seizures in one of the authors' (M.F.W.) AD patients and aggravation of preexisting seizure disorder in another. Our clinical impression is that Hydergine increases energy, interaction with others, and attention span without increasing memory.

Piracetam

Piracetam is a cyclic γ-aminobutyric acid (GABA) derivative without GABA-like side effects. It is available in Europe as Nootropil. Studies of doses ranging from 2.4 to 9.5 g qd have shown no consistent positive effect (Branconnier 1983; Schneck 1983; Wittenborn 1981).

Drugs Affecting the Cholinergic System (see also Chapter 14)

Precursors of acetylcholine (ACh), cholinomimetics, and anticholinesterases have been used in the treatment of AD. Their use is based on the discovery of reduced cholinergic function in AD (P. Davies and Maloney 1976) and on research on the effects of anticholinergic and cholinomimetic drugs on memory. Drachman and Leavitt (1974) showed scopolamine impairment of information storage in long-term memory with relative sparing of recall and retrieval from long-term memory—a finding that resembles the impairment of normal aging. The effect of scopolamine on memory is reversed by physostigmine (Granacher and Baldessarini 1976). Furthermore, physostigmine has direct memory-enhancing effects when carefully titrated in humans (Davis et al. 1978). Physostigmine at low doses also enhances memory in nonhuman primates (Bartus 1979). Based on these findings, three main strategies have been employed to increase cholinergic transmission: increasing substrate available for the biosynthesis of ACh, using cholinomimetics to augment ACh activity, and blocking the degradation of ACh to prolong its activity at the receptor site.

Precursors

ACh is produced in the brain by the acetylation of choline through the action of the enzyme choline acetyltransferase and the cofactor coenzyme A. In rats, increasing the amount of substrate available increases the concentration of ACh in the brain (Cohen and Wurtman 1976). Thus, studies have been conducted using choline chloride or phosphatidylcholine (lecithin) to augment ACh production. Fovall et al. (1983) reported mild improvement in cognition and behavior in patients treated for less than 2 months with choline in doses ranging from 1 to 16 g qd but that this finding was consistent with fluctuations in functional level often seen in the course of the disease. Lecithin administration had no effect on AD patients in another study, despite a two- to fourfold increase in plasma choline concentration (Etienne 1983). Thus, there is little evidence for the effectiveness of lecithin.

Acetyl-L-carnitine has been marketed in Italy as Nicetile since 1985. It is a naturally occurring substance that may help in the formation of acetyl coenzyme A or acetylcholine. It has been used in AD and VaD (Ravizza et al. 1988). A placebo-controlled pilot study suggested modest efficacy in AD (Sano et al. 1992). At a dose of 2 g qd, side effects are minimal. They include increased excitability, insomnia, abdominal discomfort, itching, vomiting, and diarrhea.

Anticholinesterases

Tacrine was marketed in the United States in 1993 for the treatment of mild-to-moderate AD. It is a reversible cholinesterase inhibitor that has been in use for more than 40 years. It is taken orally, reaches maximal plasma concentration in 1–2 hours, and has a half-life of 2–4 hours. It is metabolized principally by the cytochrome P_{450}-1A2 system. Age does not appear to affect tacrine clearance, but plasma concentrations are higher in women than in men. Smoking lowers plasma tacrine concentrations by one-third, presumably through induction of the cytochrome P_{450} system. Its multiple possible mechanisms of action are discussed in Chapter 15.

Outcome of therapeutic trials.   Therapeutic effects are dose related but modest. Response is not usually seen with doses below 80 mg qd (Davis and Powchik 1995). Early large trials were conducted with low doses (40–80 mg qd) because of liver toxicity, but a 30-week randomized, placebo-controlled trial of 40 mg qid has been reported (Knapp et al. 1994). In keeping with findings of earlier treatment studies (Davis et al. 1992; Farlow et al. 1992), only 28% of mildly to moderately impaired outpatients were able to remain on the drug for the entire 30 weeks. Reasons for noncompletion included liver enzyme elevations to three times the upper limit of normal (28%) and cholinergic side effects (16%), primarily nausea and vomiting. Of patients who developed liver enzyme abnormalities, in the 30-week study, 87% were successfully restarted and carried on the drug over 3 months in the open-label phase of the study. Clinicians rated 42% of tacrine-treated patients who completed the 30 weeks as improved, compared with 18% of placebo-treated individuals. Placebo-treated patients declined an average of 2 points on the Alzheimer's Disease Assessment Scale (Rosen et al. 1984), compared with a mean improvement of 2 points (of 70) for patients treated with 160 mg tacrine qd.

Toxicity and side effects.   Liver toxicity as documented by serum alanine aminotransferase (ALT) elevation above the upper normal limit occurred in approximately 50% of 2,446 study patients (Watkins et al. 1994). ALT levels greater than three times the upper normal limit were observed in 25% of the patients and greater than 20 times upper normal in 2% of the patients. The majority (90%) of the ALT elevations above 3 times the upper normal limit occurred within the first 12 weeks of treatment at a mean of 7 weeks. Women were more often affected than men. Discontinuation of treatment led to normalization of liver function within 4–6 weeks, and there was no case of death due to tacrine-induced liver toxicity.

Other side effects commonly associated with tacrine were nausea, vomiting, abdominal distress, anorexia, bradycardia, myalgia, and ataxia.

Dosing.   Tacrine is dosed for the first 6 weeks at 10 mg qid. Liver enzyme levels (ALT) are checked biweekly for the first 6 weeks, then monthly for 2 months, and afterward can be checked every 3 months. Tacrine is titrated upward every 6 weeks to a maximum of 40 mg qid. Nausea can be eased by administering tacrine with meals, but lower blood levels result. Maximal absorption can be achieved by giving the drug at least 1 hour before meals.

The manufacturer recommends reduction of tacrine dose by 40 mg qd if ALT rises to three to five times the upper limit of normal and drug discontinuation for enzyme elevations greater than five times the upper limit of normal. Patients may be rechallenged when ALT level returns to normal but not if jaundice occurs or bilirubin rises to > 3 mg/dl. The drug should be discontinued gradually, because severe worsening of cognitive impairment may accompany sudden withdrawal.

Contraindications.   Important drug-drug interactions occur with theophylline and cimetidine. Tacrine elevates theophylline levels, and cimetidine raises tacrine levels (Watkins et al. 1994). The drug should not be administered to persons with active peptic ulcer disease, asthma, significant bradycardia, or compromised liver function. The drug produces direct hepatocellular damage.

Length of treatment.   It is unclear what is an appropriate trial of tacrine after a total dose of 160 mg qd has been achieved. If obvious deterioration has occurred, it is probably pointless to continue the drug. If there has been no change or an improvement in the patient's condition, it seems reasonable to continue the drug for at least a year or until significant further decline occurs. Withdrawal of tacrine treatment needs to be gradual. There are many anecdotal reports of significant cognitive worsening following sudden tacrine withdrawal.

Serotonin Uptake Blockers

Because of evidence that patients with alcoholic amnestic disorder have low brain serotonergic activity (Branchey et al. 1985), treatment of this disorder with a serotonin uptake blocker was instituted. The serotonin uptake blocker fluvoxamine in doses of 100–200 mg qd administered over 4 weeks produced significant improvement of memory tests involving vigilance, free recall, and recognition in six patients with alcoholic amnestic disorder and no change in three patients with alcohol-related dementia or in one patient with compensated alcoholic liver disease (P. R. Martin et al. 1989). There was an inverse relationship between plasma fluvoxetine level and cerebrospinal fluid 5-hydroxyindoleacetic acid (5-HIAA), as would be expected.

This finding must be regarded as preliminary because of the small numbers of patients involved and the much more severe impairment of the patients with alcoholic dementia.

Summary

Physicians have at their disposal many effective drugs for the amelioration of dementia-related emotional states and behaviors and of emotional states or behaviors that are worsened by dementia. The dosage of these medications depends in part on patients' general physical state and in part on the nature of the dementing illness. Many effective drugs have important side effects and toxicity. Neuroleptic malignant syndrome, paradoxical hypertension from MAOIs, and withdrawal from minor tranquilizers can be life threatening. Parkinsonian symptoms and tardive dyskinesia from neuroleptics or tremor from lithium can be disabling. Thus, although drugs do much to enhance the quality of life of some patients, they may also do much damage if prescribed inappropriately or not monitored adequately. In progressive dementing disease, different medication regimens may be required at different stages of the illness. Early on, an antidepressant may be indicated; later, an antipsychotic may be needed to deal with restlessness; and ultimately, stimulants may be necessary to combat apathy and withdrawal. An anticholinesterase drug that has modest effects on cognitive deficit has been marketed for treatment of AD, and more are in development.

CHAPTER 7

Neuropsychological Evaluation of Dementia

Ronald G. Paulman, Ph.D.
Elisabeth Koss, Ph.D.
William D. MacInnes, Ph.D.

Identifying cognitive deficit in moderate to severe cases of dementia is easily accomplished by the experienced clinician through mental status examination. However, in many persons with early presentation of mental processing difficulties, memory decline, or behavioral change, comprehensive neuropsychological evaluation is indicated (McKhann et al. 1984). Unlike traditional clinical psychological assessment, clinical neuropsychological evaluation employs techniques with a demonstrated relation to brain function. Therefore, the clinical neuropsychologist assumes an important role in the diagnosis of dementia, particularly in its early stages, by providing inferences concerning likely etiology and by characterizing cognitive abilities to assist patient management and disposition planning.

Specific Goals of Neuropsychological Assessment

Describing Adaptive Cognitive Functioning

Neuropsychological assessment describes cognitive function in behaviorally relevant terms. Traditional mental status examination does not assess many abilities related to everyday function such as taking medications properly, remembering appointments, managing money, cooking safely, or driving a car. However, comprehensive neuropsychological evaluation can give useful, objective information regarding these common questions (Moss and Albert 1988; Zec 1993). Neuropsychological testing places patients in a structured situation requiring effortful processing of both new and previously acquired information. By examining learning and performance on tasks, neuropsychologists are able to ascertain how patients will perform in the occupational or psychosocial setting. For example, does a business executive continue to possess the complex organizational abilities required to manage a large department with multiple, simultaneous needs? At the other end of the spectrum, is a widowed, elderly woman able to meet her needs in an independent living situation, or does she require placement in a structured setting?

Thus, neuropsychological assessment provides a quantified, comprehensive picture of problem-solving behavior that may confirm and extend observations made by family and other caregivers.

Diagnosis and Characterization of Dementia

An understanding of the cognitive patterns associated with "normal aging" (Lezak 1983) is an important prerequisite to identifying mental declines associated with dementia in older adults. Intellectual deficits do not become apparent until the seventh decade for many persons (Schaie 1983) and are primarily manifested for activities requiring executive function, visual-spatial processing, mental speed, and motor facility (M. S. Albert and Heaton 1988; Libbon et al. 1994). Moreover, physical health and education are typically associated with greater retention of intellectual abilities later in life (Friedland 1993; Heaton et al. 1986). Memory declines associated with aging have been described as "benign senescent forgetfulness" (Kral 1978) and "age-associated memory impairment" (Crook et al. 1986). However, criteria for applying these terms are not uniform, and there remains a high degree of individual variability in memory functions among elderly individuals.

Cognitive changes observed as part of the natural process of aging are trivial compared with those observed in persons with dementia (Koss et al. 1991). Memory loss is the common abnormality in all the dementias. Also present are varying degrees of disturbance in awareness, orientation, insight, general behavior, general information, language function, praxis, visuospatial function, topographical orientation, problem-solving ability, judgment, calculation, and emotion. These nonspecific dysfunctions cover all cognitive domains and are associated with normal aging as well. Their intensity, qualitative differences, unique symptom constellation, and progressive nature all serve to distinguish them from normal aging.

As noted in Chapter 1, diagnostic criteria for dementia include impairment in short- and long-term memory and at least one of the following: aphasia, apraxia, agnosia, and impairment in executive functioning (American Psychiatric Association 1994). These deficits must also cause decline in social or occupational functioning.

Multilevel assessment of cognitive changes in an individual patient offers the best opportunity for discriminating age-related from disease-related changes in cognitive status (Albert 1988). A patient's performance on neuropsychological tests is thus combined with historical, developmental, educational, and medical information to assist in the diagnosis of dementia. Both the age and education of patients must be taken into account to make a diagnosis. For example, low performance by an individual of limited premorbid intelligence, education, or occupational attainment may not suggest a dementing condition. Conversely, average performance of cognitive tasks by a university professor may signal the onset of a dementing illness. The inability to use level of performance alone to diagnose dementia necessitates integration of all information relevant to a patient's past and present functioning.

Recommendations for Intervention

In addition to describing cognitive function and assisting diagnosis, neuropsychological evaluation leads to specific recommendations concerning further evaluation and treatment. These might include considering neuroimaging studies (if not yet performed); giving behavioral prescriptions to compensate for specific cognitive deficits such as memory, language, or visual-spatial impairments; or designing strategies for management of the living environment.

Components of a Comprehensive Neuropsychological Evaluation for Dementia

A comprehensive neuropsychological evaluation assesses several converging areas through 1) compiling the patient's developmental, medical, social, and educational historical data; 2) interviewing the patient and at least one family member, friend, or caregiver familiar with the patient's recent and past functional abilities; 3) examining a wide range of both general and specific cognitive abilities; and 4) evaluating emotional and personality functions. Elements of these examinations are described in depth in the following sections.

History

The past and present context of a patient's life influences interpretation of evaluation results. Though the objective score on a particular test is exactly the same for two individuals, its meaning may be different based on cultural background and educational or professional achievement. Neuropsychological assessment therefore begins with a systematic inquiry into a patient's early medical and developmental history; language acquisition; school grades, including any special programming; military record (if relevant); occupational experience; and acquired insults to the central nervous system (CNS) such as head trauma, toxin exposures, or neurological conditions. Present medical history is also important in that conditions such as diabetes, hypertension, cardiac problems, kidney or liver disease, and chronic obstructive pulmonary disease can all influence neuropsychological function (see Chapter 4). Past psychiatric history and treatment are also important, particularly current medication regimen. Functions such as attention and memory are susceptible in the elderly to disruption by medications such as anxiolytics or antidepressants with anticholinergic side effects (Weiner and Davis 1986).

Interviewing

The clinical interview of a patient with suspected dementia is covered in Chapter 1 and is therefore not discussed at length here. The availability of external sources of information is critically important in corroborating the information gathered during a patient interview for dementia. Although observational data from the patient's physical appearance, motor function, level of awareness, sensory impairments, and speech are easily obtained in interview, the content of a dementia patient's self-report is often unreliable. Persons coming for a dementia evaluation may be uncooperative, give unreliable (sometimes confabulated) answers to questions, or simply have memory difficulties. It is always important to have a close relative or caregiver present when conducting an initial mental status examination or clinical interview. Such caregiver appraisals concerning memory deficits in Alzheimer's disease (AD) patients frequently correlate well with objective test measures (Koss et al. 1993).

Intellectual Assessment

Intelligence testing is frequently a component of the cognitive workup for dementia. The Wechsler Adult Intelligence Scale—Revised (WAIS-R; Wechsler 1981) evaluates academically acquired knowledge in addition to many global verbal and visual-motor problem-solving skills important in daily life. As such, it can often provide a standardized index of general cognitive function compared with age peers, an estimate of a person's new learning capacity, and often (in nonaphasic individuals) an indication of premorbid level. Results of intelligence testing may suggest a diagnosis of dementia but are often not sufficient to make such a diagnosis.

Neuropsychological Testing

Several assessment strategies applied to the neuropsychological evaluation of dementia include the use of standard neuropsychological batteries, individual tests in a "process" approach, and specialized dementia batteries (Koss et al. 1993). The Halstead-Reitan Neuropsychological Battery (HRB; Reitan and Wolfson 1993) is a well-validated tool for assessing general neuropsychological function that has seen recent application to dementia (Hom 1992). However, its length (5 or more hours), limited memory assessment, and lack of specificity for dementia (Moss and Albert 1988) limit its value for patients with more than mild impairment, despite recent upward extension of norms to the elderly population (Heaton et al. 1991).

The Luria-Nebraska Neuropsychological Battery (LNNB; Golden et al. 1986) is a standardization of Luria's clinical neuropsychological approach that takes less time (3 hours) to administer than the HRB. Although the LNNB provides a useful cross section of selected cognitive abilities in normal elders and dementia patients (Gillen et al. 1983; MacInnes et al. 1983), it does not provide a comprehensive assessment of memory.

The individual test or "process" approach to neuropsychological assessment (Milberg et al. 1986) includes tests chosen according to patient characteristics and referral question. As testing progresses, instruments may be added that follow up specific areas of difficulty seen on initial measures. Although the process approach may not employ standardized batteries, tests from such batteries are frequently included. Consistent with the battery approach, interpretations are partially based on age- and/or education-corrected scores. However, the process through which solutions are achieved by patients is critical to conclusions concerning cognitive function. Assessment is therefore tailored to the needs of each individual and situation. The process approach has the disadvantage, however, of not always allowing comparison of test results across different subjects in research.

Attention and Concentration

The capacity to attend to salient environmental stimuli is a prerequisite of adaptive behavior in all organisms. In humans, attention and concentration underlie all higher neuropsychological processes (Albert 1988). Although often thought to be a volitional activity, attention is a highly complex activity involving the reticular, thalamic, and frontal systems of the brain (Wilkins et al. 1987). In dementing conditions, the fine-tuned balance between vigilance to all novel stimuli and the focus on those stimuli most relevant to survival is frequently disrupted. Thus, impaired selective attention in dementia patients leads them to be either highly distractible or excessively focused, thereby missing important environmental cues. Accompanying problems in sustaining or dividing their attention are also usually present (Albert 1988; Butters et al. 1987; Lines et al. 1991).

Selective attention may be assessed in numerous ways. The ability to track digit sequences and perform mental arithmetic problems on the WAIS-R is associated with selective attention. Moreover, selective attention is also required in the discrimination of rapidly paced auditory patterns (Seashore Rhythm Test) or visual stimuli in the presence of distractors (i.e., Stroop Color Word Test). Sustained attention may be evaluated through requiring patients to be vigilant for recurrent target stimuli in a long auditory or visual sequence. Divided attention tasks may require patients to add numbers presented on audiotape (Paced Auditory Serial Addition Test; Gronwall 1977), perform two tasks simultaneously (Paulman and Kennelly 1984), or alternate responding on a number-letter sequencing test (i.e., Trail-Making Test).

Because attention is frequently a hierarchically ordered ability, patients with mild dementia may demonstrate little impairment in simple selective or sustained attention though unable to divide or alternate their attentional focus. Conversely, patients with moderate to severe levels of dementia may have difficulty with all levels of attentional processing.

Conceptual and Executive Abilities

The capacity to think abstractly and flexibly is one of the early cognitive functions to become impaired in dementia (Holden 1988; LaRue 1988; Strub and Black 1988). A loss of executive processing abilities, such as organizing, planning, and evaluating one's problem-solving behavior, is also common early in the dementia process, even before memory deficits manifest (Baddeley et al. 1991; J. T. Becker 1988; Morris 1994). Executive brain functions are thought to be primarily mediated by the frontal lobes and are measured by neuropsychological tasks with ambiguous instructions such as the Wisconsin Card Sorting Test (Heaton 1981) or the Halstead-Reitan Category Test (Reitan and Wolfson 1993). These tasks require patients to generate and test hypotheses while using success-failure feedback to flexibly alter responses with changing task requirements.

Memory

Memory difficulties are among the most common problems reported by dementia patients, depressed individuals, healthy elderly adults, and their families. The clinician is faced with the task of determining whether a patient's memory problem is due to a neuropathological process, a psychiatric disturbance, or a normal variation. Memory is a higher-order process that includes the collection, storage, and retrieval of information. Memory is also a reconstructive process; hence, it is influenced by the emotional state of the individual and the congruity of the event with more established memories. As such, memory is an extremely complex construct and represents the integration of many functional systems of the brain (Squire 1992). Some inconsistency exists in the terminology used to describe memory functions. For example, neurologists often classify memory as immediate, recent, and remote; psychologists frequently refer to immediate memory as short-term or *primary memory*, recent memory as long-term or *secondary memory*, and remote memory as *tertiary memory* (Russell 1981; Zec 1993).

Memory involves a number of sequential cognitive processes. Information initially enters sensory memory, an extremely short-term storage modality measured in hundreds of milliseconds. From sensory memory, information is transmitted to short-term memory (also called primary memory, immediate memory, working memory, and attention span)

(Baddeley 1991; Hunt 1986). Short-term memory is a limited-capacity system in which information is maintained by continued attention and rehearsal. Short-term memory lasts only 20–30 seconds, with stored information replaced by new material unless rehearsal or some other retention strategy is introduced. Transfer of new information into long-term memory begins within the first second of exposure to the stimulus, providing for a 20- to 30-second overlap between short-term and long-term memory. The consolidation of material in long-term memory takes much longer and involves a gradual strengthening of the memory trace during a period of several minutes to several hours. This trace is highly unstable and easily subject to loss, as illustrated by anterograde amnesia in a postconcussive syndrome. Once information has entered long-term memory (of virtually unlimited capacity), it is maintained by repetition or organization through meaning and association (Albert 1988; MacInnes and Robbins 1987).

Memory retrieval is the process of locating and accessing information from long-term storage. Retrieval can be of two types: 1) direct verbatim access to memory storage traces, and 2) access to a general idea or gist of the original material with final output representing a reconstruction of this idea (Russell 1981). Another important distinction related to retrieval is between recall and recognition. Free recall is required on an essay test, for example, whereas recognition memory is evaluated in a multiple choice test. Problems in recognition memory often relate to faulty storage. This distinction can be very useful in differentiating the cognitive impairment associated with depression from dementia. Patients with a dementia syndrome such as AD often exhibit difficulties in both free recall and recognition memory (i.e., storage and retrieval problems), whereas depressed patients and normal elderly more frequently show only deficits in free recall (retrieval problems) (Albert 1988; Kaszniak et al. 1986). Two of the major forms of storage are episodic memory and semantic memory. *Episodic memory* refers to memories that have been given a temporal and spatial coding (Tulving 1972). This type of memory is associated with when and where something occurs (i.e., birth of one's first child). *Semantic memory* is a verbally mediated memory that lacks a spatial or temporal context (i.e., factual knowledge).

Both episodic and semantic memory have been categorized under the term *declarative memory. Nondeclarative memory* (sometimes called implicit or procedural memory) involves memory for overlearned skills and automatic perceptual or semantic processes that are not factually oriented (Zec 1993). Other memory distinctions include *verbal* versus *visual memory* and *retrograde* versus *anterograde amnesia* (Zec 1993).

None of the current measures of memory assesses all of the dimensions of memory. Nevertheless, formal memory tests, particularly those assessing verbal memory, better discriminate dementia patients from normal elderly than mental status exams or language tests (Christensen et al. 1991). Verbal memory measures include the Selective Reminding Test (Buschke and Fuld 1974) and the California Verbal Learning Test (CVLT; Delis et al. 1987). Such instruments have the advantage of multiple learning trials (versus one-time exposure to stimuli), adequate length to require secondary (long-term) memory, a delay condition, and a recognition trial. These are believed to be minimum criteria for the assessment of memory in AD (Zec 1993).

In contrast to the preceding list-learning verbal memory tasks, the Wechsler Memory Scale—Revised (WMS-R; Wechsler 1987) assesses paragraph-length information (stories). A disadvantage of the WMS-R and most other memory instruments is the lack of norms for the "old-old" (i.e., individuals above age 74 years in the case of the WMS-R).

Visual memory is evaluated by the WMS-R and by the Rey-Osterreith Complex Figure Test (Visser 1985). However, the required figure drawing on both tests frequently confounds the assessment of memory with motor skills. The Warrington Recognition Memory Test (Warrington 1984) is an excellent measure of both verbal and nonverbal memory (names and faces, respectively). It requires no motor output but lacks norms beyond age 70 years.

Visual-Spatial Functioning

Visual-spatial processes are complex and involve a variety of functional systems in the brain, particularly in the right hemisphere. Visual-constructional functioning is frequently evaluated through use of the WAIS-R Block Design task or figure drawing, with characteristic declines in quality seen as dementia progresses (Kirk and Kertesz 1991; Moss and Albert 1988; Zec 1993). Drawings of AD patients exhibit oversimplification, poor angulation, and impaired perspective (Kirk and Kertesz 1991). They may also display poor planning in their layout and presentation. In addition to central brain mechanisms, primary visual impairments and motor deficits may complicate the interpretation of constructional dyspraxia in the elderly.

Visual-spatial awareness may also be impaired in dementia and be manifested through agnosia. *Agnosia* is often defined as an inability to recognize sensory input despite the intactness of the sensory system itself (Holden 1988). Visual or object agnosia is an inability to name or demonstrate the use of common objects without some other sensory stimuli, such as touching the object or hearing its use. There is often a total lack of recognition of the object's meaning or character. *Spatial agnosia* is the inability to find one's way around even familiar places. Other agnosias include *color agnosia* (black-and-white or gray vision), *tactile agnosia* or *astereognosis* (inability to recognize objects by touch alone), and *autotopagnosia* (inability to localize, name, or correctly orient different parts of the body).

Problems with visual inattention or diminished self-awareness can also confuse the assessment process of the more complex aspects of visual-spatial analysis. In its extreme form, anosognosia, a patient may ignore a particular limb or state that it belongs to someone else. Visual inattention difficulties can represent a danger for the patient and must be assessed carefully.

Language

Receptive and expressive language abilities can be disrupted by a number of neurological disorders including dementing illnesses. Receptive language involves the comprehension of oral and written communication. Comprehension deficits may involve individual words or sentences. An individual may not be able to attach semantic meaning to words or understand their syntactical meaning within a sentence, that is, "lost woman's purse" versus "woman's lost purse." Visual comprehension of written material is based on auditory mastery and is also often disturbed when an individual has auditory comprehension deficits. In dementia, the appreciation of nonverbal components of language, such as tone, inflection, and facial or body movements, may also be impaired (Zec 1993).

Expressive language disturbances (disorders of production) can take numerous forms as well. These include disturbances of articulation, word finding, and paraphasia and the loss of grammar, syntax, repetition, verbal fluency, and writing (Kolb and Whishaw 1980). Speaking requires the ability to articulate individual vowels, consonants, and syllables and then combine them in the appropriate order to make interpretable words and sentences. To speak a word, it is necessary to locate it among the large repository of words previously learned. A dementia patient can often describe the use of an object but cannot name it. This dysnomia may be assessed through procedures such as the Boston Naming Test (Goodglass and Kaplan 1972). Paraphasia is the production of unintended syllables, sounds or words, such as substituting *knife* for *night* or *mother* for *woman*. Loss of grammar and syntax can also be affected and may manifest as the inability to string more than two or three words together in spontaneous sentences. Similarly, patients may be able to produce spontaneous normal speech but be unable to repeat words or sentences spoken by others.

Verbal fluency, the ability to produce words and sentences in uninterrupted strings, is affected by numerous factors including dysnomia associated with frontal and temporal lobe lesions. AD patients appear to have difficulty early in their illness in generating objects within a class (category fluency) yet remain relatively intact in generating words beginning with specific letters (letter fluency) (Binetti et al. 1995; Monsch et al. 1992, 1994; Zec 1993). Writing may also be disturbed in patients with dementia, although this may not be related to other language problems (LaBarge et al. 1992).

Motor Abilities

Motor abilities are graduated from simple functions such as strength and speed to more complex skilled movements (praxis). Basic motor deficits occur commonly in vascular and subcortical dementias and rarely in AD. An evaluation of motor functions is therefore an important component of neuropsychological testing. Simple motor strength is often assessed through use of a hand dynamometer, whereas manual speed may be tested through procedures requiring finger touch, rapid alternating hand movements, and finger tapping. Losses in motor strength and speed beyond expectations from a person's age and sex deserve further follow-up, particularly when lateralized.

Disorders of complex skilled movements that do not arise from basic motor difficulties are known as *apraxias* (Heilman et al. 1985). Patients may be unable to carry out a motor response on command that is easily performed spontaneously (ideomotor apraxia). Alternatively, they may be unable to sequence known motor acts toward a specific goal (ideational apraxia). These impairments in the production and organization of skilled behaviors are frequently present in advanced AD (Zec 1993). Evaluation of praxis may often involve instructing the patient to complete a series of common activities (i.e., preparing a cup of coffee) through both verbal command and pantomime.

Sensory-Perceptual Abilities

The interaction between performance on cognitive tests and perceptual deficits must be evaluated carefully. A substantial number of persons with dementia complain of visual problems for which no physical causes can be found. These complaints are often dismissed by clinicians and family members. Yet, several studies suggest the presence of prominent visual distortions in many AD patients in one or more of the following domains: color vision, depth perception, detection of movement, eye movements, low-contrast sensitivity, and higher order visual perception (Cronin-Colomb et al. 1991; Mendez et al. 1990). These complications, which can occur early in the disease process, are likely to affect reading and successful performance on visually related tasks that are common in a typical test battery.

Auditory comprehension difficulties likewise may be present and adversely influence performance, above and beyond the negative effect of the dementing process. Aphasic-like difficulties, of the Wernicke type, are not uncommon even in the early stages of dementia (Au et al. 1988). Comprehension deficits may arise also from attentional deficits, difficulty in changing tasks, and perhaps general slowness of neurological responses (Obler and Albert 1981). Finally, although of less immediate relevance to cognitive testing, prominent olfactory sensory dysfunction may occur early in the disease process in a majority of AD patients (Koss et al. 1988).

Cognitive deterioration may thus appear to be exaggerated because of undetected deficits in sensory function. Conversely, sensory distortions should be recognized as they present additional challenges to an already weakened system of cognitive processing.

Through medical record review, history taking with caregivers, and direct observation of the patient, the clinician frequently identifies primary sensory impairments before onset of neuropsychological testing. Formal assessment of sensory-perceptual functions may by undertaken in patients without severe sensory impairments to provide information concerning lateralized brain dysfunction, potentially useful to identification of focal vascular or neoplastic conditions. The Reitan-Kløve Sensory-Perceptual Examination (Reitan and Wolfson 1993) and the LNNB Tactile Scale (Golden et al. 1985) are two procedures that assess several basic receptive functions.

Specialized Dementia Batteries

A number of instruments have been developed with the primary purpose of identifying dementia. The Mini-Mental State Examination (MMSE; Folstein et al. 1975) (see also Chapter 1) stands in a category of its own, as a short composite screening instrument for dementia, without pretense of measuring separate cognitive functions. This test has gained such wide popularity that MMSE scores have become a convenient means to assess dementia severity. Screening instruments such as the MMSE have the merit of being brief, easy to administer, reliable, and sensitive but lack specificity.

An early successful attempt to develop a battery directly geared toward the cognitive problems of AD patients can be found in the Mattis Dementia Rating Scale (1988). In this scale, the items are administered in order of decreasing rather than increasing difficulty. By giving the most difficult item first, credit can be given for less taxing items, with a considerable time saving for intact subjects. Nevertheless, this scale takes about 45 minutes with a moderately impaired AD patient and does not provide reliable estimates of the different areas of cognition evaluated.

The Consortium to Establish a Registry for Alzheimer's Disease (CERAD), a federally funded research effort supported by 21 sites in the United States, has adopted a basic neuropsychological battery evaluating memory, language functions, and constructional praxis. This test battery evaluates acquisition of new information (with a list learning task), secondary memory (through delayed recall and recognition), language functions (with a semantic retrieval task and a shortened version of the Boston Naming test), and constructional praxis (by copy of simple geometric figures). This standardized approach, combined with appropriate medical and laboratory examinations, has increased the specificity of the diagnosis of AD, with an autopsy-confirmed hit rate of 80%–90% (Morris et al. 1989).

With progression of AD and other dementias, scores quickly "bottom out" (floor effect), and patients are untestable with traditional techniques. It then becomes necessary to resort to clinical observation or to the informant for obtaining some information about the progression of the disease and the pattern of cognitive ability decline. The Severe Impairment Battery (SIB; Saxton et al. 1990) was developed to evaluate the cognitive functioning of patients who are untestable by standard neuropsychological tests. This 20-minute test incorporates downward extensions of standard instruments. The subscales are attention, orientation, language, memory, visuospatial ability, construction, praxis, and estimation of social interactions skills. As with all new tests, the SIB will require further research to determine its validity and reliability. This test, however, stands alone in its assessment of more advanced dementia and in its clever incorporation of social interaction skills in the testing situation.

Personality and Emotional Assessment

Clinical interviewing of patients with suspected dementia is sometimes difficult because of expressive language impairments, lack of insight into internal mood states, or uncooperativeness. The use of standardized clinical psychological tests can provide the additional structure required by some patients by allowing them to respond through a written, less personal modality. Instruments such as the Minnesota Multiphasic Personality Inventory—2 (Hathaway and McKinley 1989), Beck Depression Inventory (Beck et al. 1961), and the Geriatric Depression Scale (Yesavage et al. 1983) allow a patient's emotional functioning to be compared to that of peers of the same age and sex. These findings can often provide the neuropsychologist with important information not immediately available from either the patient or other informants. Assessment of psychological functioning is therefore an integral part of the neuropsychological evaluation for dementia.

Reporting Neuropsychological Results

Results of a comprehensive neuropsychological evaluation for dementia are presented in three ways. A verbal report is frequently given to the referral source immediately on completion of the assessment. This allows for immediate scheduling for any necessary medical tests or other procedures suggested by neuropsychological findings. This initial report is followed by an extensive written report containing the patient's relevant history, clinical interview data, and intellectual and neuropsychological results. Conclusions are made concerning the presence of dementia and its likely etiology, if possible. A description of adaptive functioning in a variety of areas is also made and prognostic statements offered concerning relationships with personal, occupational, and psychosocial functioning. Specific recommendations are made for further medical and psychological testing, treatment, disposition, or further reevaluation. Finally, a reporting session is held with the patient and/or primary caregiver. At this session, findings are presented in everyday language with frequent use of real-life examples to illustrate an individual's strengths and deficits. Families or other caregivers are also given help in devising a strategy for patient management in the home, along with the names of resources in the community from which to seek further information or assistance.

Cognitive Patterns of Various Types of Dementia

Alzheimer's Disease

AD accounts for between 50% (Albert and Moss 1988) and 80% (Evans et al. 1989) of all dementias in adults. The heterogeneity in the behavioral manifestations and speed of progression of AD frequently complicate its early identification (Friedland 1988). Early or mild AD is associated with losses in recent (secondary) memory, with problems seen eventually in all stages of memory, including storage, consolidation, and retrieval (Kaszniak et al. 1986; Morris 1994). Associated symptoms may include declines in abstract reasoning, attention, word finding, and visual-constructional skills in the absence of significant sensory-motor deficits (Hom 1992; Zec 1993).

For family and caregivers, memory deficits and withdrawal from previous interests often constitute their earliest observations of change in persons with AD. The early AD patient may initially have decreased episodic memory for events of the past few months or weeks. He or she may forget significant recent life activities and display lapses during conversations. This retrograde amnesia progresses to loss of information from preceding days, hours, and minutes as the disease advances.

In early AD, patients are often acutely aware of subtle declines in memory. They may resort to written reminders though frequently cannot keep up with these or forget to refer to them. During this period of heightened awareness, AD patients may experience significant dysphoria. With increasing difficulty in remembering and following conversations comes a tendency to withdraw further from activities that bring exposure to embarrassing and/or perplexing situations. Eventually, these patients do very little. Often, they do not leave their homes and do not watch television, read, listen to the radio, or participate in conversations at mealtime. Their memory deficits hinder their ability to connect the present with the past few minutes, shrinking their world to the immediate present. The paranoid ideation developed by some AD patients may partially reflect an attempt to make sense of their confusing, unpredictable, and frightening world.

Language impairments may begin with word-finding problems and ultimately progress to highly paraphasic or incoherent speech. Visual-spatial deficits may also become apparent, with patients losing their sense of direction or constructional skills. Apraxias eventually develop, with patients unable to perform once-familiar tasks such as sewing, dressing, athletics, or driving an automobile. These problems usually occur in the context of normal motor strength and speed. All of the preceding impairments lead to significant impairments in the ability of the individual to live safely without supervision. The following case example illustrates some of these points:

> R.M. was a 65-year-old retired merchant with a history of increasing memory impairments over the previous 12 months. R.M.'s computed tomography (CT) brain scan showed mild cortical atrophy with mildly enlarged lateral ventricles and somewhat prominent sulci. His regional cerebral blood flow studies and neurological and physical exams were all within normal limits. R.M.'s initial performance on the neuropsychological evaluation showed a variety of deficits for an individual of his age and education. He demonstrated moderate to severe short-term and intermediate memory deficits in both verbal and visual modalities. R.M. also displayed some difficulty in repeating simple words and phrases, but this did not appear to be an articulation disorder. He had difficulty processing complex verbal information. When instructions were longer than one sentence, R.M. had a difficult time following them and often had to have them repeated. His performance on both fine and gross motor tasks and his ability to discriminate pitch patterns and rhythmic relationships were intact. R.M.'s basic reading, writing, and arithmetic skills were within the expected range, although he did have some problems with spelling. Novel material was especially difficult for him to grasp. Throughout the test administration, R.M. was alert, oriented, responsive, and was able to attend to the tasks quite well. It was also observed that in the testing context, R.M. was acutely aware of his difficulties in remembering and following instructions. He consistently sought reassurance that his responses were acceptable. He did not exhibit significant signs of depression but appeared anxious, particularly when he was having cognitive difficulty.
>
> When R.M. was reevaluated 12 months later, he clearly exhibited a significant cognitive decline, showing additional memory deficits and visual-spatial deficits, including visual naming difficulties and visual-spatial organization deficits. He began having more serious receptive language deficits that affected his ability to follow lengthy conversations. He also exhibited problems with relational concepts and logical-grammatical relationships. Simple arithmetic was also now difficult for him. Lastly, there was increased slowing in speed of mental processing. These measurable neuropsychological declines coincided with his family's report of overall functional declines at home. R.M.'s pattern of cognitive deficits, prior history, current medical data, and clear progression of slow, steady cognitive decline made AD the most likely diagnosis. Because of the decline in objective neuropsychological measures, his family was able to make informed decisions about his care and management. A guardianship was established for him soon after his second evaluation, and he was moved to a facility providing 24-hour supervision.

Vascular Dementia

Vascular dementia (VaD) accounts for 15%–20% of dementia cases (Cummings and Mahler 1991). This dementing disease, which may have both cortical and subcortical manifestations, includes the presence of neurological signs (i.e., gait abnormality, weakness in extremities, bradykinesia). Neuropsychologically, there is considerable overlap between the cognitive impairments of AD and VaD. This is further complicated by the fact that AD and VaD may coexist (Tomlinson 1977). Intelligence and memory deficits are frequently identical in the two groups when clinical severity of dementia is equivalent (Metter and Wilson 1993). Neuropsychological evaluation may nevertheless assist the diagnosis of VaD through the identification of asymmetries in sensory-motor performance more commonly seen in VaD than in AD. Moreover, unstructured neuropsychological tasks have shown promise in identifying the frontal-subcortical system impairments of VaD compared with the relatively greater temporal-limbic and posterior association area deficits of AD (Mendez and Ashla-Mendez 1991). Serial neuropsychological testing can also help to characterize the pattern and severity of decline in such patients over time.

Subcortical Dementias

Subcortical dementias are pervasive cognitive losses seen in several conditions involving subcortical brain regions, such as Huntington's disease, Parkinson's disease, progressive supranuclear palsy, and Binswanger's disease (Albert et al. 1974; Rom n 1987). Neuropsychological findings overlap considerably with those seen in the cortical dementias, with several distinct differences. Subcortical dementias frequently involve a slowing in general information processing; executive, memory, and visual-spatial deficits; and sensory-motor dysfunctions (Huber and Shuttleworth 1990). Marked language deficits are often absent, and these patients may continue to communicate very well, particularly early in the disease process. Nevertheless, they frequently present signs resembling frontal lobe dysfunction (Benson 1985; Strub and Black 1988). This may be manifested as a deficit in the organization of problem-solving behavior and psychiatric symptoms resembling affective or schizophreniform illnesses (Brandt and Bylsma 1993; Mahurin et al. 1993).

Posttraumatic Dementia

Patients who have sustained closed head injuries may exhibit significant residual neuropsychological impairment despite initial improvement in their neurological status (Levin et al. 1982). The course of recovery for patients who have sustained a closed head injury is highly variable. Although structural brain damage as seen on CT or magnetic resonance imaging (MRI) is usually associated with greater neuropsychological deficit, this is not always the case (Bigler 1984). After a closed head injury, serial neuropsychological evaluation is particularly important to determine the extent of recovery in both general and specific cognitive ability areas (Reitan and Wolfson 1993). Although the syndrome of posttraumatic dementia is not well defined, progressive cognitive deterioration with repeated head traumas (dementia pugilistica) has been identified (Strub and Black 1988).

Alcoholic Dementia (Alcohol-Persisting Dementia)

Chronic abuse of alcohol is associated with documented changes in brain morphology, blood flow, electrophysiology, and neuropsychological function (Parsons et al. 1987). There has been much neuropsychological focus on the amnestic deficits seen in Wernicke-Korsakoff syndrome. Such memory deficits occur within the context of preserved intelligence and most other neuropsychological functions (Salmon et al. 1993). However, chronic, heavy alcohol abuse may also result in a generalized cognitive deterioration characterized as alcoholic dementia (Wilkinson 1987). The condition is not reversible and is associated with increasing declines in cognitive ability, degree of self-care, and occupational and psychosocial function (Strub and Black 1988). Losses in abstraction, problem solving, and memory are particularly significant and may be accompanied by visual-spatial deficits. Although cognitive deterioration may slow with a cessation of drinking in some alcoholic patients (Wilkinson 1987), irreversible brain changes occur in both alcoholic dementia and Wernicke-Korsakoff syndrome (Salmon et al. 1993). The following case example illustrates alcoholic dementia:

> R.A. was a married, 52-year-old man who worked for most of his life as a sales representative, and then sales manager, for an oil drilling equipment company. R.A. held a bachelor's degree in marketing and had performed well throughout his years of formal education. At age 18 years, however, R.A. began to abuse alcohol. This continued during nearly 34 years of employment, many of which were spent traveling to oil drilling rigs throughout the Southwest. R.A.'s drinking pattern consisted of episodic "bingeing" with periods of somewhat lighter usage between binges. R.A. was moderately obese, had mild hypertension, and had smoked one pack of cigarettes per day for 35 years. He had no

history of CNS disorder, head injuries, or psychiatric conditions.

R.A. was initially brought by his wife to see their family physician. For much of their marriage, she had been quite tolerant of his alcohol usage, particularly since much of it occurred while he was on the road. However, she noticed that during the previous few years he had become less attentive to their discussions at home, had decreased interest in many leisure activities, and appeared to be highly forgetful around the house. He constantly misplaced his car keys and glasses and neglected to pay important bills. In addition, R.A.'s wife noticed that his attention span was shorter and that he was slow to catch on to new things. Similar problems were being observed by R.A.'s department head at work. R.A. had greater difficulty keeping track of company field operations and let important deadlines slip by without comment. During this time, R.A.'s alcohol usage actually decreased somewhat as he found himself becoming more sensitive to its effects. R.A.'s recovery after these less frequent binges also took much longer.

Medical examination revealed that R.A. was in generally good health except for laboratory signs of impaired liver functions and mild hepatomegaly. An MRI revealed mild cortical atrophy and ventricular dilation.

On neuropsychological evaluation, R.A. was found to have a high average verbal IQ yet a low average performance IQ. The patient displayed impaired attention and concentration, was concrete and slow on problems requiring new learning and abstraction, and exhibited moderate visual-spatial deficits. Memory testing further indicated a nearly 70% loss in retention of both verbal and visual material 30 minutes following exposure to test stimuli. All neuropsychological deficits were most apparent on complex tasks requiring organization and integration of multiple problem elements.

Concurrent personality evaluation suggested that, although R.A. had several characteristics of a personality disorder, he was not now significantly depressed and actually manifested few neurovegetative symptoms of depression. A diagnosis of dementia associated with alcoholism was subsequently made, and R.A. entered an inpatient alcohol treatment program. Alcohol treatment in the acute setting was initially altered to provide more structure and require less complex new learning in light of his neuropsychological deficits. Daily aftercare follow-up took place, and R.A. was reevaluated with a limited number of neuropsychological measures after 2 months of abstinence. At that time, he manifested slight improvements in attention and mental tracking ability but was still markedly impaired. A medical leave of absence was advised, with recommendations for monitoring of his medications by his wife, cessation of driving, less responsibility for household budgeting and bills, and consideration of entry into a local day hospital program. One year after his initial evaluation (and continued abstinence), R.A. was reevaluated neuropsychologically and continued to display significant cognitive impairments. Medical retirement was subsequently recommended and obtained.

Acquired Immunodeficiency Syndrome

As indicated in Chapter 4, advanced acquired immunodeficiency syndrome (AIDS) patients may develop what has been termed *AIDS dementia complex* (ADC) (Navia et al. 1986). More recently, the terms *HIV encephalopathy* (Van Gorp et al. 1993) and *HIV neurobehavioral dysfunction* (Bornstein 1994) have been used to describe human immunodeficiency virus (HIV) seropositive individuals manifesting less severe declines. Although variability exists, the pattern of observed deficits in ADC and HIV encephalopathy frequently resembles that of the subcortical dementias (Navia et al. 1990; Tross et al. 1988). Indeed, neuroimaging studies have implicated changes in subcortical white matter, thalamus, and basal ganglia, followed by frontal-temporal dysfunction, progressing to widespread brain involvement (Van Gorp et al. 1993). Cognitive symptoms may include declines in information processing speed, selective and sustained attention, verbal and visual memory, mental flexibility, and fine motor control (Bornstein et al. 1991; Heaton et al. 1995; Maj et al. 1994; Van Gorp et al. 1993). Neuropsychological evaluation frequently assists in identifying remaining areas of strength and weakness that may be used to formulate compensatory strategies in the work setting or assist in the management of these patients in the home.

Other Dementias

Description of all disorders leading to dementia is beyond the scope of this chapter. *Frontal lobe dementia* (see also Chapter 1) (Brun 1987; Neary et al. 1988) includes cognitive declines associated with diseases with frontal deterioration (i.e., Pick's disease) as well as conditions with affinity for frontal lobe involvement such as Creutzfeldt-Jakob disease (Sungaila and Crockett 1993). Characteristic symptoms include deficits in abstraction, executive function, self-awareness, and behavior.

Intracranial neoplasms have also been found to lead to generalized neuropsychological declines and dementia (Hom 1993).

Pseudodementia or the *dementia syndrome of depression* (Folstein and McHugh 1978) has typically referred to reversible cognitive deficits experienced by depressed patients (Wells 1979). The fact that dementia patients may experience depression complicates attempts to distinguish pseudodementia from structural brain diseases (Gilley 1993). Individuals with pseudodementia frequently resemble patients with subcortical dementia in their slowed information processing and failure to spontaneously employ learning and memory strategies (King and Caine 1990).

They have intact memory storage and significant retrieval problems, in contrast to AD patients, who have both impaired storage and retrieval (Kaszniak et al. 1986; Lachner et al. 1994; Lamberty and Bieliauskas 1993). Moreover, rapid onset of cognitive symptoms and the presence of patient complaints are also more common in depressed patients. However, persistence of deficits following recovery from depression may signal an irreversible dementia. Serial neuropsychological evaluation may therefore be useful to monitor progression or remission of memory impairments in depressed patients with equivocal signs of dementia.

When a Neuropsychological Evaluation Should Be Requested

The value of the neuropsychological examination to the physician is as 1) an aid to diagnosis, 2) an evaluation of the cognitive and emotional effects of medical treatment, and 3) an aid in designing rehabilitative or intervention strategies in the patient's overall treatment (Golden 1976).

Neuropsychological evaluation can contribute important information in diagnosing cases where 1) there is a discrepancy between the patient's self-report of difficulties and the family's assessment; 2) the physician wishes additional confirming evidence of a tentative diagnosis before recommending procedures such as MRI or angiography that may be frightening or uncomfortable or carry high morbidity; 3) emotional factors such as depression or anxiety may contribute to the symptoms; and 4) a basic screening of cognitive functions is needed.

Several examples illustrate these points. Family members often become concerned about an elderly parent's behavior. However, in a short office visit, elderly patients may deny or minimize difficulties. A neuropsychological evaluation often provides valuable diagnostic information as well as useful practical recommendations to the physician and family regarding degree of independence. Or the physician may suspect that a patient is declining cognitively but also appears to be withdrawn and slightly depressed. The neuropsychological evaluation can often help to identify the various factors contributing to the apparent decline and quantify them for future reference. A short neuropsychological screening exam can also be useful in the busy office or inpatient setting to help identify patients who warrant further evaluation for dementia and/or other emotional disorders and to do so quickly and cost-effectively.

The neuropsychological evaluation can also help to assess the cognitive effects of various medical treatments. These evaluations can be employed in a pre-post design to assess the effects of treatments such as electroconvulsive therapy, shunts for normal-pressure hydrocephalus, antidepressant or antianxiety medications, and endarterectomy surgery. Results may yield valuable objective data on patients' cognitive response, allowing the physician to make decisions on whether to continue, change, or drop a particular form of therapy.

Finally, the detailed analysis of a patient's cognitive abilities may be used to plan comprehensive interventions that focus on patients' strengths and weaknesses. This can be done in conjunction with or following termination of medical therapy and includes attempts to minimize the effects of cognitive deficits from dementing disorders. It often involves continuing education and support of the family to maximize the use of the available support network to help maintain safe, independent functioning for as long as possible. This can be particularly useful in progressive dementia cases, in which there is often little direct medical intervention possible and planning and structuring an individual's environment is the most useful intervention.

CHAPTER 8

Dealing With Family Caregivers

Myron F. Weiner, M.D.
Doris Svetlik, B.S.N., R.N., M.S.

In the long-term management of dementia, especially in progressive illnesses such as Alzheimer's disease (AD), the clinician's primary relationship is with the family of the dementia patient. Families bear the burden of understanding and of managing the patient's person and property. Therefore, after making a diagnosis and instituting what medical treatment is available and appropriate, the most important issues to address are the education and physical and emotional support of family caregivers.

Education About the Illness

Caregivers need (and want) to learn about the cognitive and behavioral effects of the illness, its anticipated course, and the various social and financial consequences of the illness. Many lay-directed guides are available for families of dementia patients, especially those with AD. The best resource is *The 36-Hour Day* (Mace and Rabins 1991). Other useful guides have been written by Powell and Courtice (1983) and D. Cohen and Eisdorfer (1986).

Family members need to understand that their patients have a reduced capacity to encode, process, integrate, communicate, and act on information that in turn impairs the ability to act appropriately in response to certain situations or information. The use of medical jargon needs to be avoided and, when used, needs to be explained. For example, the term *dementia* requires explanation. Concrete examples are important, such as the following:

233

> Your husband becomes lost when trying to find his way to the bath-
> room at night. This is a frequent symptom of dementia. Because his
> memory is impaired, he has to rely on his eyesight to help him make up
> for that loss. When he can't see well, his memory is no longer good
> enough to guide him.
>
> Your mother probably burns food on the stove because she is hav-
> ing difficulty with her concentration and her memory. Dementia pa-
> tients' attention wanders easily, and they forget what they are doing.
> They give the appearance of becoming careless when they are actually
> performing as well as they can at the moment.

Sometimes the cognitive impairment of dementia is best conveyed by
analogizing the patient's inability to reason and understand to that of a
small child—including a child's need for simple directions and for direction by example.

> You told me how you dealt with your own children when they were
> young—showing them instead of telling them. Instead of telling your
> mother to stir the soup for you so that it won't burn, show her how you
> want the soup stirred, help her to do it for a few moments, and then let
> her do it on her own. When she gets confused on the way to the bath-
> room, guide her to it. If you tell her where the bathroom is, she won't
> remember. She'll be less irritable if she's helped to do what you want
> her to do or what she wants to do instead of being told what not to do
> or that what she's doing is wrong.

Irritability requires explanation as well.

> Your observation that your father is more irritable goes along with
> the diagnosis of dementia. His irritability is due in part to the fact
> that he is no longer able to suppress minor irritation as you and I do
> when we get upset over something that we know is trivial. It is also
> partly due to his irritation with himself because he is unable to con-
> centrate and remember.

The phenomenon of disinhibition also needs to be explained, for example, so that a dementia patient who accidentally exposes his genitals is
not believed to be manifesting potentially dangerous hypersexuality.

The specific cognitive and behavioral problems in each case can be
communicated by including caregivers in the mental status examination
of the patient and by reviewing that examination with them afterward.
Performing the digit span test shows that defects in concentration make
it difficult to remember and that information must be presented in small
increments. Testing remote memory and immediate recall can demonstrate that recall is the type of memory that is most seriously affected—

that what was encoded long ago may be partially intact. Understanding that there are different types of memory deficit helps caregivers deal with the logical inconsistency that a person can easily remember something from long ago but not something that happened only a few minutes ago. Failures in simple mathematical operations point also to difficulty in concentration. Impairment of abstract reasoning can be demonstrated through the use of similarities and proverbs, and impaired judgment can be demonstrated by asking simple questions involving social judgment. Observing the clinician's management of the patient's irritability or inappropriate social behavior can be translated by caregivers into useful management strategies. Caregivers learn how to avoid increasing patients' irritability by observing the examiner.

Families often want to know what element of cognitive functioning or behavior will be affected next and whether there is a predictable pattern of loss. In the case of progressive dementing illnesses, families can be told that there will be progressive impairment of the ability to learn new skills and ideas, so that the patient will have to rely increasingly on what he or she already knows how to do. They can also be told to expect impairment of abstract thinking and reasoning ability, as indicated in the following example:

> If you were to tell your wife that it is raining cats and dogs, she might be puzzled and say that she doesn't see any cats or dogs. She also wouldn't understand what you meant if you said that a place was only a hop, skip, and a jump away. She'd think you were talking about hopping, skipping, and jumping.
>
> Her impaired judgment is likely to show up in driving. She will probably stop at a red traffic light and go when the light turns green but may not take into account that somebody may still be crossing the street.

Families of AD patients in particular are becoming more sophisticated and educated. Many want to discuss the pathophysiology of the illness to find out what areas of the brain and what neurotransmitters are involved. They become able to understand why anticholinergic drugs are prone to cause delirium in AD and to guard their patients from the antihistamines and other medications with significant anticholinergic properties. Educating families about the potentially toxic side effects of medications is also helpful. They need not be given a list of delirium-producing medications. Instead, they can be encouraged to always consider the possibility that a new medication or an increase in dosage of a long-standing medication may be responsible for a change in mental status. Families also need to be cautioned about the potential paradoxical excitatory effects of minor tranquilizers in all forms of dementia.

Families can be taught that difficulty with new learning makes it unwise to introduce their loved one into new situations and that it is wiser to involve that person in familiar activities in familiar places. They can be taught not to remind patients of their deficits and to serve as memory and a social buffer for their patients.

Prognosis

Prognosis is a very important issue for families, from both practical and emotional points of view. Families want and need to know the anticipated course of the illness. Most families can tolerate being told that a disease is expected to progress but that the exact course cannot be predicted. They can be told that there may be long periods of no apparent decline. They generally appreciate being told the worst as well as the best possible outcome. Generally speaking, it seems unwise to suggest that the course of the illness may at any time involve agitation or violence. Such a suggestion makes families wary of their affected loved ones and may cause them to overreact to trivial events. Families of acquired immunodeficiency syndrome (AIDS) patients can be told that there may be significant remission of cognitive symptoms with treatment of the underlying disease. In cases of patients with vascular dementia (VaD), the family may be offered the hope that the dementia may be slowed by the use of a single 325-mg aspirin tablet per day (Meyer et al. 1989) but that there still remains a good likelihood that the dementia will progress and that plans should be made accordingly. In cases of AD, families can be told that the disease will progress but that its rate of progression is uncertain. When families ask about the ultimate outcome of AD, they can be told that, if the patient lives long enough, this disease may result in complete inability to communicate or to care for him- or herself; but it is also useful to state that other illnesses usually supervene long before the dementing illness has run its course.

Our general policy is to suggest to families that they live one day at a time rather than live in anticipation of symptoms or behaviors that may never arise. When we are asked when nursing home care will be needed, we indicate that need for such care depends on the ability of families to deal with and to tolerate behaviors such as wandering and incontinence, and that families generally know when their tolerance has been exceeded.

Family Risk

Some of the dementias involve risk to family members. In the case of Huntington's disease and AD, the risks are genetic. In the former, which expresses in midlife, the pattern of dominant inheritance poses serious threat to siblings and offspring, and great sensitivity is needed in dealing with the issue of heritability. The situation in AD is quite different. Even if AD were carried by a dominant gene with late-life expression, that would mean an approximately 50% risk at age 90 years (Mohs et al. 1987), an unlikely life span for most persons. Therefore, it is best to respond to concern about the heritability of AD by stating that not enough is currently known to enable sound counseling but that the risk increases for siblings and children of affected persons and that transmission as a Mendelian dominant trait is relatively rare. In the instances of familial AD with onset as early as the fifth decade, families can be reasonably counseled that the risk approaches 50% for offspring of an afflicted person should they live to the age of usual disease onset in the family. When presenting data concerning the heritability of illness, clinicians need to be alert to the impact of this information on family members. An open-ended discussion following the communication of this information usually brings to light fears, misgivings, and potential negative effects.

When counseling about infectious disorders such as Creutzfeldt-Jakob disease or AIDS, the clinician indicates that these diseases can be communicated only from body fluid to body fluid, suggesting that appropriate precautions be taken. In the case of the former, blood-to-blood transmission would only be likely in the event that a caregiver punctured him- or herself with a needle contaminated with the patient's blood. In the latter case, contact with blood and seminal fluid is to be avoided.

Other Major Issues

It is important to deal with certain concrete issues. One issue is who will be the primary caregiver and/or conduit of information to and from the patient and family. The designated primary caregiver, in consultation with the clinician, the patient, and the rest of the family, needs to consider what supervision is necessary and how supervision is to be arranged. If the person is living independently, is independent living feasible or desirable? If so, how independent? Can the patient be allowed to continue driving? Buy groceries? Cook? Must eating and personal hygiene be supervised? In many instances, dementia patients can continue to live in their own accustomed residence, with once- or twice-a-day supervision by friends, relatives, and neighbors. If independent living is not feasible from the standpoint of safety or convenience, where can the dementia patient be accommodated best? Could the patient live with a friend or relative? Would a day-care program ease the burden?

For patients with more advanced disease, the issue of nursing home care arises. With near-terminal cases in nursing homes, the issue is whether to institute tube feeding. Financial and legal issues must be raised (see Chapter 9). Has a will been made? If not, is the patient able to indicate his or her true wishes? Is the patient able to transact business or enter contracts, such as for the sale of property? Does another family member have the type of power of attorney that can be used when the patient is no longer able to grant power of attorney? Is guardianship necessary to ensure impartial supervision of the patient's assets? If guardianship is needed, should it be full or partial? In anticipation of the need for Medicaid coverage of possible prolonged nursing home placement, is it best that the patient's property be transferred to other family members?

Imparting a Psychological Point of View

It is also useful to impart a psychological point of view to a patient's caregivers. Family members are often confused by daily fluctuations in cognitive ability and behavior and tend to see the dementia patient as arbitrarily deciding to forget and consciously manipulating others. Both may be true to a certain extent. However, it is more often true that what appears willful and arbitrary is the patient's attempt to avoid becoming overwhelmed, based on each person's own style of coping with or adapting to stress.

Caregivers often see dementia patients as unreasonably irritable, failing to recognize how frustrated patients become by the inability to reason, to remember, and to perform simple activities of daily living. When caregivers' attempts at orienting patients are met with apparent indifference, the caregivers must be reminded that this apparent indifference is both a product of the disease and a psychological protection against overwhelming anxiety, not indifference to the caring of others.

Family members, out of their own needs, often prefer to see loved ones with dementia as intact persons who are concealed behind a confused exterior. They can be reminded that fragments of their loved one may exist intact but that the individual's ability to integrate all the pieces into a whole person has been lost. Nevertheless, persons with dementia should be shown the same respect as human beings as cognitively intact persons are shown. Attention must also be given to certain prominent mechanisms of defense in dementia.

Dealing With Denial and Projection

Two of the most important mechanisms of defense, as pointed out in Chapter 2, are denial and projection. They need to be explained to caregivers as normal means of dealing with the emotionally overwhelming situation of literally losing one's mind and control over one's behavior. Caregivers need to be told how frightening it is to be unable to maintain a sense of self, how all persons use denial to avoid dealing with their own finiteness, and how blaming others helps each person avoid full awareness of his or her deficits or limitations.

It is often necessary for caregivers to respect patients' need for denial while addressing their realistic inability to cope with certain aspects of the environment. For example, it may be better to say that the car is being repaired or has been borrowed by another family member than to tell a dementia patient that he or she may no longer drive. One woman dealt with her concern about her husband's driving by telling him that she wanted him to supervise her driving.

Projection is more difficult for caregivers to tolerate than denial because they are usually the object of projection. When a wallet or purse, house keys, or items of clothing cannot be found, caregivers are the ones usually blamed. We tell caregivers that it is not useful to argue that one has not borrowed or stolen a particular object. It is more useful to institute a search for what is missing, accompanied by the patient if he or she is willing. It is also useful to note where commonly used objects or possessions are kept and to see that they are kept in those places if at all possible.

Delusional projection is even more difficult for caregivers because it frequently ties in with their own wishes and concerns. Thus, a dementia patient may express concern that caregivers are trying to steal his money. That may be true, in the sense that the family is attempting to control spending so that the dementia patient will not lose all of his or her financial resources, but it may also be true that the beneficiaries are trying to protect their inheritance. Their own emotional entanglement may lead caregivers into vigorous denials that further heighten mutual suspicion.

Caregivers find it easier to cope when, instead of being blamed themselves, they are told that strange-looking little people are entering the house and stealing money. When something specific is missing, caregivers need only institute a matter-of-fact search and produce what is missing, if they can. Many times, what is missing has been concealed by the patient, who can no longer remember where it is concealed. For that reason, it may be useful to periodically search the environment as a matter of routine to find such hiding places. When accusations are made that cannot be controverted, such as, "I know you are stealing my money," it is best to give a brief assurance to the contrary and to then engage the patient in some distracting activity. A reasonable reply to the foregoing accusation would be, "No, I'm not stealing your money. Breakfast is ready. Let's eat." If delusional projection does not abate and results in great perturbation for the patient or family, the use of antipsychotic medication may be temporarily indicated.

At times, the clinician may suspect that the patient's suspicions of family or other caregivers are well founded. If the family is suspected of financial or other abuse, Adult Protective Services can be contacted to investigate the situation. The family or proper agencies can be notified if abuse by professional caregivers is suspected.

Maintaining Self-Esteem

In the early stages of a dementing illness, patients have difficulty maintaining their self-esteem because they can no longer live up to their own notion of whom they ought to be and at what level they ought to function. They also recognize that they cannot do for themselves what they have been able to do since childhood: perform simple calculations, follow directions, maintain orientation in time and space, button garments, and tie shoelaces. As dementia progresses, the capacity for self-awareness and communication diminishes, and maintenance of self-esteem becomes less of a problem, both in terms of patients' self-assurance and their ability to communicate concern about themselves.

Most people define who they are by what they do. Loss of capacity to work or to carry out one's usual activities leads to a sense of uselessness. It is therefore useful for families to help patients with mild cases of dementia to find activities at which they can feel competent. These may include activities as simple as dusting the furniture or helping to fold the laundry. Patients who enjoy and are kept occupied by housekeeping chores can be encouraged to do those chores daily, it making little difference whether the house needs cleaning again or whether the laundry really needs to be folded again. Playing simple games such as bingo can be pleasurable. Each person is unique in the activities that are meaningful to him or her. Helping to discover those activities can be a positive experience for both caregiver and patient. The Pleasant Events Schedule (Teri and Logsdon 1991) mentioned in Chapter 5 is a useful tool for discovering such activities.

Impact of Dementia on the Family

The development of a dementing illness affects different families and family members in many different ways. It affects spouses, companions, children, grandchildren, and (as in the case of AIDS) parents. Mild declines are frequently unnoticed or glossed over by spouses of elderly dementia patients. In many elderly couples, there is an automatic compensation by one for the other's deficits. A husband will begin cooking as the wife becomes less competent in the kitchen, or the wife will take over household repairs from the husband. In our experience, it is not unusual for one member of a spousal pair to be physically handicapped but cognitively intact, whereas the other spouse is cognitively impaired and physically intact. In this situation, the physically disabled member guides the cognitively disabled person in doing the daily chores. Often, the first person to comment on the cognitive deficit of an elderly person with dementia is a son or daughter who lives at a distance and visits infrequently. Many times, it is difficult for the adult children to convince the intact parent that the parent with dementia needs a medical evaluation.

When dementia begins to markedly reduce a couple's quality of life, the unaffected spouse or partner feels frustration, anger, sadness—and, sometimes, frank depression. A common reaction in elders is a sense of having been robbed of one's golden years. Many elders postponed pleasures earlier in life for the sake of their careers or their children, in the expectation that retirement would bring comfortable leisure. They become frustrated at their inability to enjoy a time when they are no longer burdened by work or family responsibilities, angry at having lost the opportunity, and sad for their spouse's loss of quality of life. They become depressed as they look forward to their situation deteriorating further and eventually losing their spouse as a person.

Spousal caregivers experience difficulties in many areas. Although many individuals with dementia are indifferent to their loss of cognitive function, others strive to maintain their premorbid level of functioning and autonomy. A key area of conflict for many couples is driving. A wife will note that her husband's judgment is becoming impaired and that he not only becomes lost while driving but also changes lanes without looking or makes left-hand turns from the right-hand lane. Although she does not want her husband to feel less of a person, she fears for his and others' safety. Furthermore, she does not wish to engage in the endless arguments that dementia patients often participate in concerning intensely emotional issues, such as relinquishing driving. In situations where a spouse has difficulty saying no, we often suggest that the blame be assigned to the physician by saying, "The doctor doesn't want you to drive right now." Our female patients frequently insist that they can still cook, despite their forgetting how to carry out simple recipes and ignoring food burning on a stove top. Many strategies are employed here, including turning off the gas supply or electricity to the stove unless there is someone who can directly supervise the cooking process.

Another key area of difficulty for spouses is in coping with suspiciousness or outright delusional blaming. Being accused constantly of stealing and lying is demoralizing at best. Although spouses can be educated to not challenge suspicions and delusions, it is difficult for them not to feel unappreciated.

In our experience, two situations most often precipitate nursing home admission. They are the advent of total incontinence in the dementia patient and the caregiver's inability to get adequate sleep. Spouses seem able to tolerate occasional urinary incontinence. They are often able to manage toileting their spouse frequently and restricting fluid intake after supper to prevent "accidents" or placing their spouse in incontinence pads. Prolonged fecal incontinence is not well tolerated. The emotional transition from spouse to nurse often cannot be accomplished. When persistent incontinence appears to be a result of the dementing illness and not a result of factors such as urinary tract infection, bladder prolapse, fecal impaction, or improper diet, we begin raising the question of institutionalization with the now-exhausted spouse. The same is true when the dementia patient's nighttime agitation or wandering make it impossible for the caregiver to sleep.

Dementia affects both adult children and grandchildren. The adult children who are particularly compromised are those still actively raising their own children. They are sandwiched between caring for the generation ahead of and behind them. Our experience and that of others is that daughters and daughters-in-law are affected more than sons or sons-in-law. Brody (1989) suggests that this is so because women have more nurturing expectations of themselves than men do, but it may also have to do with the fact that men are more often employed full time outside the home than women. However, this may change as more women enter the work force.

It is often painful for children when their parents become less than fully competent. For many adult children, having an active, decisive parent is so important that they want to continue following that parent's judgment and have difficulty substituting their own judgment for that of their parents. A surprisingly large number of adults continue to be emotionally and financially dependent on their parents and experience the onset of a dementing illness as a threat to their own integrity. There are also children who want to protect parents from the consequences of dementia but whose parents' suspiciousness or need for autonomy is so great that they reject help offered regarding adequate nutrition or proper clothing. Many of our patients are widows who have lived and managed on their own for many years and are fiercely independent. In this situation, we try to help the children achieve a reasonable balance between safeguarding their parents and interfering with their parents' much-needed sense of autonomy. Adult children are understandably upset that meals-on-wheels delivered to the home are uneaten, that ice cream and cookies are preferred to a balanced diet, that clothing goes unwashed, or that the house is not kept clean. Our general stance is that, as long as fiercely independent dementia patients are able to maintain their nutrition and personal hygiene fairly well, they will have a higher quality of life living on their own than in an institution, and it may be worth taking the risk that they can still care for themselves.

Tensions also develop between the adult children of a parent with dementia. Ordinarily, one adult child assumes the majority of the burden of care. This primary nonspousal caregiver is usually self-selected and is most often the child who has maintained the strongest attachment to the parents over the years. At times, the role of primary caregiver falls to the child who is geographically closest or who is not employed outside the home. The primary caregiver's closeness to the parent is often envied by the other siblings, who respond to their envy by criticizing the primary caregiver's quality of care. He or she is seen as too domineering, too harsh, or too easy on the affected parent. Despite their willingness to criticize, envious siblings who act out their rivalry by criticism are often difficult to engage as helpers.

Grandchildren are generally not strongly affected unless grandmother or grandfather comes to live with them. At times, there is a comfortable relationship, with the grandparent enjoying the interaction with grandchildren and grandchildren tolerating their grandparent's deficit well. Often, however, grandparents with dementia regress significantly and feel competitive with grandchildren for their parents' attention. Children, in turn, may have difficulty with their grandparents' incapacity and may claim that the elders are faking. Children who feel deprived of nurturing by the presence of a grandparent in the house may also act against the older persons and attempt to discredit them or drive them out of the house.

Dementia in an adult child also poses problems for parents. Many parents appreciate the opportunity to do what they can for a child of any age. Others feel that their freedom from child rearing has been hard-won and are resentful of intrusion on their middle-age or late-life style of living. They feel a wish to care for their children, as well as guilt because they would now like to conserve some of their energy for themselves. In the case of patients with AIDS, many parents of homosexual children or intravenous drug abusers are resentful of the child's lifestyle, believe their child has caused his or her disease, and feel still further alienated. Having reached adulthood, many children are resentful of parents reentering their lives in a decision-making capacity. This is especially true for immature adults or adults for whom autonomy from parents has been a significant and poorly resolved struggle.

Caregiver Stress

It is clear that living with or coping with dementia patients can be extremely stressful. In fact, there is now a large literature on caregiver stress in AD (Light and Lebowitz 1989). Many authors suggest that caring for mentally impaired elders is more stressful than caring for the physically disabled (Brody 1989). Also, institutionalization does not totally relieve caregiver strain. Families maintain their supportive activities even when loved ones are institutionalized. They visit nursing homes frequently, interact with nursing personnel, help with feeding, feel sad about their loved one's condition, and feel guilty because they were not able to maintain their loved one at home. They also feel helpless to complain about suboptimal care for fear that staff will retaliate against their loved ones. George (1984) found that stress symptoms were as prevalent in caregivers whose loved ones with dementia resided in nursing homes as they were in caregivers who maintained their loved ones at home. As dementia progresses in AD, most AD patients appear to lose awareness of their deficit. To the family, the deficit becomes increasingly apparent as it results in a heavier work and emotional load (Pratt et al. 1985; Zarit et al. 1985). Despite the heavy emotional burden and frequent signs of emotional and physical overload, several questionnaire studies show no strong relationship between duration or severity of illness and indices of caregiver burden (George and Gwyther 1986; Zarit et al. 1980). Patient and caregiver factors such as health status and problem solving seem to have greater impact on burden (Zarit and Teri 1992). Dysphoria is extremely common. In a survey of primary caregivers, Rabins et al. (1982) found that 87% reported chronic depression, fatigue, and/or anger when asked about their emotional state. Coppell et al. (1985) found that 40% of 68 AD caregivers were experiencing depressive symptoms. Only 1 caregiver, however, met criteria for major depression.

Before recommending means to partially relieve the physical and emotional distress of caregivers, the particular stressors need to be identified. This requires spending time with the family. In the setting of our dementia clinic, this is done during the initial interview with the psychiatrist, in which the family is seen apart from the patient by both the psychiatrist and the clinic nurse. Caregiver stress is also assessed at the reporting interview, to which all concerned family members are invited. Aside from diagnosis and direct treatment recommendations, our clinic team tries to help families arrive at a management plan that is optimal for them and the patient. We state that our aim is to maintain the highest quality of life for all members of the family and that planning for a dementia patient's care involves balancing that person's needs against the needs of the rest of the family. On rare occasions, we recommend supportive counseling or active psychiatric treatment for a family member. So far, we have not suggested family therapy, but we would not hesitate to recommend it for the cognitively intact family members if we felt it were indicated. We also give active support to professional caregivers caring for dementia patients at home. They are liable to intense buffeting between family members with divergent points of view and often stand between an irritable, nonunderstanding spouse and the dementia patient. Frequently, elderly spouses are only slightly less affected by dementia than the primary patient and thus cannot fathom why the husband or wife cannot understand. We offer continued advice and support by telephone and through annual revisits, and we suggest active involvement with the educational programs and support groups of the local Alzheimer's Association. Other sources of community support are indicated in Chapter 10.

Sexuality

One area that is rarely addressed with regard to dementia patients and their spouses is the effect of the disease on their sexual feelings and behaviors. Aronson (1988) states that basic human needs for affection and intimacy persist well into the illness. For spouses, however, the sexual act with a partner who no longer recognizes the meaning of intimacy becomes a parody of lovemaking (Volicer et al. 1988). In our clinical experience, these statements hold true for many couples. In most couples in which the onset of dementia is after the age of 70 years, sexual involvement has already diminished and does not present a problem; but for younger couples with active sex lives, problems do occur. Spouses report that, as they assume a caregiver role in relation to their spouse and become more of a parent than a partner in the relationship, their sexual desire decreases. Some even report feelings of revulsion because it feels as though they are committing incest with their "child." These feelings cause great conflict, guilt, and frustration for spouses who try to deal with them alone, and they are often not comfortable bringing these issues up with professionals. Therefore, the responsibility lies with the professional to address this aspect of the disease and its impact on the relationship. In some cases, dementia patients become hypersexual.

Volicer et al. (1988) suggest that caregivers be taught how to distract or gently dissuade sexually persistent spouses. In our experience, some spouses cannot be dissuaded behaviorally nor is their sexual drive reduced through use of tranquilizers or antipsychotics. We have found medroxyprogesterone useful in reducing inappropriate sexual aggression in male dementia patients (see Chapter 6).

Nursing Home Placement

Decisions regarding nursing home placement are usually made by the family and are implemented when the primary caregiver becomes physically and emotionally overwhelmed. Chenoweth and Spencer (1986) found that 72% of caregivers indicated that being overwhelmed by 24-hour-a-day care was the most important precipitant of nursing home placement. Less frequently cited reasons were the caregiver becoming ill (21%), behavioral problems (18%), and incontinence (18%); many reported more than one reason. Two important obstacles to nursing home placement are the reluctance of dementia patients to accept nursing home care and the caregivers' guilt over "abandoning" a loved one. In general, the former is not a substantial obstacle, except as a source for self-recrimination by the caregiver. Families are usually counseled to follow the path that offers the greatest quality of life to those able to appreciate that quality. Here again, an analogy to early childhood may be useful. Thus, one can say that a patient with severe dementia is very similar to an infant: not able to recognize the source of caregiving but in need of being cared for. The source of the caregiving is far less important than that caregiving be provided.

Family scapegoating may become a difficulty in deciding about nursing home placement. The family member who is managing the problem firsthand is often told by family members living at a distance how unfair it is to institutionalize the patient. The physician can help to undercut this process by adding the weight of medical opinion to the decision.

Families also need to be counseled that, once a nursing home placement is made, the length and frequency of visits should be such that the patient comes to accept the nursing home as a permanent place of residence. Thus, families are urged not to visit daily or to visit for hours at a time. Instead, they are encouraged to visit a few times a week and for brief periods. Once the transition to the nursing home is accepted, brief outings can be arranged.

In our experience, the transition to full-time nursing home placement is facilitated by enrolling patients in day care at the nursing facility, later using the facility for respite care, and finally for full-time nursing care.

Ethical Issues for Caregivers

The primary ethical issues that arise in dealing with dementia patients occur in relation to following that person's wishes with regard to independence and maintenance of life. Many persons who eventually develop dementia express the desire to be cared for at home in the event of a debilitating illness. Their loved ones agree. However, the time comes when the dementia patient becomes an impossible burden for the primary caregiver, often because the caregiver has become physically incapacitated. At that point, the family weighs practical necessity against the earlier expressed wishes of the patient and decides whether that person's experienced quality of life is more important than state of health or length of life or whether the needs of other family members take precedence. The family may decide that the patient's quality of life would not be measurably diminished by nursing home placement, whereas the quality of life of the now-disabled caregiver might be immeasurably improved. Many dementia patients who live alone do not want to be removed from their home despite their inability to adequately maintain themselves. If failure to institutionalize would lead to the dementia patient's near-term death by starvation, it is unlikely that society at large would condone such a decision, and the family might find itself opposed by legally constituted authorities such as Adult Protective Services. In the eventuality that a severely impaired person living alone refuses needed institutionalization, Adult Protective Services can assist in arranging involuntary nursing home placement.

The conflict between maintaining life and quality of life also arises when dementia progresses to the point that the person is no longer capable of self-feeding and does not swallow spoon-fed food. Some dementia patients will have previously expressed their preference verbally or in writing to be or not to be sustained by artificial means. If they have expressed a preference to not be so sustained, and the family agrees, it is permissible to offer food and water at appropriate intervals and to let nature take its course. This position is supported by the Supreme Court of New Jersey, which held that every person has a common-law right to determine what medical interventions can be performed on him of her. That right continues after the person is no longer competent, as long as the person's previous competently expressed wishes can be ascertained (*In re Conroy* 1985). The *Conroy* court also held that, where there has been no expression of preference on the part of the dementia patient, the family and physician have the right to decide, based on their knowledge of that individual's interests and preferences, what he or she would have wanted. A decision to discontinue life-extending treatment was based by another court on the spouse's testimony concerning his wife's independent nature and dislike of physicians (*In re Colyer* 1983). Where there has been no clear statement of the patient's wishes concerning artificial maintenance of life support and where that person's probable wishes cannot be clearly inferred, decisions can be made based on what appears to be in the best interest of the patient. To continue life support using the best interests of the patient as a guide, the generally accepted formula is that the benefits the patient derives from life should outweigh the burden of the treatment (Cantor 1987). The actual weighing of these factors is highly subjective and should involve discussion between physician and family, in consultation with a legal advisor familiar with the law in that particular jurisdiction. As indicated in Chapter 9, the U.S. Supreme Court has ruled that individuals have the right to terminate life-sustaining treatment or may designate a person to represent their wishes *(Cruzan v. Director, Missouri Dept. of Health, et al.* 1990).

Summary

With no cure currently available for many dementing illnesses, an important role for health care professionals is family support. Educating families about the disease process helps lessen stress and anxiety, as does introducing families to a dynamic view of their loved one's behavior. Making referrals to other agencies encourages interaction of the families with others and helps to avoid feelings of isolation. Providing concrete management suggestions for specific behaviors and help with decisions about placement is also necessary as part of family support. Addressing intrafamily issues can also be important. Being available to listen to complaints and validate emotions when there is no specific intervention or solution to a problem is also important for caregivers. Discussions and questions should be encouraged by the health care team so that family members' knowledge and emotional comfort can be assessed and enhanced.

CHAPTER 9

Legal and Ethical Aspects of Dementia

Barton E. Bernstein, J.D., L.M.S.W.
Myron F. Weiner, M.D.

Medicine is a healing art informed by science. It differs from other healing arts such as prayer and mystical ritual in that medicine's base is in science rather than faith or the supernatural. The physician who diagnoses and manages patients bases day-to-day decisions on a complex, ever-changing admixture of science, societal and personal values, and practical considerations (Sadler and Hulgus 1992). The scientific and practical considerations are discussed elsewhere in this book. In this chapter, we deal with societal values, institutional values, and the personal values of the dementia patient, the patient's family, and the physician.

Values are expressed in societies as law and as ethical precepts. The law is society's operating manual; ethics is its conscience. The law tells us what we *must* do to facilitate the operation of our society; ethics tells us what is *best* for individuals and society. Ideally, law is based on what is best for individuals and society, but the interests of individuals and the larger societal group frequently come into conflict. Furthermore, activities that physicians, patients, or their families wish to undertake as scientifically sound or practical may be illegal or unethical.

Legal Issues

Dementia is often defined as "a condition of deteriorated mentality." Deteriorated mentality in legal terms has to do with the capacity to function within specific legal contexts. Early in the course of a dementing illness, the functions of competence and testamentary capacity may be relatively intact, and patients can continue to manage their own affairs, consent to medical treatment, and make and execute a will. Late in the course of a dementing illness, it is likely that competence and testamentary capacity will be impaired. Early in the process, it is important that clinicians call these issues to the attention of patients and their families.

Competence

In a progressive dementing illness, it must be assumed that competence will ultimately be impaired. *Competence* refers to the authority to function within a specific legal context and is defined differently according to the specific legal situation (Perr 1978). There are many types of legal competency, including competence in criminal and civil trials, in attempting to marry, in making contracts, in consenting to medical treatment, and in making a will. Each type requires specific legal tests.

Competence in a criminal trial requires that, at the time of the alleged offense, persons have had the capacity to appreciate the criminality of their conduct or to conform their conduct to the requirements of the law allegedly violated. A second but usually related issue is whether accused individuals are competent to stand trial. The criteria here include the defendants' ability to cooperate with a lawyer in the preparation of a meaningful defense, to understand the charges against them, and to operate within the guidelines required by orderly trial procedures (Shuman 1986). Expert witnesses must determine whether defendants have a rational and factual understanding of the charges against them and if they know what the crime was, why it was a crime, and that they are being tried for the crime (Bernstein and Weiner 1980; Robey 1965).

An apocryphal story concerns a mildly demented and moderately paranoid woman who lived alone and in terror of imaginary persecutors who passed her house each day, making threatening gestures. The story goes that she frequently called the local police station, where the officers would allow her to talk about her fears and calm down. One day, a new officer answered the telephone, heard her complaint, and suggested in a half-serious way that she get a gun to drive them off. The woman's next telephone call to the police station was a triumphant declaration that she had shot one of her persecutors! Had she come to trial, she would have been found not guilty by reason of diminished competence. If a dementia patient broke into a house, believing that it was his own, and took money from a dresser drawer, again believing that it was his own, he would not be found guilty of a criminal act because he failed to appreciate the criminality of his behavior—that is, he did not have the requisite criminal intent. That same person could be liable for civil damages if, when attempting to obtain what he thought was his own money, he injured another person or damaged another person's property (Lucas-Blaustein et al. 1988).

Competence in a civil suit requires the ability to understand the general nature of a particular transaction and its implications, as in the following example:

> A man with a mild cognitive defect who had been treated for heart disease stated on an application for a large life insurance policy that he was in good health. A civil trial arose after his death because the insurance company refused to indemnify the family, based on the deceased's failure to fully disclose his medical condition (although he died of a gunshot wound). His family held that because of his cognitive defect, he had probably forgotten that he had been treated for heart disease and therefore had not knowingly misrepresented himself to the insurance company. Representatives of the insurance company produced sufficient evidence of this man's ability to manage complex situations (including the ability to maintain two separate marriages and families in two cities located 100 miles apart) that the jury found for the insurance company.

Competence to enter a contract includes competence to enter a marital contract. Many marriages entered into by elderly, cognitively impaired persons are thought by these individuals' natural heirs to be poorly disguised attempts by unscrupulous persons to inherit substantial estates. Competence to consent to marriage includes an understanding of the responsibilities and obligations of marriage, for example, that the spouse might claim a portion of the estate. As far as other contracts are concerned, the test of competence is that the person understands the nature of the transaction and its implications, as seen in the following example:

> An elderly woman was examined in her home to ascertain whether it was possible for her to continue living independently, her husband having been admitted to a nursing home a month earlier. She was reported to experience visual hallucinations of children and animals running through the house, especially in the late afternoon and early evening. On one occasion, she chased an imaginary little girl into the street. The woman had a history of hypertension, excessive alcohol intake, and continued heavy smoking. Her medications included a combination beta-blocker and diuretic, 50 mg of doxepin, and 15 mg of temazepam hs. The only abnormalities revealed on a brief physical and neurological examination were a blood pressure of 180/110 mmHg and occasional premature ventricular beats. Mental status examination revealed profound defects in concentration, recent memory, remote memory, orientation, and fund of information. Although her vision was

adequate, she could not understand simple written sentences. She was also paying little attention to her grooming or to the care of her house. At that time, it was the physician's impression that she should not be allowed to live alone, especially in view of her heavy smoking and her propensity to leave lighted cigarettes around the house.

It was discovered that shortly before the physician's visit, an insurance salesman had induced the woman to withdraw half the cash value of her husband's life insurance policy ($25,000) and endorse the check to him. In exchange, she was given worthless stock in an invention that was never manufactured. In a civil hearing, the physician testified that she could not have understood the nature and consequences of the business transaction she had entered into. Based on that evidence and testimony provided by the woman's neighbors, the judge ruled against the insurance salesman.

Competence to manage property and financial matters is based on individuals' awareness of their material holdings and their ability to manage them prudently.

Competence to consent to medical treatment involves an awareness of the condition for which treatment is offered, the likely effects of the treatment offered, and the consequences of failing to accept treatment. This issue is discussed frequently and usually involves patients' resisting their physicians' suggestions or acting against medical advice, as in the following example:

A 90-year-old woman with impaired peripheral circulation was brought to a hospital for evaluation of a gangrenous big toe. Her surgeon found dry gangrene with no evidence of infection and recommended that her toe be amputated. When she refused, psychiatric consultation was obtained to determine her competence to consent or refuse treatment. The psychiatrist found her to be mildly to moderately demented but not depressed or suicidal. She was not oriented in time but knew that she was in a hospital and that her surgeon wanted to amputate her toe. She knew there was danger of an infection developing and spreading if the toe was not surgically amputated, and she knew that the toe would probably eventually fall off on its own. On that basis, the psychiatrist indicated to the surgeon that she was mentally competent to refuse surgery.

Consent to Participate in Research

Many studies of cognition-enhancing drugs are under way. In these studies, the issue arises of capacity to consent to an experimental treatment and to understand what is meant by receiving a placebo treatment in a double-blind study. All patients who undergo nonemergency medical treatment need to furnish informed consent to treatment. In its simplest form, informed consent requires that the physician impart sufficient information regarding the proposed treatment so that the patient is able to consider all of the relevant information and the consequences of refusing treatment (McLean and Maher 1983). In practice, federal regulations require eight specific elements of informed consent (U.S. Department of Health and Human Services 1981):

1. A statement that the study involves research, an explanation of the purposes of the research and the expected duration of the subject's participation, a description of the procedures followed, and identification of any procedures that are experimental
2. A description of any reasonably foreseeable risks or discomforts to the subject
3. A description of any benefits to the subject or to others that may reasonably be expected from the research
4. A disclosure of appropriate alternative procedures or courses of treatment, if any, that might be advantageous to the subject
5. A statement describing the extent, if any, to which confidentiality of records identifying the subject will be maintained
6. For research involving more than minimal risk, an explanation as to whether any compensation and medical treatments are available if injury occurs and, if so, what they consist of or where further information may be obtained
7. An explanation of whom to contact for answers to pertinent questions about the research and research subjects' rights and whom to contact in the event of a research-related injury to the subject
8. A statement that participation is voluntary, that refusal to participate will involve no penalty or loss of benefits to which the subject is otherwise entitled, and that the subject may discontinue participation at any time without penalty or loss of benefits to which the subject is otherwise entitled

When the informed-consent document is drawn up, it is usually too complicated for dementia patients to understand. As a consequence, a brief explanation is made by the investigator at the patient's level of comprehension. Applebaum and Roth (1982) suggest hierarchical steps to consent for research, the first being that of evidencing a choice and the second being that of showing a functional understanding of the issues. By these minimal criteria, most dementia patients living at home are able to give informed consent.

Experimental treatments require balancing potential harm to patients against the need for biomedical research. Therefore, patients must be informed that such treatments are experimental. They must be told what is known about the potential dangers and positive effects, and effort must be made to be certain that patients understand to what they are consenting. Patients or their legal representatives must understand the possibility of being in a placebo group when enrolled in a double-blind study.

Testamentary Capacity

Testamentary capacity is the ability to create a valid and enforceable will. The legal requirements for testamentary capacity is that individuals know they are making a will and that they are able to determine the natural objects of their bounty (i.e., to whom one usually leaves one's property and possessions) and to know the nature and extent of their estate and/or acquired properties. If it is established that these standards are met, individuals have the absolute right to will their property to any person or entity, be that spouse, children, a stranger, a beloved cause, or an organization.

Undue Influence

A frequent issue with regard to both competence and testamentary capacity is *undue influence.* This is the influence of one person over another to cause that person to act in a way that he or she would not act without that influence. Vulnerability to undue influence occurs on the basis of the patient's cognitive impairment, physical or emotional dependence on another person, or all three factors. Is the testator easy prey to designing others? In the following cases, the first illustrates emotional dependence; the second, dependence based on physical and cognitive impairment:

> **Case 1.** Mr. A., an elderly man with a history of marked emotional dependence on his wife and on alcohol, lost his wife after a year-long illness. He then asked his wife's paid companion to remain in his employ and to look after him. She did so and, over a period of a year, induced him to pay $10,000 to repair her house, to buy her a $40,000 automobile, and to make her the beneficiary of a $100,000 certificate of deposit. This man's cognitive impairment was minimal, but it was obvious that his emotional makeup made him susceptible to undue influence (i.e., a designing other).

Case 2.   Mrs. B., a wealthy elderly woman, had hired as a companion a woman who had formerly worked as a beautician. Mrs. B. had broken both hips a number of years previously; they had not healed well, and she was confined to a wheelchair. She had not left her bedroom in 5 years. Meals were brought to her there, she transacted her business there, and she was visited there three times a week by a masseuse. Over the course of a few years, Mrs. B.'s companion took over the hiring and firing of household help, hiring several members of her own family. She alienated her employer from her family and ultimately convinced her employer to make her the director of the employer's substantially endowed charitable foundation. The old woman's family then filed a motion for guardianship in the probate court. A psychiatrist was appointed by the court to determine her competence to manage her own affairs prudently.

The psychiatrist interviewed Mrs. B. on three separate occasions. He found her to be physically feeble and to have poor vision. She was alert and oriented to time and place. Although mildly cognitively impaired (her Mini-Mental State Exam score was 20), she was able to perform simple calculations, could remember three of three objects in 5 minutes, could read and understand a simple paragraph, could reason abstractly, and knew a great deal about her personal affairs. She did not know the exact salaries paid to her employees but did know the extent of her wealth and could give good reasons why her family members should not run her personal and financial affairs. The examiner concluded that she understood in principle the nature of her business affairs and the extent of her property but did not think she was capable of independently gathering the information she needed to manage her own affairs. The court then rejected the family's petition for guardianship and instead appointed her attorney ad litem as a limited guardian. In that capacity, with appropriate consultation and occasional court approval, he was to make her major financial decisions while she managed her everyday affairs. Her companion was discharged.

When a dementing illness is identified with reasonable certainty, patients, their families, and other potential survivors need to consider undertaking certain legal steps and both legal and financial counseling (Overman and Stoudemire 1988). The time to take those steps is when dementia patients are still sufficiently lucid to understand and to communicate their wishes. The first step is to create a power of attorney; the second is to create a will.

Power of Attorney

A *power of attorney* is a written and notarized or witnessed instrument that authorizes another to act in one's behalf. It can be a general power of attorney, which authorizes another to act fully on behalf of the grantor, or a specific power of attorney, which limits the grantee to certain acts, such as the selling of a house or an automobile or managing a piece of property in the absence of the grantor. The power of attorney may also be limited as to time and may be drafted so as to terminate either on the happening of an event or after a particular date. It may also be terminated at any time by the grantor. Further, the power of attorney may provide that "this instrument and the powers given thereunder shall not terminate on the mental or physical incapacity of the grantor." Thus, this instrument, often called a durable power of attorney, becomes an irrevocable power of attorney when dementia becomes incapacitating. When recorded in the county deed records, anyone dealing with the grantee has the right to rely on the recorded instrument. Likewise, when a revocation is filed, or on the death of the grantor, the power of attorney is null and void.

The durable power of attorney is vital in many situations. Unattended securities or real estate investments may fall precipitously in value; partnerships, sole proprietorships, and all manner of financial ventures including privately held colorations may suffer without guidance. A business partner who worked well under a partner's observation may prove less than trustworthy working with or for the widow or widower and when unobserved. The danger of granting a power of attorney is its possible unwitting or deliberate misuse by the grantee because the grantor is liable for all the acts of the grantee in his or her name. The grantee stands in the legal shoes of the grantor.

Durable Powers of Attorney for Health Care

Often, persons with progressive dementing illnesses or their families realize that important decisions will have to be made concerning health care and medical treatment. Nevertheless, many persons are leery of authorizing a general power of attorney and surrendering control over a substantial part of their personal and financial lives. To remedy this problem, many states have established a procedure for executing durable powers of attorney for health care. In Texas, the law provides that competent patients may now designate persons and successors (in case of death, disability, or unwillingness to serve) who can act as their legal surrogate for health care decisions. The power of attorney would be used when the patient lacks capacity to make health care decisions or to offer informed consent to medical treatment. The physician would not act under the power if the patient objects, regardless of the patient's capacity.

In such statutes, the person holding the power of attorney cannot be the patient's physician or an employee of the treating hospital except if such person is also a relative of the patient. Witnesses are required. A physician or hospital cannot require a person to execute a health care power of attorney in order to receive services. Such laws also provide that physicians and hospital employees are not liable for acts done in good faith under the terms of the power or directives of the agent appointed under the power of attorney unless due care was not exercised. States with these laws also provide sample forms.

At times, especially as the result of a stroke or head injury, severe, incapacitating dementia may be an accomplished fact before adequate protective legal steps can be made. In that instance, a fiduciary may be required.

The Fiduciaries: Guardianship, Conservatorship, and Trusteeship

Fiduciaries serve a broad and vital role in financial and other types of assistance. When individuals cannot protect themselves or their estate, courts may, upon application and order, appoint a guardian, conservator, or trustee, or the parties, by written instrument, may establish a guardianship, conservatorship, or trusteeship. These terms are defined as follows, although there are minor differences from state to state.

Fiduciary

A *fiduciary* is a person entrusted to act on behalf of another, usually in the conduct of the latter's business, for example, an attorney, a broker, or a director of a corporation.

Guardian

A *guardian* is a person lawfully invested with the power and charged with the duty of taking care of the person and managing the property and rights of the person who, because of some peculiarity of status, physical or mental incapacity, or other reasons, is considered incapable of managing his or her own affairs. Guardianship may be limited to business affairs only (American Bar Association Commission on the Mentally Disabled 1979), as illustrated in the case of Mrs. B. The court may appoint a guardian of the person or of the estate. One guardian may perform one function only or both functions.

Trustee

A *trustee* broadly means a person standing in a fiduciary or confidential relationship with another. Narrowly, it applies to a person appointed or required by law to execute a trust. Management is entrusted to the trustee for the use and benefit of the beneficiary.

Conservator

A *conservator* is essentially the same as a guardian. A conservator manages the person and property of an individual found incapable by a probate court of managing his or her own affairs. Management of the person and the property may be divided into two separate functions.

In legal theory and practice, these procedures separate individuals from their estates and business dealings and allow a competent friend, relative, attorney, or financial institution to manage the estate or business transactions on behalf of the individuals involved. They act in a fiduciary or trust capacity and must exercise scrupulous good faith in their dealings. As indicated previously, guardianships can be partial or limited, allowing individuals to continue managing those aspects of their affairs that they are competent to handle. Likewise, a revocable living trust is a popular option when dementia is diagnosed and the patient and/or family wishes to select their own competent management. The trust department of most banks can serve as trustee. Trustee fees are set out in published fee schedules.

Procedures are well established to provide due process under the federal and state constitutions (i.e., notice of the application and an opportunity to be heard).

The application for appointment of a guardian, conservator, trustee, or fiduciary of any type sets forth the nature of the problem and the reason court intervention is needed in concise and descriptive terms, together with a brief narrative of facts that support the legal relief sought. This is an outline for the court to consider. Further evidence is presented to the court at the time of the hearing.

The application also states the nature of the property, the status and condition of the individual involved, and a suggestion as to how the person or property should be protected and managed. It also indicates all parties by name, address, and other identifying information, setting forth who should be notified and how the notification should take place. Any person whose rights may be affected has a right to be notified and must be granted an opportunity to be heard. Once filed, the application must be served on all necessary parties, or the parties themselves may file a waiver of service and enter their appearance in the case.

Having accomplished notice, the court sets the case for a hearing. There is also a provision for ex parte emergency hearings (i.e., orders of the court without notice). These emergency orders are issued when undue delay will cause irreparable damage to the person or property. They are designed to protect and preserve the status quo or preserve the property until a full and open hearing is held.

The court has broad latitude. It can dismiss the application; it may grant the application, giving the fiduciary broad powers of control and management; or it may grant limited and closely supervised authority designed to preserve and protect the property or person in the least intrusive way. Normally, if a fiduciary is appointed, the court will require a fidelity bond that guarantees the faithful performance of the fiduciary's duties and that indemnifies the estate in the event of any failure in the performance of the assigned duties and obligations.

Substituted Decision Making

In 1985, New York State enacted a surrogate decision-making program for persons with mental disabilities who reside in state-operated or state-licensed facilities as a means to maximize patient autonomy and reduce delays in obtaining judicial authorization for medical treatment. Specifically excluded are issues related to emergency procedures and withdrawal or discontinuance of life-sustaining treatment. A panel of volunteers with specifically mandated composition ascertains, by direct questioning of the patient, whether he or she is competent to make the needed health care decision and also decides if the patient has an able and willing surrogate decision maker. If three of the four panelists find the patient unable to make the needed decision and also find that there is no suitable surrogate, the panel then decides whether the proposed medical procedure is in the patient's best interest. This procedure has reduced the decision-making time from an average of 135 days when judicial hearings were required to an average of 14 days (Herr and Hopkins 1994).

Massachusetts allows cognitively impaired competent persons to execute a health care proxy in which their agent must attempt to make health care choices the principal would have made if he or she were still competent (J. W. Fisher 1994).

Wills

Although it is beyond the scope of this presentation to delineate the specific contents of a will, certain specific questions can be asked of the patient and/or the family, together or separately:

1. Does the individual have a will?
2. Are all assets and liabilities known and easy to locate? Many dementia patients hide what they deem important.
3. Are all important papers in a convenient place?
4. Is the will up-to-date and satisfactory? When and by whom was it last reviewed?
5. Does the individual have any wish with regard to maintenance of life by artificial means, that is, to execute a living will or directive to physicians?
6. Does the individual wish to donate body parts to science or to be an organ donor?

Often, patients will have already expressed their wishes with regard to life maintenance by artificial or extraordinary medical means. It is usually not necessary to specify this in a will, and, in fact, it is difficult to specify what is meant by artificial means. Such means can range from tube or intravenous feeding to mechanical ventilatory support. Patients and their families can be alerted to these issues and discuss them if they feel them to be important. The *living will* is a separate instrument executed with will formalities. Each state uses a different form. To designate the cessation of life-sustaining efforts requires a formal instrument witnessed by two uninvolved adults and a notary. When a living will is executed, statutes and medical traditions provide numerous safeguards, including the following:

1. An independent verification of death is made by the attending physician and often by a colleague.
2. The person requesting or using the organs may not be the physician who determines the moment of death. When organ donation is involved, separate teams of physicians determine death and remove the organs.
3. Organ donation is usually waived if any family member objects.
4. The living will may be revoked at any time by the declarant.

In addition to raising the issue of donating body parts, the issue of a postmortem examination can also be raised. In research settings, a postmortem examination is a crucial link between clinical and basic science researchers. But does the patient or family wish a postmortem examination? Often, such an examination is important to family members who are interested in a precise diagnosis and a prognostication as to whether they or their children may be affected. Some family members may favor autopsy for altruistic reasons, but other family members may object on religious or personal grounds. The principal objections to autopsy are concerns about disfigurement of the body, extra expense to the family, and possible delay of funeral services. In some states, autopsy permission may be given by patient or family in advance of death, but in many jurisdictions, autopsy permission may be given only after death. It may be useful in promoting autopsy to have patients and families state their intent to have an autopsy in writing; however, the next of kin (their spouse or a child) always has the right to refuse after death.

Ethical Considerations

The management of dementia patients is replete with ethical considerations (Melnick and Dubler 1985), some of which were mentioned earlier in Chapter 8. Four primary ethical issues must be addressed in medical decision making: 1) autonomy (respect for the person and the freedom of an individual to choose), 2) justice or equitability (equal treatment for all), 3) beneficence (doing what will benefit the patient or society), and 4) nonmaleficence (the Hippocratic notion of doing no harm, especially if no good can be done) (Beauchamp and Childress 1989). It is much easier to violate considerations of justice or equitability in dealing with persons who often cannot judge for themselves what is fair or who are subject to inordinate influence and domination by others. Dementia frequently causes individuals to lose their personhood in the eyes of their caregivers, and it is easy to lose sight of their rights as human beings.

Research with dementia patients also has its ethical issues. The need for ethical guidelines in dealing with human subjects for research was given impetus by the world's awareness of abuses that occurred in Nazi Germany during World War II. This gave rise to the Nuremberg Code (1949). Patient abuses in the United States led to forming the National Commission for the Protection of Subjects of Biomedical and Behavioral Research in 1974 and the publication of the Belmont Report (1978), which set forth the four fundamental ethical principles and guidelines for research involving human subjects and the requirements of informed consent set forth above.

Autonomy

Issues related to autonomy are frequent in patients with early dementia and arise in relation to driving automobiles and living independently. Many individuals equate their ability to drive with their personal autonomy. For these individuals, not being able to drive means becoming a prisoner in their own or someone else's home. From the ethical standpoint, it would seem reasonable to allow driving until a person becomes a danger to him- or herself or others. Unfortunately, the damage may have been done by that time, but in our experience that is rarely the case. The most common occurrence is for a person with dementia to become lost while driving. Less commonly, as the result of poor depth perception or poor judgment, accidents occur. Although tests of driving skill exist (Carr et al. 1992), we do not know how well they predict whether an automobile operator is a danger to self or others. Ultimately, physicians must rely on the accounts of concerned family or others in making a recommendation concerning driving. When a person with dementia who has not been lost or in an accident drives only a circumscribed route in familiar surroundings, we urge families to wait. We weigh danger to self and others against autonomy needs and make a reasoned judgment. With some patients, in the presence of family members, we make a direct recommendation to not drive. Patients who do not recognize their impairment are not usually confronted, because that sets physician and family against the patient. Means are found by the family to get the car out of the patient's hands in such a way that the denial is not challenged.

Living independently is important to many dementia patients. Often they are women who have been single, who have raised their families as single parents or who have been widowed for many years. Their living conditions are repugnant to their families. Rugs smell of pet urine and feces; food rots in the refrigerator; dust and old newspapers gather. It is obvious in dealing with many of these individuals that their freedom is their most precious possession. They have often resisted moving in with family members and have refused living in a protected environment. They are usually adequately nourished, although their particular food preferences might seem bizarre. In such situations, physicians together with families and patients weigh the cost-benefit ratio of safety and possible prolongation of life to loss of freedom. In most cases, a compromise is possible; the elderly dementia patient continues to live alone but with unobtrusive supervision and occasional house and refrigerator cleaning.

The same issue arises in relation to diagnostic workups. If all clinical evidence points to an irreversible dementia, how far do physicians go in advocating a "complete" workup? In these situations, the patient's wishes should be respected unless there is good reason to suspect a treatable cause of dementia. The refusal of a diagnostic workup by a person with a clinical course characteristic of Alzheimer's disease (AD) should be given more weight than the refusal of an HIV-positive person to undergo such a workup. In the former case, the likelihood is not great that a treatable condition will be found. In the latter case, it is very likely.

Freedom to refuse treatment is a less frequent issue, largely because there is so little treatment currently available for dementia-producing conditions. When treatment is available and it is refused, the issue raised is what is best for the particular patient. What, for example, is to be done if a person with a diagnosed subdural hematoma refuses surgery? The danger to life may not be immediate, but the condition is life threatening, and its treatment is likely to improve cognitive function. Given this scenario, physicians are less likely to heed patients' wishes and are more likely to pursue the coercive means that are available, such as requesting a court or a relative to assume guardianship. Such would be true also in the case of central nervous system syphilis. The situation would be quite different in the case of surgery for normal-pressure hydrocephalus, in which the likelihood of reversing the cognitive deficit is small and the complication rate is great. In this instance, more weight could be given to the patient's wishes.

The situation may differ considerably, however, when patients' behavior intrudes on the rights of others or when their dementia-related behavior is so self-destructive that it will cause loss of life or severe damage to person or property if not interrupted. Where there is immediate danger to self or others, it is imperative to seek means to modify the behavior. Instances of this sort are frequent in nursing homes, in which the agitated behavior of patients with dementia places others in danger or poses a danger to the dementia patients themselves through exhaustion and failure to eat. The use of medications to control such behavior is called treatment. The control of behavior by mechanical means such as restraints or geriatric chairs is not regarded as treatment but if short-term and infrequent may be more humane than exposing patients to the acute and chronic risks of neuroleptics or keeping them heavily sedated with other medications, as in the following examples:

A frail 83-year-old man with dementia frequently attacked, with minimal provocation, the staff and other residents of a special care unit. He was treated with up to 10 mg qd haloperidol, 2 mg qd lorazepam, and 400 mg qd trazodone, with no alteration in his behavior. Because he was a significant danger to others, the staff decided, with the family's agreement, that the most humane and safe way to deal with him was to confine him to a geriatric chair when out of his room and to keep him out of reach of other residents. At mealtimes, he was seated at a table by himself as a means to keep him from reaching out and trying to break others' fingers. At the same time, his doses of haloperidol and lorazepam were reduced.

Is it appropriate to place individuals in a situation that would seem less than humane to keep them from hurting themselves? Consider the following example:

An elderly AD patient had become so demented that he could no longer speak intelligibly or respond to ordinary verbal communication. Despite the use of bed rails to prevent him from falling out, he would fall in attempting to get out of bed by climbing over the rails. He would also become quite agitated when in his room and would throw or destroy pieces of furniture. The use of both high- and low-potency antipsychotics in modest doses resulted in profound extrapyramidal effects.

The psychiatric consultant suggested that he be treated like a violent person with a psychosis. His bed and all other furniture except for a mattress and bedding were removed from his room for several months. He became calmer as his dementia progressed, and his bed and furniture were replaced in his room.

The Omnibus Reconciliation Act (OBRA) regulations of 1987, which went into effect in October 1990 and were published in final form in September 1991, hold that nursing home residents should have the right of freedom from chemical or mechanical restraint (Health Care Financing Administration 1991). Physicians are now required to justify the use of neuroleptics by making an appropriate psychiatric diagnosis. Agitation is not a sufficient justification because it is not a diagnosis; delirium is. Tightening the requirements for neuroleptic use have led to a considerable reduction in the number of nursing home patients receiving these medications without significant increase in the use of other psychotherapeutic medications (Rovner et al. 1992).

Freedom to die is still another important issue. Patients are free to die through the natural course of an irreversible, progressive illness if they so choose. In the final stages of dementia, patients are not able to express the wish to die. In this instance, the physician must rely on patients' previously expressed wishes, often contained in a living will. Without such a directive, who is to decide? Do physicians have an obligation to maintain life when ability to communicate and to understand, mobility, bowel and bladder function, and the ability to eat are lost? Many persons will have indicated at an earlier time that they do not wish to be kept alive by artificial means or that a gastrostomy or a nasogastric tube would be repugnant. Does that also apply to intravenous administration of water to maintain hydration and kidney function? When there has been no previous indication by an individual as to the life-support measures that are acceptable, who is to decide? Usually, family members are available to suggest what might have been desired, based on what is known of the individual in question. However, in the case of very elderly persons, family members may not have known the person, or there may be no family member available. No definitive answers can be given for these questions. They clearly need to be decided on an individual basis and predicated on what is best for the individual. What is best for individuals in this circumstance might be judged by the quality of life they would experience if they continued to live balanced against the pain and indignity of being assisted in surviving beyond the point that their natural functions would allow, given an irreversible illness (Thomas and Waluchow 1987). A Massachusetts court held that no judicial review is necessary for a "no-code" order for an irreversibly, terminally ill AD patient in the event of cardiac or respiratory failure (*In re Dinnerstein* 1978).

The New Jersey Supreme Court (*In re Conroy* 1985) has provided guidelines for withdrawal of life support from incompetent nursing home residents. First, there must be a judicial finding supported by at least two examining physicians that the patient is incompetent to make treatment decisions. A guardian, appointed by a court that has examined the guardian's qualifications and good faith, can make the initial determination to withdraw treatment. Before implementation, that decision would require support from two physicians independent of the nursing home, from the patient's close family, and from a state employee charged with safeguarding the interests of institutionalized persons.

The U.S. Supreme Court addressed the issue of the right to die in a 1990 decision (Cruzan v. Director, Missouri Dept. of Health, et al. 1990). In this case, parents of a long-comatose 33-year-old woman had been refused permission by the State of Missouri to discontinue their daughter's gastrostomy feedings. The Supreme Court held that states may require rigorous proof of an individual's wish to not have life prolonged by artificial means; however, if adequate proof is produced, states may not interfere with a person's wish to discontinue life-sustaining treatment.

Beneficence

Truth telling is held to be good, and U.S. physicians are increasingly admonished to tell patients their diagnosis and prognosis. Indeed, in most instances, telling patients the truth seems the best course of action. The good that telling the truth does is to allow patients to participate in directing their treatment and in directing their lives (Drickamer and Lach 1992). It also gives patients who are able to understand an explanation for the difficulties they have with their memory, communication, and understanding (Fisher 1994; Post and Foley 1992). A diagnosis of a progressive dementing illness can stimulate an individual to get business and family affairs in order and to provide for a transition to others making judgments. Some patients, however, are ill prepared to learn such news and may react with great emotional turmoil and suicide attempts. Where there is substantial evidence that such will occur, the physician is justified in withholding a diagnosis from the patient (but not from a responsible family member) (Pellegrino 1992). We have also had the experience of an evaluee in our dementia clinic stating that she did not wish to know her diagnosis. She was willing for our staff to discuss the diagnosis and to make a treatment plan with her family so long as she did not have to hear the dreaded words *Alzheimer's disease*.

The principle of beneficence also applies to treatment. If there is no great likelihood that a treatment will help an individual or that extrapolating the results of that treatment to others will be of benefit to society, the physician advocates less strongly for the treatment. A conflict of interest occurs, however, when the physician is a clinical researcher interested in the outcome of a new treatment whose efficacy is unknown. It is here that the principle of informed consent described earlier in this chapter comes into play. Although there are guidelines for informed consent, it seems unlikely that a person who is desperate for hope looks beyond the assurances and promises of the investigator and quite likely that consent is based primarily on trust in the institution or the investigator. Human beings are seldom placed at great risk so that trivial scientific questions can be answered. Institutional review boards are very attentive to certain risks, including physical well-being and confidentiality.

Subjects are also solicited frequently for research aimed at understanding the pathogenesis and clinical course of a disease; such research offers no immediate benefit to the subjects themselves. Here, the risk-benefit ratio is important, with the risk to the patient weighed against the potential benefit to society. Although a friend or family member may be empowered to make such decisions and, for example, may volunteer a severely ill dementia patient for a research project, ethical issues arise. Would the proposed subject have wished to be a participant in such research? Is it fair to involve a person who is not able to understand or give consent in potentially harmful research?

Justice

Institutional review boards are less sensitive to other ethical issues such as selection bias and the fairness of studies. Selection bias may involve the exclusion of certain individuals because they cannot afford transportation to the research site. Veatch (1987) avows that it is unfair to withhold an active drug from persons applying for a study who do not want to lose the opportunity to receive the active dug. Indeed, placebo-controlled studies are potentially unfair unless all subjects studied have access to active medication. On the other hand, if the study drug is ineffective or has unsuspected harmful effects, subjects in the control group would have avoided the harmful effects. In addition, there is much evidence from cognitive enhancer studies that crossover designs confound the effects of active drug and placebo and that parallel designs are preferable. Furthermore, in the case of AD, the criterion for positive outcome is shifting from improved cognitive status to slowing of deterioration. Thus, parallel studies may need to last as long as a year. This has been partially compensated by reducing the proportion of placebo-treated patients to 20% of the entire sample.

Sudden changes in the cognitive status of dementia patients often herald other illnesses. To what extent should physicians go to rule out every possible cause of other illness before concluding that the worsening observed was part of the dementia process? Failure to exhaust every avenue may deny an AD patient treatment for another illness. Should a decision not to pursue the cause of worsened mental status be made on the basis that the person is no longer a productive member of society or because treating the second illness would prolong the burden of care for the family and society? Can different worth be assigned to different persons and treatment decisions be made on the basis of such decisions concerning worth? On the other hand, do society and families have the right to prioritize their resources so that the greatest good is done for the greatest number or for those who can give in return? Is it just to expend an entire family's resources on sustaining a life that is barely human at the cost of educating children?

Finally, is it just to let "nature take its course" and to allow the enfeebled dementia patient no longer capable of self-feeding or self-hydration to die of starvation or dehydration? Where does allowing to die end and killing begin? Is it ever just to withhold food and water from an incompetent person whose wishes on the subject are not known? This method was the subject of an entire conference (Lynn 1986), and it can be reasonably concluded that nutrition and hydration by medical means (intravenous fluids, nasogastric tube, gastrostomy) need not always be provided (Lynn and Childress 1986), but once initiated, they must be regarded as part of the medical treatment. Issues such as these are clearly best addressed by raising them before the situation arises, as is now being done on admission to hospitals under the provisions of the Patient Self-Determination Act of 1990 (Public Law 101-508 1990).

Nonmaleficence

We do not wish to administer treatments that produce effects more harmful than the symptoms they alleviate. The use of neuroleptics to control mild agitation or to promote sleep may lead to disastrous consequences, including disabling tardive dyskinesias or falls due to the extrapyramidal effects of the drugs. The federal government has attempted to address these issues by mandating that physicians prescribe antipsychotics only to treat specific conditions (rather than behaviors) and that residents who use antipsychotics receive gradual dose reductions, drug holidays, and behavioral programming in an effort to discontinue such drugs (Health Care Financing Administration 1991). A position statement by the American Geriatrics Society and others seeks to place the use of antipsychotic medications within a rational treatment framework with other psychotherapeutic medications, indicating that in addition to addressing abuse of psychotherapeutic medications, consideration must also be given to their appropriate use and monitoring (Board of Directors 1992). Other issues with regard to side effects occur in drug research. How can cognitively impaired persons report side effects accurately? In attempting to ascertain side effects, we are forced to rely heavily on the accounts of caregivers and objective tests such as blood pressure and blood chemistries. Other side effects that are not detectable by such means but that may significantly reduce quality of life may go undiscovered.

Summary

Legal and ethical concerns appear to add complexity to the already difficult medical and practical issues in the care of dementia patients. On the other hand, knowledge of legal issues allows clinicians to know what the law allows them to do. Reflection on ethical issues can help provide a frame of reference for deciding with patients, families, and concerned others what is best to do. From the legal standpoint, attention must be paid to potential or actual changes in capacity for reasoning and decision making. If ignored, patients, their loved ones, responsible family members, and business associates and enterprises will all be adversely affected. Also, legally enforceable means are the best means for every person's expression of will concerning his or her own fate or the fate of his or her possessions. Questions concerning wills, living wills, and power of attorney for health care or financial decisions need to be addressed, despite the wish of all persons to avoid contemplation of death or mental incapacity. Ethical issues must also be faced. Is the patient's autonomy being respected without endangering the patient or others? Is the patient being dealt with as someone less worthy of treatment than other persons? Is the patient and the patient's family receiving benefit from the treatment, and is one benefiting at the expense of the other? Such decisions must be faced not only for the individuals concerned directly but also for the welfare of society as a whole. It is out of single decisions about single individuals that the ethical fabric of society is woven.

CHAPTER 10

Mobilizing Community Resources

Valerie Stephenson, L.M.S.W.-A.C.P

Doris Svetlik, B.S.N., R.N., M.S.

As noted in Chapter 1, most of the dementing illnesses seen clinically are not reversible, and many are progressive. For that reason, health care providers' role in the ongoing care of dementia patients includes helping families cope with their emotional reactions and physical stressors, supporting families in making complex care decisions, and facilitating use of appropriate community professionals and resources.

The purpose of this chapter is to help physicians and other clinicians support caregivers in mobilizing community resources. This is a difficult job for many reasons. The needs of families change constantly because the needs of patients change as their diseases progress. Options for care and support of dementia patients and families are everchanging and expanding. Whether families use community resources depends on family and patient attitudes, and the availability, accessibility, and acceptability of such resources. Often, families do not know what services are available in the community or how to access them. Even if families know what services are available and how to access them, the services themselves may not be acceptable for a variety of reasons. It is the responsibility of clinicians not only to inform families and patients of available services but to provide them with resources that can assist in making informed decisions.

Resource Needs and Factors Influencing Utilization

A variety of services and care options may be needed for dementia patients and their families, depending on the stage of the disease, the cognitive and self-care deficits, psychiatric and behavioral problems, and informal social supports available to families. Table 10–1 lists services that may be needed for persons with dementia and their families.

It is important to link dementia patients and their families to community and long-term care resources because of the special needs and problems that present frequently in regard to patients with dementing illnesses. The existence of caregiver burden in families of dementia patients is well documented (Zarit 1989). The degree of burden is variable and depends on patient characteristics and caregiver factors such as age, health status, sex, personality, coping characteristics, amount of social supports, problem-solving ability, and the relationship between dementia patient and caregiver (Zarit and Teri 1992), but there is little debate that caregiver burden is more severe for dementia caregivers than for other caregivers (Brody 1989). Although the effectiveness of care and support services in reducing caregiver burden is unclear (Zarit and Teri 1992), the need for these services is well documented (Caserta et al. 1987). Likewise, needs and problems of dementia patients who live alone and without the assistance or availability of family are of special concern to health care providers. Approximately 20% of dementia patients live alone in the community; 10% of these live alone without outside support

Table 10–1.   Services that may be needed for dementia patients and their families

Medical care including treatment of coexisting medical conditions	Financial/benefits counseling
	Protective services
Psychotropic medications	Home health aide
Multidimensional assessment	Homemaker
Skilled nursing	Paid companion/sitter
Physical therapy	Shopping
Occupational therapy	Home-delivered meals
Speech therapy	Chore services
Day care	Telephone reassurance
Respite care	Personal emergency response system
Caregiver education and training	Recreation/exercise
Caregiver counseling	Transportation
Family support groups	Escort service
Patient counseling	Special equipment (ramps, hospital bed,
Legal services	geri-chair, etc.)
Nutrition counseling	

Source.   Reprinted from Office of Technology Assessment: *Losing a Million Minds: Confronting the Tragedy of Alzheimer's Disease and Other Dementias.* Washington, DC, Office of Technology Assessment, 1987.

(Office of Technology Assessment 1990). Mobilizing care and support services for these individuals helps to reduce safety and health risks and helps to maximize their functioning so that they can remain at home as long as possible.

Although a need for services may be clear, dementia patients and their families do not always use the services that are available. An example of this comes from a 3-year respite care demonstration project conducted in four North Carolina counties. The project was developed in response to needs identified in earlier studies. Although the majority of families who used the respite services reported they were helpful, only a small percentage of the families who were eligible for services actually used them (Office of Technology Assessment 1990). This example fits with other data from 11 studies summarized in the Office of Technology Assessment (1990) report and followed by these conclusions:

1. Only one-fourth to one-half of all noninstitutionalized persons with dementia use any paid in-home or community services other than physicians' services.
2. Among those with dementia who do use services, many use very few services or use them infrequently.
3. Many persons with dementia only use services very late in the course of the disease.
4. On average, dementia patients use fewer paid services than noninstitutionalized persons with physical impairments.

The most frequently identified reasons that caregivers and patients do not use community resources include lack of knowledge about services and inability to pay for services (Office of Technology Assessment 1990). There are numerous personal reasons for not using available services. On the part of caregivers, they include denial of the patient's illness, embarrassment over the patient's behavior, fear of disapproval by friends or relatives, viewing caregiving as a personal responsibility, being too overwhelmed with work or by their emotions to enlist outside help, not wishing others in the home, and feeling uncomfortable making decisions for the patient. Patient issues include unawareness of need for services, inability to arrange for services, fear of others recognizing their cognitive deficits, fear of being exploited, and cost of services (Office of Technology Assessment 1990). Health care professionals can facilitate the use of resources for patients and families by informing them of resources and by assisting in overcoming personal resistances to their use.

Availability of Resources

Depending on the type of services needed, information can be obtained from several different levels of resources. For example, printed educational information is typically found through state and national resources, whereas information for specific services is generally found at the local level.

Knowing that services exist does not always enable access to those services. The clinician needs to provide patients and families with key links to national, state, or local information resources that can assist patients and families over time as needs change.

Although resources are abundant, both resources and family needs change continually, necessitating a "lifeline" for tracking resources. It would be ideal if there were one central resource for all information and services in all locations, but that is not the case. However, there are a number of key sources of information. They are listed in Appendix 12. These sources should enable health care professionals to support caregivers in becoming service conscious and service knowledgeable.

Accessibility

Several factors influence the accessibility of resources and services, including finances, logistical considerations, eligibility requirements, and physical ease of access. As noted earlier, cost is one of the main deterrents to use of services. This is seen especially in middle-income situations in which patients' and/or families' income disqualifies them for subsidized programs, but their income is insufficient to pay out of pocket for needed services. The financial issues are compounded when viewed from the perspective that Alzheimer's disease (AD) and other dementing illnesses require long-term care that may exceed 10 years, during which caregivers lose their employment because of increasing caregiving responsibilities. Additionally, some family caregivers may view it as selfish to pay for services that are geared toward providing relief and support for themselves instead of direct care for the patient. Finally, Medicare and other insurance coverage for most dementia care services is limited, at least with regard to the nonskilled services that are frequently needed.

Logistical problems, such as transportation needs, location of services, the ability to cut through red tape, and so on, can mean the difference between using or not using resources and services. Ease of access to services becomes of paramount concern when the lives of people become as unpredictable, disrupted, and frustrating when families deal

with a dementing illness. For example, adult day care might provide respite for the caregiver and/or allow the caregiver to continue working, but
the location of the center and transportation difficulties may prevent use
of the service. Even if transportation services are available, many caregivers report that the stress of trying to get the patient ready in time to
meet the transportation schedule may prevent use of the service. Issues
such as whether the transportation resource can provide door-to-van
service or only curb-to-van service can become critical. Families may
abandon resources too early if it seems that negotiating or working
within the "system" is too complex or if they are not prepared to deal
with these types of issues. Health care professionals can help by preparing families to deal with potential barriers. If families know what to expect, it may help limit or remove potential logistical barriers to service.
This also underscores the importance of maintaining the lifeline so that
caregivers have someone to call for additional information and support.

Acceptability

Services and care must be acceptable to patients and families. This may
have as much to do with becoming comfortable with the idea of accepting outside services as with approval of and satisfaction with a specific
service. From this perspective, clinicians can help encourage service use
by 1) facilitating the recognition and acceptance of the need for services
and 2) facilitating involvement in informed decision making regarding
services.

Accepting the Need

Helping patients and families accept needed services and convincing
them that they require additional care or services is an important issue
in that many families may not seek outside assistance until there is a
crisis (Zarit and Teri 1991). In most instances, we cannot and would not
force services on families or individuals. Some strategies, however, may
be useful in facilitating families' acceptance of assistance. A thorough
assessment of dementia patients enables families to see their patients
more objectively, especially if they can observe part of the assessment
(see Chapter 1). When health care professionals present specific information to families concerning their patients' strengths and weaknesses, it
enables families to make informed decisions about care needs and appropriate matches between the patient's needs and services. Such information helps to minimize misinterpretations of the level of care needed

by patients and prevents premature decisions regarding services or care that may be unnecessary at the patient's current level of functioning. This information helps families answer the question, How will we know what services we need and when?

The importance of obtaining a good assessment also applies to the family. In dementia care, the patient and family are viewed as an integral unit. It is equally important to obtain information concerning the family, especially the primary caregiver, to assist the patient and family in coping with the disease. We know that many factors influence the level of burden that an individual caregiver experiences. Obtaining information about the caregiver and family system combined with the assessment of the patient's needs will aid the professional in identifying caregiver needs. Whether the health care professional performs this assessment directly or refers to another professional to carry this out, the importance of this assessment cannot be overstated. This process can strengthen the relationship between the health care provider and family and sets the tone for recognition of the importance of the caregiver's health and well-being. It can also lay the foundation for family members' acceptance of help in the future. Also, the process of obtaining objective data from families on their informal support systems, caregiving skills, health status, strengths, and limitations may help them realize more clearly what their needs are. When people are asked specific questions in these areas, they may be better able to view their situation more objectively and in the context of the total picture of patient as well as caregiver needs.

Health care professionals, especially physicians, have much influence over the decisions of their patients and families. The health care provider can use this advantage by formally giving patients and families "permission" to use medically related and social support services. Some physicians write respite prescriptions for family members who evidence difficulty accepting the need and importance of time off from their caregiving responsibilities. Acceptance of care services is a *process* in the same way as acceptance of the disease. Helping patients and families to work through this process by providing emotional support and encouragement are valuable interventions.

Informed Decisions

In general, services and care are evaluated in terms of

- Quality of care
- Level and types of services provided

- Staff characteristics and dementia-related skills
- Philosophy of dementia care and program goals
- Physical plant and atmosphere
- Location/convenience
- Fees
- Dependability
- Safety and security
- Reputation

Patients and family members may have their own standards by which they evaluate potential and current services. They may also have their own mechanisms to evaluate services. These may include information obtained by word of mouth, their own personal feelings, reactions and judgments during a site visit, and/or communications with the service providers. Some patients and family members, however, feel ill-prepared to make decisions about care and services. Feeling more knowledgeable about evaluating services may help them be more accepting of various services. Being an informed consumer of services also enables persons to feel empowered to advocate for improved care and/or choose another provider if personal standards are not met. Patients and families will be more willing to use services if they feel they have some amount of control and are not helpless or powerless in these difficult decisions. Multiple guides, checklists, and other items available from sources in Appendix 12 can aid consumers in precare decisions as well as ongoing monitoring.

Conclusion

Effective resource referral requires more than giving patients and families a list of services. It requires the availability of health care providers to patients and their families for both routine planning and for family crises. It is the responsibility of health care providers to understand the issues that affect service utilization and to recognize their role in facilitating timely and appropriate use. Health care providers do not need to have a comprehensive knowledge of all services. They need, instead, to serve as a critical link in the chain that empowers patients and families to mobilize community resources.

CHAPTER 11

Nursing Care of Patients With Dementia

Linda A. Gerdner, M.A., R.N.
Jacqueline M. Stolley, M.A., R.N.C.
Geri Richards Hall, M.A., R.N., C.S.
Linda Garand, M.S., R.N., C.S.
Kathleen C. Buckwalter, Ph.D., R.N., F.A.A.N

Caring for persons with dementia is a challenge, whether they are in a hospital, in a nursing home, or at home. Nursing interventions aim to promote optimum quality of life for caregivers and recipients and to manage problems frequently seen in this population. Such problems include agitation and confused behavior, inadequate nutrition and hydration, falls, and incontinence. Problem behaviors of dementia patients are stressful to both patients and caregivers. Over time, this frustration may lead to reduced empathy and a less positive attitude toward patients, especially for nursing staff (Astrom et al. 1991) and may affect quality of care. Effective management of problematic behaviors may therefore not only improve the quality of life for dementia patients but also reduce stress levels in health care personnel.

In this chapter, we describe a conceptual model of care, the progressively lowered stress threshold (PLST) model (Hall and Buckwalter 1987), that assists formal and informal caregivers in providing patient care. We illustrate the application of this conceptual approach with problem behaviors.

Progressively Lowered Stress Threshold Model

The PLST model, based on the theories of Larazus (1966) and Selye (1980), has the following underlying assumptions:

1. All humans require some control over their person and their environment.
2. Everyone needs some degree of unconditional positive regard.
3. All behavior has cause and meaning.
4. Confused, agitated patients are best regarded as frightened and uncomfortable.
5. Patient care plans should consider patient needs throughout a 24-hour day rather than 8-hour working shifts.

Persons who are cognitively intact have a relatively high and constant stress threshold. In contrast, persons with progressive dementia have diminished ability to process sensory stimuli and to communicate with their environment. Consequently, these individuals have heightened potential for anxiety and dysfunctional behavior. Ideally, dementia patients deal calmly with their cognitive and conative losses and remain socially and cognitively accessible. Anxious behavior occurs when dementia patients experience stress (Hall and Buckwalter 1987). Dysfunctional or catastrophic behavior occurs when stress levels become intolerable; communication deteriorates as patients become unable to deal appropriately with their environment and become socially and cognitively inaccessible (Wolanin and Phillips 1981). Stress levels for patients vary throughout the day depending on many factors, including fatigue, inappropriate stimuli, physical distress, changes in routine or environment, and excessive demands (Hall and Buckwalter 1987). Nursing interventions include modification of the environment, reducing stimuli that appear to cause dysfunctional behavior, whether they be radio, television, or mirrors, while maintaining sufficient stimulation to prevent the effects of sensory deprivation (Barnes and Raskind 1980).

Agitation

Agitation is a dysfunctional behavior frequently seen in dementia patients. One definition of *agitation* is "inappropriate verbal, vocal, or motor activity that is not explained by needs or confusion of the individual per se. Although agitation probably results from a combination of needs and confusion, these antecedent conditions are not always apparent" (Cohen-Mansfield and Billig 1986, p. 712). Agitation includes aggressive behavior (i.e., hitting, kicking), physical nonaggressive behavior (i.e., restlessness, pacing, inappropriate disrobing), and verbal behaviors (i.e., complaining, negativism, repetitive phrases) (Cohen-Mansfield and Marx 1989).

Nursing care of agitated patients is complex and challenging. Interventions for agitated behaviors are most effective when used prophylactically (Hall and Buckwalter 1987). This method requires determining when agitation is most likely to occur during the day, under what circumstances (e.g., bathing, dressing), and interrupting, postponing, modifying, or finding alternatives to activities that cause agitation. Caregivers need to break down complex tasks into simple steps and determine whether activities of daily living require motor, perceptual, and cognitive skills that are beyond the patient's ability. Attempts should be made to engage patients in activities that are meaningful and at which they are likely to succeed.

Methods for Reducing Dysfunctional Behavior

The following sections address means to reduce dysfunctional behaviors, including sleep promotion, monitoring physical comfort, use of psychotropic medications, dealing with sensory deficits, creating a sense of safety, maintaining communication, increasing patients' sense of control, dealing with delusions and hallucinations, and reminiscence/reassurance techniques.

Sleep Promotion

Disruption of diurnal rhythms in dementia patients may result in sleep loss. For patients whose sleep is interrupted and whose daytime sleepiness contributes to irritability or other problem behaviors, caregivers can arrange for short, regular rest periods or quiet time reading or listening to music midmorning and midafternoon (Hall and Buckwalter 1987). Satlin et al. (1991) noted that exposure to bright lights in the evening may diminish sleep-wake cycle disturbances. Regular exercise helps diminish fatigue and promote a more stable diurnal rhythm (Hall 1994). If the in-home caregiver selects the same time to rest, the care recipient may be more likely to rest. It is preferable, however, for patients to nap in reclining chairs rather than in bed to reduce the likelihood of them thinking that a new day is beginning. A back massage may promote relaxation and facilitate rest.

Monitoring Physical Comfort

Caregivers need to continually assess patients' level of physical comfort (Curl 1989; Ryden 1992). Bowel movements need to be monitored to be certain that normal elimination patterns are maintained. Routine checks for skin irritation, ingrown toenails, or adverse medication reactions, and so on, are important, because patients may be unable to report their discomfort and may express it only in the form of agitated behavior.

Psychotropic Medications

If nursing staff is allowed discretionary management of psychotropic drugs prescribed for problem behaviors, nurses should start with the lowest dose and observe its effects before increasing dosage. Nurses need to ensure that medications are swallowed and need to monitor both positive and negative effects of medications. A realistic goal of pharmacological management is to reduce problem behaviors to tolerable levels rather than completely eliminate them (Curl 1989). Medication sufficient to totally eliminate problem behaviors may significantly compromise patients' quality of life.

Sensory Deficits

Sensory deficits may result in misinterpretation of environmental stimuli. When eyeglasses and hearing aids are needed and can be tolerated, they should be used. Appropriate communication techniques help to compensate for visual or hearing impairment, for example, the use of touch with visually impaired patients and gestures with the hearing impaired. Speaking in a louder voice may be useful for hearing-impaired patients but does not help overcome cognitive deficit. When increasing speech volume, it is best to lower the tone, so as to avoid shouting.

Safety

It is important to provide an environment in which patients feel safe. One element is the provision of a predictable daily routine. Another is the use of nonthreatening postures and movements and establishing eye contact when attempting to communicate. A calm, friendly tone of voice and gentle, unhurried touch and demeanor contribute to a sense of safety. Nurses can briefly explain what they wish to do before moving into patients' personal space to implement care (Ryden 1992). It is probably best to make positive statements such as "Let's go this way" rather than negative statements such as "Don't go that way," unless there is an immediate safety issue. In this way, patients feel guidance and support rather than criticism. Patients can be reassured directly that they are doing a good job of cooperating with nursing care by saying "good" or "that's right" during the interaction.

Determine to the extent possible which sense dominates the patients' perception of the world (auditory, kinesthetic, olfactory, or gustatory) by listening to the descriptive words used by the patient and communicating with them through their preferred sense. For example, if the patient says, "I feel like such a burden," the kinesthetic sense is being used and the nurse can respond with "feeling" words. If the patient says, "Things don't look good," the nurse would explore with visual words such as, "How do you picture things?" This approach promotes a feeling of trust (Feil 1992).

It is useful to avoid asking questions that begin with "why," because this often requires a response that patients are unable to provide (Feil 1992), leading to frustration. A better approach is offering an explanation and giving them a chance to respond with "yes" or "no." For example, instead of asking a patient why she is tugging at her dress, it might be better to ask if she needs to go to the toilet.

Patient-patient interactions may lead to agitation. In those instances, patients need to be removed firmly and quickly from each other's territory. Patient-staff interactions may lead to dysfunctional behavior when staff are attempting to engage patients in social activities or self-care, especially if done in a hurried manner and if patients' tolerance is exceeded. In those cases, it may be necessary to make a judgment as to which is more important, engaging the patient in the activity or avoiding a disturbance.

Communication

There are many communication-related issues in dealing with dementia patients. Frequently, it is not possible to understand what patients are attempting to communicate. Patients may be asked to repeat themselves, or nursing staff can offer a suggestion as to what is meant. If communication fails, it is appropriate to take a brief break, try again, and have another staff member listen. At times, family members will be able to help nursing staff understand names or phrases that patients call out, and this will facilitate an understanding of the expressed meaning.

A useful assumption is that patients know what they need and what makes them uncomfortable. If a patient refuses to participate in an activity, it is fair to assume that there is a reason. In many cases it will be necessary to deduce the reason from the patient's past behavior, such as a woman being uncomfortable around male patients or an avoidance of competitive activities. General principles for communicating with dementia patients include the following (Bartol 1979):

- Identifying oneself and addressing the patient by name
- Using short words and simple sentences
- Asking one question at a time
- Giving adequate time for response
- Repeating when necessary
- Using nouns (chair, bathroom) instead of pronouns (it, there)
- Speaking slowly and enunciating clearly
- Accompanying speech with clarifying or reinforcing gestures
- Sharing successful strategies with other staff

Nonverbal communication becomes increasingly important as the ability to receive and express verbal language deteriorates. Feil (1992) found that gently stroking patients from earlobe to chin often has a calming effect.

Control

Opportunities can be provided for patients to experience a sense of control over themselves and their environment. Examples include offering simple choices of food, clothing, and recreational activity whenever possible.

Dealing With Delusions and Hallucinations

Validation is preferable to confrontation or reality orientation in patients who are hallucinating or delusional. Validation is communicating understanding and acceptance of the patient's feelings (Feil 1992). In the case of an individual who smells fumes, it is reasonable to say, "I don't smell the fumes, but I can see that you are upset, and we will keep you safe from anything that might harm you." In addition to accepting the patient's feelings, it is useful to distract patients and redirect them into some reality-based activity. An elderly nurse, for example, was allowed to sit at the nurse's station in the middle of the night writing nursing notes (dated 1932) until she became tired and went to bed (M. Smith et al. 1993). Instead of contradicting a woman who states, "Papa's coming to get me," the patient can be encouraged to talk about her feelings for her father and what a good person he was. Attention should also be paid to circumstances under which misperceptions seem to arise or be aggravated and to avoid those situations. For example, dementia patients who are frightened by their perception of television actors as being in the room can be kept from watching television.

There is a role for reality orientation of dementia patients. It is quite appropriate in helping to deal with the acute confusion that occurs when many dementia patients are admitted to health care facilities. Staff and all visitors should identify themselves to the patient and indicate to patients where they are and that they have not been abandoned by their families.

Reminiscence/Reassurance Techniques

Encouraging patients to reminisce and tell stories about themselves also helps to increase socialization and quality of life. As noted in Chapter 5, reality orientation of patients with progressive dementing illnesses may embarrass, irritate, and agitate patients. Activities that elicit pleasant memories from earlier times may help patients feel comfortable; these activities include review of photo albums, personal memorabilia, listing favorite food items, playing a musical instrument, or listening to favorite music. Gerdner (1992) studied the immediate and 1-hour residual effects of music preferred by patients when they were younger on the frequency of agitated behaviors in confused nursing home residents. There was a reduction in agitated behaviors during the 30-minute implementation of music in four of the five subjects, with a statistically significant reduction in behaviors in the hour immediately following the presentation of music.

Baily et al. (1992) used dolls and stuffed animals to provide comfort and companionship for Alzheimer's disease patients. This was particularly effective with a woman who talked repeatedly about her need to return home to care for her husband and children, and made subsequent attempts to escape from the nursing facility to do so. This behavior frequently required the use of physical and chemical restraints. The patient was given two teddy bears, one pink and the other blue, which she named "Pinky" and "Blue Boy," and sat happily in her room holding and talking to the toy bears while she was watching television. With the implementation of this intervention, there was no further need for the use of restraints. However, care needs to be taken in the use of dolls and toys to be certain that patients cannot harm themselves with them.

Nutrition and Hydration

The multiplicity of behavioral symptoms in dementia patients poses numerous threats to nutrition and hydration. Weight loss may be ignored in community-dwelling patients who were initially overweight but may indicate depression or the development of an unrelated disorder, such as a malignancy. A 10-pound loss of weight over a 6-month period or less is significant and needs to be pursued (Nutrition Screening Initiative 1991). Patients who live alone may buy inadequate or inappropriate food, become unable to cook, or simply forget to eat. Overeating and excessive weight gain may also occur in dementing illness and may be dealt with by providing sufficient activity and structure to the patient's day.

Community-dwelling patients may need community services to help with transportation, shopping, meal planning and preparation, and safe use of utensils. Care needs to be taken to discard spoiled food. Congregate meals may be helpful inducements to eating for some patients. For others, home delivery of meals may stimulate eating, but this is often ineffective because patients may reheat containers on the stove top or simply refuse the meals (Hall 1991). Patients need to be monitored for their ability to heat prepared foods. Although microwave ovens are safer than conventional ovens, patients may be unable to use them.

In progressive dementing illnesses, patients become unable to prepare foods, may no longer perceive food as food, may have difficulty settling down to eat, or may have motor apraxia, tremor, or rigidity sufficient to interfere with self-feeding. In addition, the use of antipsychotics or antidepressants may cause difficulty with chewing or swallowing (Hall 1991).

Advanced dementia patients seem to eat best if offered culturally appropriate foods; small, frequent feedings; and high-calorie finger foods. Foods that are refused may be eaten if they are taken away and placed on different-colored plates. Consistent with the PLST model, consumption is increased by serving one food at a time with one utensil. Table settings are best kept simple, with a place mat contrasting with the color of the table to enhance perception. Care needs to be taken that nonfood items such as styrofoam cups and plants are not consumed (Hellen 1990).

Nursing Home Residents

Cognitive loss leads to significant risk of undernourishment in institutionalized elders (Durnbaugh et al. 1993; Keller 1993). Residents are often placed in large dining rooms where stimuli are overwhelming. Van Ort and Phillips (1992) characterized nursing home dining rooms as chaotic, becoming noisier and more active when food arrives. Dementia patients often require twice the feeding time of cognitively intact persons. Because nursing staff spend more time feeding the impaired residents than the minimum time allocated for daily care specified by most state laws (Durnbaugh et al. 1993), meal times may become hectic and stressful to staff and patients alike. Van Ort and Phillips (1992) suggest intake can be improved when feeding residents by 1) placing the residents' food in front of them instead of in front of the person feeding them, 2) not mixing foods together, and 3) having the same person feed the resident throughout the entire meal.

Dining groups should be small and controlled for noise and other distractions. Hall et al. (1986) found that feeding cognitively impaired nursing home residents in groups of three or four resulted in increased food intake, weight gain, or stabilization; increased socialization; and decreased dysfunctional behaviors. Medications should not be administered at mealtimes, because this turns a social occasion into a medical treatment. Medicating at mealtimes distracts residents from eating, may ruin the taste of the food, and adds additional confusing stimuli. When possible, patients should be seated in dining chairs instead of geri-chairs or wheelchairs to increase socialization and minimize "sick role" behavior.

Meals should be presented with attention to color and normal food appearance. If culturally specific foods have been part of the patient's history, family can be encouraged to provide them. Nursing home residents may also benefit from a belt pack filled with high-calorie finger foods (Hall 1991). Serving the largest meal at midday may have the advantage of patients eating when they are less fatigued. Sweetened food, finger foods, verbal cuing, and soft foods may all be of help in different situations. Nutritional supplements are useful in maintaining weight, and vitamin supplements ensure meeting daily requirements but are not a substitute for an environment conducive to eating.

Nursing home residents who hesitate to eat for fear they cannot pay for the food may be given meal tickets that can be stamped at each meal. Those who imagine themselves awaiting a family member may begin to eat if a place is set for that family member (Hellen 1990).

Late-stage dementia patients may need a period of rest before feeding. They may require plate guards and nonskid surfaces to facilitate their eating and rubber-coated spoons to decrease mouth injury (Hellen 1990). Feeding is best done one-on-one to avoid distraction. Persons with dementia may have distortion in depth perception. Therefore, utensils should be brought from the side of the face rather than directly in front to minimize fear of being poked. Attention must be paid to food consistency, sufficient time needs to be allotted for feeding, and patients should receive their largest meal at their best time of day (Siebens et al. 1986). Hydration is an important issue in late-stage dementia patients. Many patients must be helped to drink every 2–3 hours to prevent constipation and urinary tract infections. Sweet liquids such as lemonade or powdered drink mixes may assist, and fluid intake should be maintained at approximately 1,500 ml qd (McCormick et al. 1988).

A diet order of "consistency as tolerated" allows dietitians to work closely with family and nursing staff to determine the most appropriate foods as patients' needs change. Bite-sized foods eventually give way to blended foods, and spouted drinking cups and straws facilitate swallowing. Patients should also sit up to eat and drink and should remain sitting for a period of time following meals to prevent both esophageal reflux and aspiration. Families are often willing to help with feeding in the later stages, when much individual attention is required. Some caregivers have had success with large-nipple baby bottles, but bulb-syringe feeding should be avoided because of the danger of aspiration.

When patients are no longer able to take foods by mouth, the issue of enteral feeding arises, whether by nasogastric tube or gastrostomy. Volicer et al. (1989) found no difference in mortality between residents who were hand fed with a spoon and those receiving enteral feedings. Problems associated with nasogastric or gastrostomy feedings include the resident pulling the tube out, nasal irritation, and aspiration resulting from the tube being dislodged due to restlessness. Interestingly, living wills that preclude the use of extraordinary measures may not preclude the use of nasogastric tubes, because the provision of food and water is not regarded as an extraordinary measure (Hall 1991). In most states, the health care team assists the family in dealing with this issue, and families should be encouraged to consider their preference before the need arises. There is no difference in nutritional supplements used for enteral feedings (Riley 1990).

Falls

Persons with illnesses such as Huntington's disease and Parkinson's disease are at particular risk of falling. In other dementia patients, sensory deficits may lead to falls. Many medications increase the risk of falling, especially those effecting the cardiovascular system, the central nervous system, and laxatives (Stolley 1992).

Falls occur more frequently among cognitively impaired elders than cognitively intact elders (Hernandez and Miller 1986; Lund and Sheafor 1985). Falls also increase with progression of cognitive impairment (Morris et al. 1987; Reinboth and Gyldevand 1982; Swartzbeck 1983). Wandering, poor judgment, and agitation are also risk factors for falls.

Fall prevention includes assessment for postural hypotension with correction or compensation. Measures to judiciously increase blood volume or muscle tone help to correct postural hypotension. Means to compensate for orthostatic hypotension include support hose, exercising of legs before arising, and gradual assumption of upright posture. Impairment of gait due to various factors can be compensated by use of handrails, walkers, and canes. Supportive footwear with nonskid soles can also prevent falls.

Unneeded medications should be discontinued and needed medications administered at the lowest possible dose. The association of laxatives with falls is due to the bowel urgency that such agents may cause. For this reason, among others, high fiber intake, adequate fluids, and exercise are preferable to laxatives for maintaining bowel regularity.

Restraints

The use of restraints has become a focus of attention for elders in all settings. Initially, the Omnibus Budget Reconciliation Act of 1987 (OBRA) targeted the use of physical restraints and set forth criteria for their use (Health Care Financing Administration 1992). These criteria include

- Performing a thorough assessment of the behavior requiring restraints
- Using alternatives to physical restraint

- Consulting with experts such as physical and occupational therapists
- Obtaining a physician's order
- Obtaining informed consent from the patient or a responsible other
- Continually assessing the need for restraint

Additionally, OBRA set forth stringent requirements regarding the documentation and assessment of need when restraints are employed (Health Care Financing Administration 1992). More recently, the Food and Drug Administration published similar guidelines for the use of restraints in all health care facilities (U.S. Food and Drug Administration 1992).

Patients are often restrained to protect them from falling or pulling out tubes or to prevent wandering or aggressive behaviors. Although restraints can protect patients, they can also be harmful, causing both increased agitation, dependency, and demoralization. They also lead to problems associated with immobilization, such as bone loss, nosocomial infections, decubiti, and reduced functional capacity (Strumpf and Evans 1991). Patients have strangled in attempting to free themselves from restraints (Dube and Mitchell 1986), and restraints contribute to prolonged hospitalization by promoting immobility (Creditor 1993). Restraints do not necessarily reduce the frequency of falls, and elders are more likely to suffer serious injuries if they do fall while restrained (Tinetti et al. 1991).

There are many alternatives to restraints. Interventions to prevent falling should be implemented first. Aggressive, agitated dementia patients should be evaluated before restraints are used. With the PLST model, the various potential stressors (fatigue, change, multiple competing stimuli, excessive demands for performance, and physical discomfort) should all be considered with appropriate intervention.

Regular walking on a predictable route can help reduce wandering or agitated behaviors. If patients do wander, the route may be so ingrained that staff can easily find them. Environmental cues such as red or yellow tape form effective boundaries when placed on the floors in circumscribed areas (Hall 1991). Wedge cushions and posturing devices can prevent falls by supporting patients and by deterring them from leaving their chairs. In this way, struggling with restraints is reduced. Placement of chairs at regular intervals can cue patients to sit and rest, thereby reducing falls associated with fatigue. Allowing patients to sleep on mattresses placed directly on the floor enables them to sleep unrestrained.

Devices such as nasogastric tubes and indwelling catheters are undesirable in dementia patients. If a feeding tube is needed for a prolonged period, a gastrostomy tube causes considerably less discomfort. The gastrostomy tube can be camouflaged with a binder or by clothing to reduce the likelihood that it will be pulled out. Interventions to prevent or deal with incontinence (see next section) can eliminate the need for a urinary catheter. If an indwelling catheter is needed, garments can be worn to prevent access to the device instead of restraining the patient's hands or wrists. Routine perineal care can prevent skin infections that irritate the perineal area and that may precipitate the patients pulling out catheters.

Incontinence

In dementia patients, incontinence can result from the interacting effects of the cognitive impairment and the environment. The effects of dementia include disinhibition, difficulty connecting physical stimuli with the appropriate social behavior, and failing to understand the meaning of physical stimuli (including pain). Incontinence in dementia patients warrants medical investigation, especially if urinary or fecal incontinence is sudden in onset or occurs early in the course of an illness.

Functional incontinence, the most frequent type of urinary incontinence in dementia patients, is due to failure to reach the bathroom in time due to environmental barriers or disorientation (Williams and Pannill 1982). The dementia patient may not be able to adequately interpret the environment and may therefore void in inappropriate places. Well-lighted hallways and bathrooms, keeping bathroom doors open, or providing bedside commodes may be helpful. Using a toilet seat that differs in color from the toilet bowl may facilitate its recognition. Patients with dementia may be unable to recognize their own reflection in a mirror. Bathroom mirrors may lead dementia patients to believe that others are watching them, and the patient may choose a more private area, such as their own room, in which to urinate.

Interventions for functional incontinence include labeling of bathrooms to provide cues to appropriate places in which to urinate (McCormick and Burgio 1984). Prompted voiding or regular bathroom scheduling has been implemented successfully (Schnelle 1990), and modification of clothing (e.g., Velcro versus buttons) for quick, easy removal can be especially helpful.

The bladder may be underactive or acontractile due to medication, fecal impaction, neurological impairment, or prostatic hypertrophy, causing overflow incontinence or urinary retention (Agency for Health

Care Policy and Research 1992). Interventions for overflow incontinence include use of environmental cues such as running water or flushing the toilet, toileting at regular intervals, and providing enough time for bladder emptying (McClosky and Bulechek 1992). Overflow incontinence may also occur in patients receiving anticholinergic drugs. Discontinuing or reducing the dose of the offending drug is an option in the case of medications for behavior disturbances, especially if environmental modification can be substituted.

Urinary frequency and incontinence may occur in diabetic patients and in patients with excessive water intake. Detrusor instability and stress incontinence are common in elders. The former may be alleviated with low doses of oxybutynin. However, extreme caution must be taken when prescribing anticholinergics. Careful deliberation of the risks and benefits must be assessed for use in the elderly, particularly those with compromised cholinergic activity. In dementia patients, mild stress incontinence is probably best dealt with through the use of small pads such as panty liners. Urinary tract or vaginal infections also cause urinary frequency and incontinence. When a normally continent patient becomes suddenly incontinent, a urine specimen should be obtained to determine whether a urinary tract infection is present.

There are many aspects to fecal incontinence (reviewed in Winograd 1988). Change in diet or eating habits may lead to diarrhea. Medications may constipate or increase gastrointestinal mobility. Fecal impaction can also lead to seepage of liquid stool. Fecal impaction should be suspected in the absence of regular bowel movements. Adjusting the patient's diet or removal of an impaction may solve the problem. When there is no underlying medical problem, attempting to ascertain the time of the patient's regular bowel movements may enable caregivers to establish a schedule of toileting.

Total incontinence occurs in the late stage of dementing illnesses as patients no longer respond appropriately to urges to urinate and defecate. Underpads and disposable incontinence pads may be used to provide containment (Brink 1990). Pads should be absorbent and changed frequently. It is essential that areas exposed to urine be kept clean and dry; moisture barrier cream can be used to prevent excoriation (Doughty 1992).

Bathing

Safety is an important consideration during personal hygiene and should be adapted according to the person's level of independence. In the early stage of dementia, the person may only require supervision or assistance. The thermostat on the hot water heater should be adjusted so that it is not possible for persons with dementia to burn themselves. Safety items may be installed to decrease the risk of falls; these include nonskid strips on the floor of the tub and grab bars to facilitate getting in and out of the tub. Also, the installation of bath seats allows individuals to sit above the water, providing a greater sense of security. These items may be rented or purchased from medical supply houses, large drug-stores, and some department stores. Medicare, Medicaid, or major medi-cal insurance may pay part or all of the rental cost of equipment if ordered by a physician (Mace and Rabins 1991).

If the underlying disease progresses, the person with dementia be-comes increasingly dependent on the caregiver to provide for his or her personal hygiene, which can be extremely challenging. It is best to main-tain established habits. For example, persons who have taken tub baths throughout their lives may find a shower to be confusing and frightening. Even if they are used to taking a shower, this procedure may become stressful following the onset of dementia. A hand-held showerhead pro-vides a greater sense of control and consequently may be less frightening.

It is also useful to determine the time of day the person is accus-tomed to bathing and to maintain this routine as much as possible. Those used to bathing in the evening prior to going to bed may find it confus-ing to receive a bath in the morning prior to eating breakfast. It is also important to start the bathing tasks when the person is well rested, such as first thing in the morning or following a nap.

Individuals who are reluctant to bathe or shower may be more re-ceptive if their spouse bathes or showers with them. However, it is im-portant to note that the patient with dementia may refuse to bathe in the presence of someone of the opposite sex. Thus, a wife may not recognize her husband and may refuse his assistance. Another family member or paid caregiver may be helpful in these situations.

The bath should be prepared in advance to decrease the number of decisions required during the process (A. Robinson et al. 1988). When the bath water is drawn, the caregiver should ensure that it is an appro-priate temperature and not too hot. Filling the tub with only 2–3 inches of water may facilitate a feeling of security. Bubble baths or bath oils that make tubs slippery should be avoided. Soap, towels, and clean clothes need to be laid out. Privacy and a warm environmental temperature are also important. Following these preparations, caregivers can invite the patient with dementia to bathe using a calm and gentle approach and allowing the person to feel the water before entering the tub to assure them it is not too hot. The procedure should be explained one step at a time in simple sentences with a combination of verbal and visual cues.

During the bath, the skin should be observed for rashes or reddened areas. Patients should be encouraged to maintain as much independence as functional abilities allow. A reward after bathing (a cup of tea and a cookie) may turn the process into a treat instead of an ordeal.

If an individual refuses a shower or tub bath, it might be helpful to offer a sponge bath. If the person continues to refuse, it is best to abandon the idea temporarily and try again later.

Summary

In this chapter, we discuss briefly the psychosocial, environmental, and physical issues that require consideration in the nursing care of dementia patients. With a frame of reference that views patients and their behavior in terms of response to stress, attention is given to problems commonly encountered by nurses who deal with dementia patients living in the community, in nursing homes, or in hospitals. These include agitation, nutrition, falls, incontinence, bathing, and the psychosocial, physical, and pharmacological approaches to their management.

CHAPTER 12

Structuring Environments for Patients With Dementia

Margaret P. Calkins, M.Arch.
Paul K. Chafetz, Ph.D.

In this chapter, we address the impact of the surrounding environment on persons with dementia. Understanding the ways dementia patients interpret their environment can help physicians advise families and professional caregivers on optimal environmental design, which can enhance the quality of life of persons with dementia.

Life's activities do not exist in a vacuum—rather they occur within a physical and social context. Environmental characteristics of spaces create certain behavioral options while closing off other choices. A residential living room, a neighborhood park, and a ballroom elicit and are appropriate for different forms of behavior. Unfortunately, cognitive impairments of dementia patients make it increasingly difficult to "read" these cues, making inappropriate behaviors more likely.

Most people with mild dementia reside in their own homes or with relatives. Although at least half of all nursing home residents are demented to some degree (Office of Technology Assessment 1987), these residents account for only one-third of all dementia cases (U.S. Department of Health and Human Services 1984). Of the remaining dementia patients, four-fifths live with family. One implication of these figures is that interventions for dementia, including environmental interventions, should be energetically applied to noninstitutional settings. The counterbalancing consideration, however, is that the small percentage of dementia patients who reside in nursing homes are usually the most impaired. They are the most vulnerable to environmental barriers and hence most dependent on environmental prostheses. All settings in which persons with dementia reside should be designed according to therapeutic environmental principles. The goal of environmental design for people with dementia is to maximize their functional independence, dignity, and life satisfaction. The role of the environment in achieving these goals may not be immediately apparent, but Lawton and Nahemow's (1973; Lawton 1982, 1989) competence-environmental press model provides a means for understanding the potential therapeutic effects of the environment. This ecological model of behavioral adaptation and affective outcomes is based on earlier work by Murray (1938) and Lewin (1951). The uniting thread is the notion that optimal behavioral adaptation and functioning occur when there is a good fit between the individual's competence (defined in terms of biological health, sensorimotor functioning, cognitive skills, ego strength, and social status/resources) and the level of environmental demand. Kahana and Kahana (1983) expressed the same idea as the congruence of individual's needs and the environment's capacity to meet these needs. Their research demonstrated that high congruence correlates with positive morale. Lawton characterized the results of good person-environment fit as optimal adaptation and described a continuum of outcomes based on the degree of fit (Figure 12–1).

When environmental press is slightly below competence, the result is maximum comfort. If press is somewhat less, the individual may be-

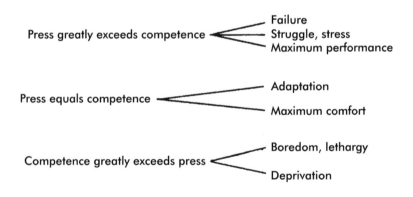

Figure 12–1.   Balance of environmental press and personal competence: behavioral and affective outcomes.
Source.   Adapted from the ecological model of Lawton and Nahemow (1973).

come bored and lethargic. Significantly lower environmental press (or sensory deprivation) results in negative affect and maladaptive behavior. When press is slightly greater than competence, the person is challenged, resulting in maximum performance. More press becomes overwhelming, resulting in stress, failure to cope, negative affect, and maladaptive behaviors. The ecological model also recognizes that although highly competent individuals can adapt to a broad range of press, individuals with less competence can deal only with a smaller range; thus, behavioral and affective outcomes are more sensitive to environmental demand in impaired individuals (Lawton 1980).

Two conclusions follow from the foregoing principles. The first is that satisfaction and good adaptation are possible at any level of competence, as long as the fit is good. This is why there is no one perfect therapeutic environment for persons with dementia (Lawton 1989). The second conclusion is that loss of competence associated with dementia leaves caregivers with more options on the environmental side of the person-environment equation than on the person side as they seek to maintain a workable balance. The environment of impaired persons can and should be made into a behavioral prosthesis (Calkins 1988; Cautela 1966).

If one accepts this theory, the task becomes one of defining the pertinent variables or characteristics on both sides of the equation. Because significant attention has already been focused on the cognitive, functional, and behavioral characteristics of persons with dementia, these only are reviewed in this chapter as they specifically relate to the interface between the individual and the environment.

Therapeutic Goals

The environment is composed of the group or social milieu, the organizational context, and the physical environment (Calkins 1993). A setting (e.g., a home or a nursing home) represents the interaction of individuals and the three dimensions of the environment. It is important to explore each of the three dimensions of the environment to understand the role of environmental press on an individual. Using Kahana's terms, one must explore the congruence between the individual and the environment and must also recognize the potential for congruence or conflict between different dimensions of the environment. For example, a nursing facility with a homelike decor that is operated with rigid a time schedule for rising and retiring, blocking of residents' schedules so they are always together in large groups, and staff-determined bathing schedules may be particularly difficult for the cognitively impaired person to understand and cope with.

Given the complexity of the environment and the unique needs of persons with dementia, the challenge of creating optimally functioning settings is significant. It is useful to develop a set of therapeutic goals based on generally accepted care goals for this population (Calkins 1988; U. Cohen and Weisman 1991). Although the literature suggests a broad range of specific therapies and various care strategies, there are some commonly accepted care goals, such as ensuring safety and security, enhancing functional independence, and minimizing disruptive behaviors and agitation. Each of the specific goals described below begins with a brief description of the relevance of the goal, considers the environmental implications of the goal, and presents a set of strategies or interventions that can be used to achieve the goal. Although the primary focus of this chapter is on the physical environment, the sociocultural milieu is also discussed, albeit to a lesser extent.

Regulate Stimulation

The brain changes of Alzheimer's disease (AD) and other dementing illnesses decrease ability to interpret and cope with stimulation (Reisberg et al. 1987). This is particularly true for multiple, competing stimuli, which can easily overwhelm the person with dementia. Thus, it is not surprising that the literature has many descriptions and recommendations for reducing environmental stimuli. Indeed, one of the most promising theoretical advances to emerge in recent years, developed by Hall and Buckwalter (1987), deals with the ability of persons with dementia to cope with stimulation. The progressively lowered stress threshold theory (see also Chapter 11) suggests that, as dementia progresses, the individual's ability to receive and interpret stimulation and information from the environment decreases. As a consequence, his or her stress threshold decreases. The authors argue that a person experiences stress when coping with the demands of the environment and that this stress accumulates, eventually exceeding the threshold for tolerating stress, which may lead to dysfunctional behavior or catastrophic reactions. This theory has provided the impetus for many low-stimulus programs and interventions. Hall and Buckwalter's model can be seen as deriving from Lawton and Nahemow's competence-press model (1973), but the competence-press model argues that too much or too little stimulation causes maladaptive behavior and negative affect. Indeed, some of Lawton's early research on sensorily deprived institutional settings indicated multiple negative consequences of low-stimulus units (Lawton 1981). Thus, the challenge is to create an environment that regulates stimulation so that it is neither overwhelming nor inadequate. Unfortunately, there is little published information about enhancing environmental stimulation.

Stimulation is not a unitary construct but can be conceptualized in terms of quantity and quality. Quantity of stimulation refers to the amount, usually in measurable terms such as decibels, footcandles, number of objects in a space, and the number of people moving through a space. Quality refers to the extent to which the stimulation is perceived as noxious (e.g., negative odors, incomprehensible sounds from a public address (PA) system, high degree of glare on the floor) or positive (e.g., visual and tactile variety throughout the unit, smell of food cooking, a fresh breeze blowing through a window on a spring day). It is significantly more difficult to measure the quality of stimulation, in part because it requires some interpretation of what is perceived as positive by people who may have lost their ability to communicate. However, it can be argued that there are sociocultural patterns that suggest what environmental characteristics are likely to be perceived as pleasant, which can be generalized to this impaired population.

Auditory Stimulation

When designing to provide regulated stimulation without stress, one goal is to minimize noxious visual, olfactory, thermal, and acoustic stimuli. Most of the literature on noxious stimulation refers to acoustic stimulation, or noise. Normal aging involves clear-cut decline in hearing acuity, especially in the higher frequencies (which includes the frequencies of most speech) (Bergman et al. 1976; Olsho et al. 1985). Dementing illness reduces ability to selectively attend to certain stimulation; hence, persons with dementia are easily distracted by noise or stimulation from their environment. This assertion is supported by the information processing model of memory, which suggests that the greatest age-related changes in memory are associated with decreased capacity of the working memory (i.e., storing and processing information) (Salthouse 1985). When working memory is overloaded, performance decreases and stress increases (Salthouse and Babcock 1991; Salthouse et al. 1991). Despite the attention in the literature on noise and stimulation (Glass and Singer 1972; Reim et al. 1971), there is little research on the exact effects of different types of noise, although many researchers and caregivers suggest that auditory distraction and overload are common (Burnside 1988; Hiatt 1987b).

It is important to eliminate unnecessary noise, such as from a PA system and loud alarms, from call systems or exit doors in long-term care settings, and from radios or TVs in all settings (except when being actively attended to). The PA system may be useful for the residents without cognitive impairment but can be confusing for dementia patients, who often do not understand where the "voice" is coming from. New call-system technology allows staff to carry individual pagers, minimizing the noise from a central panel. Other systems employ decentralized LED display monitors that make a loud, centrally located buzzer unnecessary. Loud buzzers are not needed to sound a door alarm. Reconfiguring the system so it emits a doorbell chime is an equally effective way of alerting staff to potentially hazardous egress. Different types of alarm systems are discussed in greater detail in the section on safety and security. Machinery such as ice machines and large coolers also generate significant amounts of noise that persons with dementia have a particularly hard time screening out. This type of machinery typically emits low-frequency sounds that sound even louder to the older individual and make it more difficult to hear conversation. Machinery should be located off the unit or in well sound-proofed rooms.

Noise bounces off surfaces, particularly when they are parallel and made of hard materials. Several different materials can be applied throughout the unit to provide acoustic attenuation. Carpeting is one option. Carpeting has higher friction than vinyl tile, making it somewhat more difficult for a frail older person using a wheelchair to maintain independent mobility. However, selecting a carpet with a tight weave (18- to 26-oz face weight) and a level loop surface can minimize this problem. There are also carpeting products with less resistance because they are not woven and have short, straight fibers (much like a flocked wallpaper). In the past, facilities have found it more difficult to maintain carpeting because it stained easily and smelled quickly of urine. Using a product that is solution dyed and has a waterproof barrier between the fibers and the backing has virtually eliminated these problems. Unfortunately, vacuuming of carpeting produces more noise than regular cleaning procedures for hard flooring surfaces. Carpeting on the floor is not the only acoustic option. Several carpetlike products can be applied to walls. These products have additional advantages of hiding bumps and scratches from carts and wheelchairs and of being more durable than many other wall treatments. Replacing old acoustic ceiling tiles with new ones can attenuate noise.

Not all noise is bad. If a residential unit has a kitchen, the sounds of pots, dishes, and silverware clinking together can cue residents that it is almost time for a meal (Calkins 1989). This is particularly effective for residents with limited verbal comprehension. Also, the sounds of birds (either outside or in a cage inside) can serve as a pleasant source of noise. Music can be used effectively, as long as it is appropriate for the age cohort of the individuals with dementia (Panella 1987). Many caregivers have found that persons with almost no language skills can still sing songs from their childhood. Care should be taken to avoid music that the individual with dementia would not have selected. Also, it is best not to have music playing constantly, because this is likely to be more distracting than pleasing. Music is best employed at specific times of the day, such as before a meal, in the late afternoon, or as a structured activity.

Visual Stimulation

Sensitive design also addresses the amount and quality of visual stimulation. As individuals age, a number of visual changes occur normally, including yellowing and hardening of the lens, affecting color perception, and restricting near vision (Pentecost 1984). Persons with dementia may have additional visual impairments, including impaired depth perception and difficulty in judging the meaning of visual patterns or objects. Lighting plays an important role in the quality of the visual environment. Glare caused by direct sunlight coming in windows or by unshielded lightbulbs is very hard on the eye, making it difficult to see the rest of the room. Lighting should be fairly even throughout the room to avoid darker areas that may be frightening to individuals with dementia. On the other hand, lighting design should also not be monotonous. Varying the lighting levels gradually between rooms, or over the course of the day, can add visual interest to the setting (Dobbs et al. 1988). At home, using more lamps (being careful of the placement of the cords) is generally better than a single lamp in a room. Halogen uplights, which use 300- or 500-watt halogen bulbs aimed at the ceiling, provide generous amounts of nonglare light. Finally, window treatment should be designed to avoid reflections that often occur when it is lighter inside than out. Sheers or easily pulled curtains can eliminate these reflections.

There is no best style of interior decorating, particularly for long-term care facilities. It should, however, be as homelike as possible. It is important to remember that colors are perceived differently by older individuals. Yellows and reds are easier for the older eye to perceive and stand out more in the environment. Blues and greens tend to recede and are harder to distinguish from each other. There is no evidence that color coding (using colors as an orientation cue) is effective for this population (Cooper et al. 1986). An exception may be the use of blue and pink for men's and women's restrooms (Coons 1986). However, color contrast can be used to highlight elements of the environment to which the residents should attend. For instance, plates should contrast with tables, chair seats should contrast with floors, and there should be a clear contrast between the floor and the walls. Baseboard treatment, however, should match the color of the walls as much as possible because high-contrast baseboards can make hallways look even longer than they actually are. There is no research on the amount of pattern that persons with dementia can tolerate. Some have argued for the elimination of all patterns (Shroyer et al. 1988), although this can cause the environment to appear impoverished. It is probably good to avoid the use of large, highly contrasting patterns, although smaller patterns with moderate contrast may be very appropriate.

Tactile Stimulation

Another aspect of stimulation is the presence of manipulatable objects. There are few objects to touch, pick up, and carry around in most institutional settings. Thus, residents seeking tactile stimulation may spend time going through dressers and closets, their own or others. Easily accessible objects that are appropriate to pick up and explore should be placed throughout the space. Small chests or display cases provide easily accessible storage space. The same principle can be used in home settings, by removing valuable or potentially hazardous objects and having other items easily accessible, such as figurines, photos, or towels to fold.

Maximize Awareness and Orientation

Orientation to place relies in large measure on visual input and is often impaired in AD and other dementing illnesses. Dementia patients are often disoriented and have a hard time "reading" their environment or understanding where they are in relation to where they want to go. Remembering that theirs is the fourth bedroom on the left after turning right at the end of the hall is beyond the skill of most residents of long-term care facilities. Traditional signage (with words) is difficult for this population to read and comprehend. The principle "out of sight, out of mind" is quite appropriate with persons with dementia. Thus, care settings should be designed so that the most frequently desired destinations (living rooms, bathrooms, dining rooms) are highly visible throughout the space. Several strategies have been developed for additional orientation cues. One approach is to use multiple cues that relate to different abilities and senses (Weisman 1987; Weisman et al. 1991). Words can be combined with graphics, and tactile cues (e.g., signs that can be touched) can also be used. It is important to give the greatest emphasis to those cues that are most personally important to individuals with dementia (Calkins 1989). Orientation cues to bedrooms, bathrooms, and shared public areas should be most visible. Cues do not have to be limited to signs. In a typical long-term care facility, the bedroom entrance with the resident's name on a small card and a room number (often reflecting the complexity of the whole facility) is not likely to support independent way finding. Having personalized memorabilia at bedroom entrances is more effective than personally nonmeaningful objects (Namazi et al. 1991). At home, a large sign, a picture of a bed, or a colored door can facilitate way finding (Calkins et al. 1990; Pynoos et al. 1987). Large and colorful cues at bathroom entrances (signs or canopies that are visible from down the hallway) can aid in locating bathrooms, a necessary prerequisite for maintaining continence. Whenever possible, cues should relate to the goal (Brawley 1992). For instance, a red-striped pole might indicate a barber shop or area where the men are shaved. This can be done in the home as well as in care facilities. Persons with dementia may also enjoy looking outside if the view is interesting. However, it can be frustrating if they have visual access to areas to which they do not have physical access (Calkins 1991). Orientation refers to more than spatial orientation. Persons with dementia are also confused with respect to time and activity. Placement of windows that are highly visible throughout the space can help keep some people oriented to time. Also, adjustable lights, which can be dimmed as evening approaches, can cue that it is bedtime. Using a single room for multiple, unrelated purposes is likely to confuse dementia patients. It is best to have a dedicated dining room that is used only for meals and other food-related activities (e.g., coffee klatches, afternoon tea) (Weber 1992). If this is not possible, highly visible and appropriate cues can indicate that a meal is about to be served. Setting the table with placemats and flatware cue eating and can be a meaningful activity. Predictability also enhances awareness. Constantly changing schedules can be very disturbing to the person with dementia.

Knowing that lunch is always served after a music program can be reassuring and help patients prepare for the meal.

Support Personal Continuity With the Past

Residential or *homelike* refers to what a particular individual is used to. Some people have lived in apartments, whereas others have always been in single-family, detached houses. People from different socioeconomic backgrounds may have very different experiences and expectations. Some dementia patients may revert to memories of earlier living places that are significantly different from their local place of residence. Nevertheless, some aspects of home are nearly universal. Homes are places where people typically have substantial autonomy and control over their environment and their actions. Thus, creating a setting that supports appropriate autonomy is highly desirable. Opportunities for getting up for a midnight snack, or sleeping late in the morning and having just a cup of coffee for breakfast, or taking a shower at night instead of a bath in the middle of the day are all characteristics of a noninstitutional, residential setting. Given the preponderance of women in long-term care settings, providing a kitchen on a residential unit may be one of the most important residential features available. Kitchens provide a natural setting for a variety of activities that are easily broken down into small, manageable tasks such as washing dishes, setting tables, and wiping the counters. It is easier to be successful at and derive meaning from these familiar tasks than from new and unfamiliar activities such as basket weaving or other crafts (Weber 1992). Finally, a kitchen also provides multisensory stimulation, orienting residents to the fact that a meal is about to be served (Calkins 1991). Residents should be encouraged to bring in furniture from home and hang their own pictures on the walls (Calkins 1988; Koff 1988). The presence of culturally or religiously significant symbols can help residents feel comfortable in this new setting (Lawton 1989).

Provide Secure Freedom

Persons with dementia have impaired judgment and often misuse common elements of the environment or get lost. However, there are contrasting views about how much autonomy and control are wanted by persons with dementia. Shroyer (1988) suggests that persons with severe dementia prefer not to make choices. An alternative approach, espoused by Calkins (1988), Namazi and Johnson (1992), and U. Cohen and Weisman (1991), is that persons with dementia often struggle to maintain control and should be given opportunities to make choices that are appropriate to their cognitive and functional abilities. In dealing with security issues, the former approach would seek to minimize their access to everything that is potentially hazardous. The alternative goal would be to create a setting in which they can exert self-determination in an appropriately secure way that minimizes risk.

Egress from the house or residential unit is a major concern, and many caregivers have resolved this issue by securing the doors. Results from research on home modifications (Calkins et al. 1989; Noelker 1987; Olsen et al. 1993) indicate that family caregivers are quite creative in finding ways to secure doors and windows of their homes. Examples include double locks (either installing a second doorknob or often locating a dead-bolt lock at the top or bottom of the door), hanging a curtain in front of the door, using "keep away" signs, and keeping the area by the door very dark. Many institution-based research projects have explored a variety of strategies to minimize residents' egress. One set of studies explored the efficacy of placing lines of tape in front of an exit door to keep dementia patients from reaching the door (Chafetz and West 1987; Hussian and Brown 1987; Namazi et al. 1989). The results were varied, with only one researcher finding the tape lines effective. An alternative strategy is to place fabric that is approximately 18 inches high across the door at handle height (starting 25 inches from the floor) (Namazi et al. 1989). This can be attached to the door frames with adhesive Velcro tape. The minimal pressure required to release the barrier is acceptable by many state fire codes. There are also a variety of electronic security devices for locking doors. Fire codes in many states now allow doors in long-term facilities to be secured if they unlock automatically in case of a fire. Many of these devices allow staff and visitors to leave the unit without setting off an alarm by entering a code number or simultaneously pushing two buttons to disable the alarm. Other systems only lock the door or set off an alarm when a resident wearing a tag approaches the door. Most of these approaches, however, significantly restrict the freedom of the person with dementia. A preferable alternative approach is to provide direct and unrestricted access to a secure courtyard or garden. There are some potential risks involved when dementia patients can go outside unattended, but some research has demonstrated a significant decrease in agitation when exit doors are unlocked (Namazi and Johnson 1992).

There is ample evidence of positive benefits of going outdoors and the exercise this can provide (Gueldner and Spradley 1988; Rapelji et al. 1981; Sullivan 1987). With many electronic systems, doors can be wired so they can be secured at night or during inclement weather but left unlocked during the day. Certain security precautions should be taken to minimize the hazards of an accessible kitchen. There should be locked cabinets for knives and cleaning supplies. The stove can be made safe by installing a separate power switch with a timer (so it automatically shuts off, even if the staff forget to turn it off) located in an out-of-the-way place, such as inside a cabinet. This keeps impaired persons from using the stove unsupervised. There are also new products that are significantly safer than traditional appliances. One example is the induction cooktop, in which the cooking surface does not get hot enough to burn a hand placed directly on the burner. Although this device is a little less familiar, the safety value may outweigh the benefits of familiarity.

It is generally helpful for caregivers to have easy visual access to the patients. However, given the emphasis on creating less institutional long-term care settings, the traditional large, centrally located nurse's station may not be the most appropriate solution. Having a desk incorporated into the kitchen or other central space provides a place for staff to work without residents feeling as though they are constantly being watched. At home, there are a variety of relatively inexpensive motion detector or sound monitors that can alert the caregiver to the location of the person with dementia.

Persons with dementia often have a variety of age-related impairments that can be addressed with an appropriately designed environment. Efforts should be made to eliminate or minimize changes in floor levels. Noelker (1987) found that environmental barriers such as stairs have a significant impact on caregivers' ability to provide care and on the amount of burden they experience. When level changes are unavoidable, the edge of steps or ramps can be highlighted with color-contrasting tape so it is highly visible. Handrails need to be incorporated at all level changes and anywhere else a person might fall. Counters and furniture should have rounded edges to minimize injury if someone falls against them. Furniture should be sturdy, because it is sometimes used in lieu of a handrail to steady oneself.

Enhance Positive Social Interactions

As meaningful conversation becomes increasingly difficult, the environment can help to support meaningful interaction in a number of ways.

Persons with dementia find it increasingly difficult to construct conversation about topics that are not readily seen or touched. Thus, if the environment is impoverished and there is nothing of interest to look at or do, there is little to talk about. However, a setting filled with personalized artifacts, interesting manipulatables, a variety of things to watch from the windows, and visually and tactually rich wall hangings supports conversation at a variety of levels. Meaningful interaction is also encouraged by engaging in more meaningful activities. Thus, working together with someone else on setting the table or clearing up, raking the yard, or gardening provide avenues for easy conversation.

As noted above, extraneous noise can make it more difficult to hear and interpret conversation. This includes not only noise from PA systems, call bells, and machinery and equipment but also noise from other people. Caregivers who call loudly down the hall or across the room on a regular basis can disrupt ongoing interactions. Other people in the room doing other things can also make positive interaction more difficult, given the easy distractibility of this population. Having a variety of smaller program/activity rooms, as opposed to one large, centrally located dayroom, will increase the ability of individuals to hear what is going on and encourage their meaningful participation. However, not everyone wants to be engaged in activities all of the time. Having a variety of places to sit and watch ongoing activities is important. An area with two or three chairs gives people a chance to sit together and talk about what's going on. Musculoskeletal changes associated with aging cause older people to have a harder time turning their head to look at someone sitting next to them. Therefore, chairs should be arranged in societal arrangements (i.e., at right angles to each other, instead of side by side) (McClannahan and Risley 1974; Sommer and Ross 1958).

Finally, research has suggested that there are benefits of increased resident privacy (DeLong 1970; Lawton 1970; Pastalan 1974; Proshansky et al. 1970). When people do not have access to private places, they tend to create their own privacy by withdrawing socially (often referred to as "null" behavior). Having a private place is important for the residents of long-term care facilities and for families who visit and wish to hold private conversations. It is also important for caregivers at home who need time away from their loved one. Privacy can be a challenge to provide, particularly in facilities with shared bedrooms. The so-called privacy curtain provides only visual separation, not true privacy. Therefore, extra efforts should be made to provide alternative places for privacy.

Summary

There is increasing evidence of the positive effects of the environment on the behavioral, functional, and emotional status of cognitively impaired individuals. Several investigators have identified numerous changes that family caregivers make to their homes to make caring easier or safer (Calkins et al. 1990; Gnaedinger 1989; R. V. Olsen et al. 1993; Pynoos and Ohta 1988). Long-term care facilities have increasingly recognized the unique care needs of this population and have begun to respond to these challenges. One common response is to develop so-called special care units (SCUs) that ideally combine programmatic, organizational, and physical environmental characteristics designed to meet the needs of the cognitively impaired and their caregivers. The Office of Technology Assessment recently released a report on SCUs (U.S. Congress Office of Technology Assessment 1992) that showed little consensus between facilities and across states as to what constitutes an SCU. The report demonstrates, however, that the structure of the physical and social environment can affect the functioning and quality of life of persons with dementia. The challenge is to identify the specific ways in which the environment affects individuals with dementia and their caregivers.

This chapter includes a review of five principles for environmental interventions to enhance quality of life.

1. **Regulate stimulation.** Persons with progressive dementia are sensitive to stimulation and have a hard time interpreting it or screening out undesired or unnecessary stimulation. Stimulation is not a unitary construct, and the differential impacts of quality versus quality need to be recognized. Strategies include minimizing negative or noxious stimuli and enhancing positive or meaningful stimulation.

2. **Maximize awareness and orientation.** Because of their cognitive impairments, dementia patients cannot rely on their memory to orient themselves within a space. Therefore, the environment needs to provide cues to help them maintain independence. Use of multiple cues, which appeal to different senses and cognitive abilities, appears to be an effective strategy. Making the cues meaningful, such as personalized cues at bedrooms entrances, has also been shown to be effective.

3. **Support personal continuity with the past.** Persons with dementia are most competent at skills they have practiced over a lifetime.

They benefit from opportunities to engage in long-practiced routines and activities, such as domestic tasks for housewives. They are usually more comfortable in settings that resemble home and that have recognizable items such as their own furnishings.

4. **Provide secure freedom.**   The impaired judgment of individuals with dementia renders almost any setting potentially hazardous. Limiting access, although sometimes necessary, can be executed in a way that only minimally reduces autonomy and control. The goal is to promote access to things and areas that are important and positive for the individual with dementia in an environment that is secure from unnecessary hazards. Direct, unrestricted access to a secure outside area is critical.

5. **Enhance positive social interaction.**   Because verbal communication becomes increasingly difficult, it is critical that the environment support meaningful and positive nonverbal communication. Minimizing potential distractions can encourage greater focus on activities. Providing a variety of things to look at and touch and encouraging familiar activities such as cooking or yard care are likely to induce more meaningful interaction.

It is important to recognize the potential therapeutic effects of the environment on persons with dementia. Many of the most effective interventions are relatively inexpensive and thus highly cost effective. Many facilities indicate that appropriate environmental settings decrease costly staff turnover, minimize burden and stress, and reduce accidents and catastrophic reactions, although at this time these assertions are seldom supported by empirical research. Research is growing in this vital area, and more caregiver conferences are including presentations and information about the therapeutic role of the physical environment. For more information, the reader can consult a number of excellent design guides that address in great detail the environmental needs of persons with dementia and their caregivers in great detail (Calkins 1988; Calkins et al. 1990; Cohen and Day 1993; Cohen and Weisman 1991; Coons 1991; R. V. Olsen et al. 1993; Sloane and Mathew 1991; Weisman et al. 1991).

CHAPTER 13

Advances in the Biology of Alzheimer's Disease

Steven T. DeKosky, M.D.

For many years, the major focus of research in Alzheimer's disease (AD) was on the structural and neuropathological changes occurring in the brains of patients. In the past decade, a new body of research has expanded beyond examination of structural and neuropathological changes in brain tissue (as Hughlings Jackson put it, "the thing caused") and has focused more on mechanisms by which the disease may have emerged or on mechanisms that may contribute to the pathological cascade ("the cause of the thing"). Just as the new technology of silver staining enabled Alzheimer to discover the disease bearing his name, many of our new findings through the 1970s, 1980s, and 1990s have resulted from the application of emerging technologies. In the 1970s, radioimmunoassay enabled the development of sensitive brain enzyme assays, and radioactive ligands enabled autoradiographic and homogenate studies of neurotransmitter receptors. These discoveries, beginning with the determination of the cholinergic deficit in AD (P. Davies and Maloney 1976) led to trials of medications aimed at enhancing cholinergic neurotransmission in human brain. In the 1980s, powerful computer systems enabled image analysis to be applied to brain tissue studies of both neuropathology and neurotransmitter systems. In the 1980s and 1990s, expansion and widespread availability of molecular biological techniques and development of transgenic models has enabled the testing of hypotheses about causation or pathophysiology of AD. As rational pharmacotherapy derives mainly from knowledge of etiology or pathophysi-

I thank Scot D. Styren, Ph.D., for assistance in the preparation of this manuscript. Supported by the Alzheimer's Disease Research Center (AGO 5133).

ological cascade, newer therapeutic strategies based on experimental findings will also be based on the discoveries about the mechanism of disease that these new biological tools reveal.

Structural Changes in Alzheimer's Disease

This section deals with research concerning the selective vulnerability of certain neuronal populations, neuron and synapse loss, and pathological changes in AD.

Selective Vulnerability

Earlier views of AD as due to diffuse neuron loss or cerebrovascular disease have given way to the concept of AD as a corticolimbic system disease in which the initiating pathophysiological cascades occur in vulnerable regions of the brain. In some ways, AD resembles spinocerebellar degenerations or motor neuron disease due to generalized enzyme deficits. In these diseases and in AD, only a few cases are familial, and in each, certain central nervous system (CNS) regions are devastated, whereas others are relatively unharmed. The limbic system, especially the entorhinal cortex, hippocampus, and amygdala, are among the brain regions most affected by the neuritic plaques (NPs) and neurofibrillary tangles (NFTs) that characterize AD. The association regions of the cerebral cortex, especially the inferior and medial temporal cortices but also the parietal, frontal, and occipital cortices, are affected much more than primary sensory and motor cortex. Pyramidal neurons are the major cortical cell type lost in AD (Terry et al. 1981), and the extent of pyramidal cell loss in frontal and temporal cortex correlates with cognitive decline (Mann et al. 1988).

Selective vulnerability to neuronal death is seen in neurons in the basal forebrain cholinergic nuclei, locus coeruleus (LC), and dorsal raphe nuclei in the basal forebrain and brain stem (Bondareff et al. 1982; Whitehouse et al. 1982). These nuclei include the projection systems for acetylcholine (ACL), norepinephrine (NE), and serotonin. They lose up to 90% of their cells, but nearby cell clusters are normal. In association cortices, the large pyramidal cells of lamina III and lamina V are preferentially lost (Mann et al. 1988; Terry et al. 1981). Yet such loss does not occur in the motor cortex, where spasticity and hyperreflexia would emerge if neuron loss occurred.

Although the basis for the selective vulnerability of specific neuronal systems in AD is not understood, the connection of limbic and association areas may explain the pattern of degeneration. The site of the earliest NP formation is the mesial temporal region, notably the entorhinal cortex (Braak and Braak 1991; Mann and Esiri 1988). This also occurs in Down's syndrome, in which all patients over the age of 40 years develop the neuropathological and biochemical changes of AD (Mann and Esiri 1989). Thus, a pattern of spread of the pathological changes from mesial temporal lobe to cortical association areas to projection nuclei that extensively innervate the cortex (basal forebrain cholinergic neurons, LC, raphe nuclei) provides an anatomical substrate based on connectivity (Hof and Morrison 1994). If cortical pathology led to retrograde transmission of disease to the brain stem projection nuclei that degenerate, this might account for the loss of neurons in the basal forebrain, LC, and raphe nuclei (Pearson et al. 1985). One hypothetical mechanism involves loss of retrograde axonal transport interfering with the delivery of target-derived neurotrophic factors to cell bodies of the vulnerable neurons (Tuszynski and Gage 1994). The cytoskeletal pathology in AD certainly puts such structure-dependent processes at risk, although currently we have no way to assess anterograde or retrograde axonal transport in living humans.

The large pyramidal cells affected by AD are mainly those with long corticocortical axons. This may relate to greater metabolic demands on such cells than on the relatively spared smaller interneurons. The neuronal loss appears to have strong correlation with the intracellular presence of neurofilament protein and manifestations of neurofibrillary pathology (Hof and Morrison 1994).

Synapse Loss

The final common pathway of neuronal information transfer is the synapse. Loss of synapses in AD appears to be widespread in the affected regions (C. A. Davies et al. 1987; Hamos et al. 1989; Honer et al. 1992; Masliah et al. 1991; Scheff and Price 1993; Scheff et al. 1990; Zhan et al. 1993). The extent of synapse loss correlates with cognitive deficit in living patients who have undergone cortical biopsy (DeKosky and Scheff 1990). Biochemical markers of synapses (synaptic proteins) decline in AD, and their level also correlates with cognitive status of patients prior to death (Terry et al. 1991). By comparison of synapse counts from the cortex of living patients who underwent cortical biopsy with counts from patients

who died with more severe disease, it appears that synapse loss continues as the disease progresses (DeKosky and Scheff 1990).

Neuritic Plaques and Neurofibrillary Tangles

The neuropathological diagnosis of AD rests on the appearance of the
NPs and NFTs originally described by Alzheimer in the limbic system
and cerebral cortex. Assessing the number and distribution of these
neuropathological hallmarks remains the basis of the neuropathological
diagnosis (Braak and Braak 1991; Khachaturian 1985; Mirra et al. 1991).

Neuritic Plaques

NPs are spherical tangles of neuritic processes, including degenerating
axons and dendrites, astrocytic processes, and microglial processes
(Terry et al. 1994; Yamaguchi et al. 1992) (Figure 4–1). Various proteases
are found in plaques. Whether they are part of the initiating pathology
or a reaction to the neural degeneration is not known (Fraser et al. 1993;
Hinds et al. 1994). In the center of these spheres of degenerating neuropil
is β-amyloid, a fragment of a large molecule known as amyloid precursor
protein (APP) (see the section Amyloid Metabolism and Alzheimer's Disease later in this chapter). In many areas of the brain, "diffuse" plaques
are seen, which consist of fibrils of β-amyloid without the surrounding
neuritic degeneration. Interestingly, such diffuse plaques also occur in
the cerebellum and thalamus (Joachim et al. 1989b), where the neuritic
reaction and "mature" plaques (cores of amyloid surrounded by neuritic
degeneration) are not seen. Thus, β-amyloid deposition can occur in certain regions of brain, but some other intrinsic property of specific brain
regions is necessary to produce the neuritic degenerative and inflammatory process.

Although early studies indicated a correlation between NPs in the
cortex and severity of dementia (Blessed et al. 1968; Bowen and Neary
1985; Martin et al. 1987), other studies have not reliably reproduced this
finding (DeKosky et al. 1992; Mann et al. 1988; Neary et al. 1986; Terry et
al. 1991; Wilcock et al. 1982). Although synapse counts in cortex correlate
best with dementia severity, the presence of NPs is the *sine qua non* of AD.

Neurofibrillary Tangles

NFTs (see Figure 4–2) are depositions of highly insoluble protein within
cortical and limbic neurons (Ohtsubo et al. 1990; Terry et al. 1994). Under

the electron microscope, the protein comprising tangles consists of paired helical filaments (PHF), which are highly cross-linked and very insoluble. They are believed to be composed primarily of highly phosphorylated tau protein, a normal constituent of the neuron, which is a microtubule-associated-protein. It is not known how tau protein becomes phosphorylated at multiple sites and cross-linked so excessively that it is virtually impossible to solubilize. Disruption of cytoarchitecture by the pathological process might provide the mechanism by which neurons die (Hof and Morrison 1994). "Ghost" or "tombstone" tangles are collections of NFTs that lie free in the neuropil, usually in the pyramidal shape of the neurons that contained them prior to their death. This is a testimony to the longevity of the NFTs and their cellular source. The number of neurons in a region of brain that contain PHF may correlate with duration of the pathological process, because once formed, there does not appear to be a way for the neuron to rid itself of this protein (Hyman et al. 1994). As discussed below, NFTs and abnormalities of the cytoskeleton may mark vulnerable neurons that will die or become atrophic.

Alterations in Neurotransmission

Modern advances in understanding AD began in the late 1960s and early 1970s, when researchers in Great Britain developed criteria based on numbers of NPs and NFTs to make a neuropathological diagnosis of AD and to separate AD from vascular dementia (Tomlinson et al. 1970). In addition to being important for diagnosis and understanding pathophysiology, these diagnostic criteria enabled researchers to compare neurochemical changes in AD brain with normal aged control brains and to devise therapies that, it was hoped, would restore neurotransmission in the AD brain. Alterations in markers of neurotransmission—enzymes that synthesize the neurotransmitters, concentrations of the neurotransmitters themselves, and numbers of receptors for these specific neurotransmitters—became a prime focus of research in AD in the 1970s.

Devising a drug to enhance neurotransmission in a "failing" system had been accomplished for Parkinson's disease by compensating for striatonigral dopamine deficiency with oral administration of the dopamine precursor levodopa (L-dopa). Finding specific neurotransmitter defects in AD was expected to lead to the same sort of treatment.

The Cholinergic System and Alzheimer's Disease

The first specific neurotransmitter defect to be discovered in AD was that of the cholinergic system, in which there is loss of the synthetic enzyme choline acetyltransferase (ChAT) in the cortex and hippocampus (Bowen et al. 1976; Davies and Maloney 1976; Perry et al. 1977). ChAT is found in the presynaptic boutons of the cholinergic source neurons in the basal forebrain nuclei, a group of neurons at the base of the human forebrain comprising the medial septal nucleus, the diagonal band of Broca, and the nucleus basalis of Meynert. Lesions of these cell groups in rats or monkeys lead to loss of ChAT and the ability to synthesize the neurotransmitter acetylcholine (ACh) in the cortex or hippocampus (Bartus and Dean 1982; Geula and Mesulam 1994; Wenk 1993). The loss of this enzyme was an exciting finding because the cholinergic system was amenable to manipulation by medications and because this neurotransmitter is associated with short-term or recent memory function (Bartus and Dean 1982), one of the first and most obvious functional losses in patients with AD. Further, the loss of this selective set of projection neurons appeared specific to AD (Whitehouse et al. 1982) because the cholinergic neurons of the basal ganglia and the spinal cord were unaffected by the disease.

A variety of efforts have been made to supplement or stimulate cholinergic neurotransmission in the brains of patients with AD. Age-related losses of recent memory function are common in aging mammals from rats to subhuman primates, and supplementation of their cholinergic systems by oral choline or by acetylcholinesterases (which delay the hydrolysis of ACh made at the synapse) improves memory function of these aging animals. Encouraged by these results, clinical trials of the precursors choline and lecithin and anticholinesterases such as physostigmine were performed in the late 1970s and early 1980s. As noted in Chapters 6 and 14, none of these efforts produced significant improvement in cognition of patients. In 1986, the oral anticholinesterase tacrine was reported to produce remarkable improvement in memory and cognition in a group of 17 AD patients (Summers et al. 1986). Subsequent studies have found much more modest improvement (Farlow et al. 1992; Knapp et al. 1994), but sufficient improvement was seen in patients given tacrine to enable its approval by the Food and Drug Administration for treatment of AD. As of this writing, it is the only drug so approved, but several other anticholinesterases are currently in clinical trials (see Chapter 14).

Cholinergic-Receptor Changes

Total numbers of cholinergic receptors in cortex and hippocampus appear to decrease with aging but do not differ in AD from normal age-matched control subjects. It is clear that the cholinergic M_1 receptor, which comprises about 80% of the cholinergic receptors in the human cortex, is unchanged in number in AD. The finding of normal numbers of total cholinergic receptors led to the belief that cholinergic neurotransmitter function could be aided with an appropriate supplementation strategy or with a direct receptor stimulator or agonist. Several attempts to administer cholinergic receptor agonists through the periphery have been unsuccessful, as indicated in Chapter 14. A few studies have suggested that the M_2 receptor population is decreased (Araujo et al. 1988; Mash et al. 1985). Because the M_2 receptor is found on the presynaptic bouton, loss of these presynaptic elements might be accompanied by loss of the M_2 receptors as well.

Some studies suggested that the receptor systems may not be as intact as the initial receptor-binding studies indicated (Flynn et al. 1991). A "disconnection" of the receptor from its second messenger in the cell (failure to activate a G-protein that transmits the message intracellularly) would mean that even if the surface receptor were present one might not be able to activate the neuron as effectively. This area is also under investigation; others have not found this disconnection (Pearce and Potter 1991).

One difficulty with neurochemical studies using postmortem tissue is that the studies reveal changes at end stage; there may be less total destruction of neural elements in earlier stages of disease. Biopsy studies of AD patients early in the disease confirmed that there was significant loss of ChAT in the cortex in mildly affected AD cases, with a weak but statistically significant correlation of loss of cortical ChAT with cognitive loss (DeKosky et al. 1992). Biopsy cases had significantly more ChAT activity in the cortex than patients who had died of the disease at later stages.

Noradrenergic Alterations

Decrease in the amount and uptake of norepinephrine (NE) was determined early in the course of AD research. The synthesizing enzyme for NE, tyrosine hydroxylase, is decreased in AD, and its source nucleus, the brain stem LC, is depleted of neurons (Bondareff et al. 1982; Marcyniuk et al. 1986). Interestingly, the loss of LC neurons is in the anterior and

lateral aspects of the nucleus that project to the forebrain. The more cau-
dal neurons of the LC are spared in AD. These neurons project to the
cerebellum and spinal cord, where the pathology of AD does not occur.
There is no loss of NE in those areas, and clinical symptoms referable to
these regions are not seen in AD. There is no correlation of cognitive loss
with degree of loss of LC neurons or decrease in amount of NE, but there
is some correlation between loss of this neurotransmitter and the presence of mood symptoms in patients while they were alive (Zubenko and
Moosy 1988).

Serotonergic Alterations

In AD, there is loss of dorsal raphe neurons, which are the serotonin
source neurons for the forebrain (Yamamoto and Hirano 1985; Zweig et
al. 1988). There is also loss of serotonin nerve terminals from the cerebral
cortex, based on reduced concentrations of serotonin, and its major metabolite 5-hydroxyindoleacetic acid (5-HIAA); reduced serotonin uptake;
and reduced serotonin release in cortex (Francis et al. 1994). As with NE,
there is not a strong correlation of serotonergic changes with cognition,
but noncognitive symptoms such as depression and aggressive behavior
may have some relation to loss of serotonin. As indicated in Chapter 6,
trazodone has been used to suppress aggressive behavior in AD. Serotonin reuptake inhibitors such as sertraline and fluoxetine have been used
effectively in depression in AD, although controlled trials of the effectiveness of these serotonergic (and noradrenergic) drugs have not been
performed.

Dopaminergic Alterations

In most cases of AD, there is not a significant loss of substantia nigra
dopaminergic neurons as there is in Parkinson's disease (Mann et al.
1980). In keeping with this pathological finding, most AD patients do not
have tremor, rigidity, or bradykinesia.

Glutamatergic Alterations

Alterations in glutamatergic metabolism have been proposed for years,
because elevated levels of glutamate and other excitatory amino acids
(EAAs) can cause excitotoxic neuronal death. Because the pool of glutamate associated with neurotransmission is much smaller than the pool

associated with metabolism, measurement of total glutamate would not reveal findings referable to specific changes in the neurotransmitter metabolic pool. However, the large pyramidal neurons of the cortex and the entorhinal cortex neurons that project to the hippocampus are lost in AD, and both have EAAs as their neurotransmitters. This is reflected by loss of D-aspartate binding in cortex (Proctor et al. 1988). A number of EAA receptors, specifically glutamate receptor subtypes, have been examined in AD, but no major alterations have been found (Palmer 1991). However, the possibility that dysregulation of EAA metabolism might lead to excitotoxic neuronal death has led to a number of preclinical studies examining the effects of blocking or modulating some of the various subtypes of glutamate receptors.

Other Neurotransmitters

A variety of other neurotransmitters, including somatostatin, corticotropin-releasing factor, and other peptide neurotransmitters, have been reported to be abnormal in AD cortex or in other parts of AD brain. In some cases, these losses probably reflect the loss or dysfunction of small cortical interneurons or downregulation of their function (Hof and Morrison 1994). Because we do not know the function of most of these peptide neurotransmitters, it is difficult to say how these changes reflect clinical manifestations of AD or what their relationship is with the pathophysiology of the disease.

Amyloid Metabolism and Alzheimer's Disease

The amorphous substance in the center of NPs has a β-pleated sheet arrangement and was revealed by Congo red staining to be amyloid. This amyloid is found in the center of NPs and in the walls of small blood vessels in all cases of AD. Amyloid has been cloned and found to be a small (40–43 amino acid) fragment of a larger protein (Glenner and Wong 1984). The larger protein was termed the *amyloid precursor protein* (APP) because the smaller fragment (the β-fragment, β-amyloid, or β/A4, as it was variously known) appeared to be derived from the larger precursor. APP is a cell surface protein, with a "tail" in the intracellular space, a putative transmembrane portion, and a long extracellular portion. In the pathway of normal APP metabolism, the molecule is cut at a site just above the cell membrane (Figure 13–1). The enzyme that cuts the molecule at that site (the α-secretase site) is not yet identified, but the site is in the middle of the β-amyloid fragment. Therefore, the "normal" or major pathway of APP degradation would not form β-amyloid. The normal metabolism produces a long fragment of the APP molecule, termed *soluble APP,* which appears to be protease nexin II—a substance used in cell culture research. The β-amyloid fragment consists of a portion of the

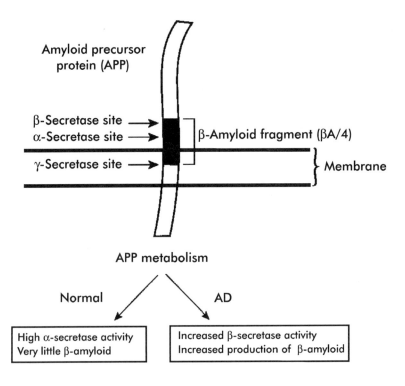

Figure 13–1.   Metabolic pathways for amyloid precursor protein.
Top: Diagrammatic representation of the amyloid precursor protein (APP) in a cell membrane. The normal predominant metabolic pathway results in α-secretase cutting the molecule at a site just above the membrane, in the middle of the β-amyloid fragment. This normal pathway does not produce the intact β-fragment. In AD, a hypothesized enzyme, γ secretase, cuts the APP molecule at a site normally within the putative membrane domain of the APP molecule. Another hypothesized enzyme, β-secretase, cuts it outside the cell to make the 40–43 amino acid β-amyloid fragment.

Bottom: The relative direction of APP metabolism is shown diagramatically. Although small amounts of β-amyloid are found in normal biological fluids, the processing appears to be almost entirely via the α-secretase pathway, transecting the APP molecule and precluding formation of β-amyloid. In AD, the metabolic pathway produces the β-amyloid fragment predominantly, thus α-secretase activity is downregulated.

APP that extends from a site in the middle of the putative intramembranous segment to just above the membrane spanning segment, which is beyond the α-secretase cut site (Selkoe 1991). Cuts at two sites produce β-amyloid. The extracellular cut site is termed the β-site (Haass and Selkoe 1993). The intramembrane cut site is termed the α-site. Neither the cutting enzymes β- or α-secretase has been identified.

Identification of the molecular structure of APP and β-amyloid led to development of sensitive antibodies to both molecules and also enabled more detailed examination of APP metabolism. For example, although it was initially felt that β-amyloid was formed by a process that was part of the metabolic abnormality leading to AD, sensitive antibodies have identified small amounts of β-amyloid in normal cerebrospinal fluid. Thus, the change in APP metabolism in AD is now felt to be a *shift* in the metabolism of APP from production of soluble APP to predominantly β-amyloid, as illustrated in Figure 13–1. It is not known how this shift occurs or what causes it. Altered protein structure produced by the point mutations (changes in single amino acids) in the APP gene may alter APP metabolism directly in some familial cases. When the APP gene is normal, the shift must occur by some other mechanism (see the section Genetics in Alzheimer's Disease in this chapter for a discussion of the interactions of amyloid and the genetics of AD). Because *amyloidogenic* fragments of APP (fragments that contain intact β-amyloid) can be found in lysosomes, it is possible that β-amyloid may be generated by a neuronal endosomal/lysosomal pathway—cut by peptidases and proteases in a lysosome and then secreted. All of these mechanisms are under active study.

Does amyloid pathology result from overproduction of APP, which then moves down the alternative pathway and produces β-amyloid? APP synthesis is upregulated in a variety of experimental injuries in rats, including cortex-denervating basal forebrain or dorsal raphe lesions (Wallace and Haroutunian 1993). Following severe head trauma in humans, diffuse plaques are seen in many cases in patients who die in a few weeks (Gentleman et al. 1993; Roberts et al. 1991). Levels of APP are also elevated in Down's syndrome. There is some evidence that APP is overproduced in AD (B. J. Cummings et al. 1992; S. Johnson et al. 1990). For example, cultured skin fibroblasts from persons with familial AD (APP mutation in codon 670-671) have been shown to overproduce β-amyloid (Citron et al. 1994). Yield of APP messenger RNA (mRNA) appears sensitive to hypoxia, which might prevent finding upregulation of APP mRNA in cases of AD in which the patients had been hypoxic prior to death, and as such perimortem hypoxia is not uncommon (Harrison et al. 1994). Studies have to be performed carefully to see if APP elevation is present in the brains of persons who die at earlier stages of the disease and without hypoxia. Finally, although experimental and human trauma studies show acute or subacute elevations of APP mRNA after injury, patients who die with end-stage AD may no longer have such elevations of APP even though it may have been present during the early and middle stages of the disease. Thus, theories of causation have to consider that amyloid metabolism alterations may occur without altered rates of APP production. The production of an abnormally long (42 amino acids instead of 40) β-amyloid appears to be pathogenic in persons with the codon 717 mutation (Suzuki et al. 1995).

Is β-amyloid a cause or a result of AD? β-Amyloid does not appear to be toxic to synapses, because synaptic density is maintained in areas where there is early deposition of β-amyloid (Masliah et al. 1990). However, there is evidence that β-amyloid is toxic to neurons (Yankner et al. 1989), and amyloid may produce neuronal death by mechanisms involving free radicals (Behl et al. 1994), apoptosis (Laferla et al. 1995), or stimulation of glia cells to produce toxic substances such as tumor necrosis factor (Meda et al. 1995).

A powerful genetic tool available to assess the effects of a gene mutation or overproduction of a gene product is the transfer of a gene into the genome of a different species. Transgenic technology has enabled amyloid constructs to be integrated into the mouse genome. One group of mice, in which a mutant human APP gene (valine at residue 717 substituted by phenylalanine) from a familial AD patient has been inserted, produce amyloid deposits in brain, develop neuritic plaques, synaptic loss, astrocytosis and microgliosis, and the number of plaques increases with age (Games et al. 1995). In another study using transgenic mice, the animals were engineered so that neurons would overproduce APP β-amyloid. The neurons in the brain regions expressing the transgene degenerated and appeared to undergo apoptosis (programmed cell death), with subsequent reactive gliosis, suggesting that intracellular β-amyloid is highly toxic to neurons and may initiate a process of programmed cell death (LaFerla et al. 1995). Finally, a transgenic mouse model has been developed that overexpresses one of the normal APP gene isoforms (a 751-amino acid molecule) in brain. These animals develop AD-type pathology and also exhibit age-related progressive deficits in memory and learning (Moran et al. 1995). Thus, it appears that we have an animal model for some aspects of AD pathology. Such animals could be used to test many types of treatment, including strategies to slow amyloid production or interfere with its pathological actions in brain. Orally administered small-molecule anionic sulphonates or sulphates have been shown to arrest inflammation-associated amyloid deposits in mouse spleen (Kisilevsky et al. 1995), making these compounds possible candidates for treating AD.

Genetics of Alzheimer's Disease

Several different point mutations on different genes are associated with autosomal dominant AD (Table 13–1). The APP gene is on the long arm of chromosome 21. All persons with Down's syndrome (trisomy 21) have a duplication of the APP gene region, and all Down's patients over the age of 40 years develop the pathological changes of AD, including NPs and NFTs, neurotransmitter deficits, and neuronal loss (Noetzel 1994; Wisniewski et al. 1985).

Table 13–1.   Genetic involvement in Alzheimer's disease

Gene	Effect	Comment
Chromosome 21 (autosomal dominant)	APP amino acid substitution	Several different point mutations are found in different families
Chromosome 14 (autosomal dominant)	Missense mutations in a putative transmembrane protein of unknown function	Accounts for the majority of familial AD cases
Volga German kindreds (autosomal dominant)	Unknown	Very small numbers of families; autosomal dominant, but neither chromosome 14 nor chromosome 21 abnormalities are present
Down's syndrome (trisomy 21)	All Down's patients develop AD pathology by the fifth decade, including NPs, NFTs, and loss of brain ChAT and norepinephrine	Trisomy 21 leads to an increased gene dosage (1.5) for APP. Does this increased synthesis of APP somehow lead to AD?
Chromosome 19 (apolipoprotein E)	E4 allele, normally with an allele frequency of 12% in the population, is found in 40%–50% of late-onset, sporadic AD	Mechanism of increased risk is unclear; E4 homozygotes have eightfold elevated risk of developing AD

Note.   APP = amyloid precursor protein; NP = neuritic plaques; NFT = neurofibillary tangles; ChAT = choline acetyltransferase.

Familial AD (FAD) is also characterized by several different point mutations in the APP molecule (St. George-Hyslop 1994). None of the mutations is within the β-amyloid span itself; they appear to flank it on either side. There are only a few families with these mutations, but the fact that the mutations occur in the APP gene strengthens the argument that dysregulation in amyloid metabolism is linked to the etiology of AD. Families have also been identified with a point mutation localized to chromosome 14 (Mullan et al. 1992; Schellenberg et al. 1992; Van Broeckhoven et al. 1992). The majority of FAD kindreds have the chromosome 14 abnormality. A gene has been found at location 14q24.3 that may account for 70% of early-onset autosomal dominant AD. The gene has recently been identified (Sherrington et al. 1995). It appears to be a membrane protein, previously unknown, in which several different missense mutations have been determined in several families. The nature of its dysfunction in AD or the relationship of such altered function to amyloid metabolism remains to be determined. If it is a gene related to the processing of amyloid, that would be powerful evidence that amyloid is involved in the etiology of some forms of AD. If the gene is unrelated to amyloid metabolism, amyloid will still be regarded as important in pathogenesis but not as the initiating factor.

Finally, there are a small number of families of Volga German descent who also have autosomal-dominant FAD but have neither chromosome 21 nor chromosome 14 defects (Schellenberg et al. 1992). Therefore, there is at least one additional genetic site associated with autosomal-dominant AD.

Genetics of Apolipoprotein E

Investigators at Duke University found a linkage between late-onset AD in families that had increased numbers of cases of AD (but were not autosomal dominant kindreds) and an abnormality on chromosome 19 (Pericak-Vance et al. 1991). The abnormality was suspected to be in apolipoprotein E (ApoE), which is on chromosome 19. Roses and colleagues (1994) subsequently showed that the E4 allele, one of the three alleles (E2, E3, E4) of ApoE, was present more frequently in patients with AD than in the general population, in both familial and sporadic AD cases (Strittmatter et al. 1993). The latter finding was especially important because the majority of autosomal-dominant AD cases occur in the fifth and sixth decades of life. The E4 allele, which is also associated with cardiovascular disease, has a frequency of 12%–14% in the general population. In older cohorts of subjects, the frequency of the allele is lower, probably due to death from cardiac disease associated with the E4 allele (Cauley et al. 1993). Thus, the overrepresentation of the E4 allele in older AD patients is even more striking. Persons homozygous for the E4 allele have an eight times greater risk of developing AD as do non-E4 carriers, and they have an earlier mean age at onset of AD (Corder et al. 1993).

Because not all E4 carriers develop AD, it may be a "risk gene," conferring added risk of developing AD but requiring some other, yet undescribed interactive factors for expression of the disease. Because not all cases of AD carry E4, the presence of the allele is not necessary for development of AD. Further, the E2 allele, which is the least common allele (with a gene frequency of 7%), appears to confer some protection against development of AD, because cases of AD with the E2 allele are fewer than expected on the basis of allele frequency alone (Corder et al. 1994; Talbot et al. 1994). A recent report suggests an association between E2 and increased risk of early AD with reduced survival (van Duijn et al. 1995, but more studies are needed to resolve this important issue.

The mechanism by which ApoE confers its risk is not known. ApoE binds to β-amyloid, and the molecule coded by the E4 allele binds more tightly to amyloid than that coded by the E2 or E3 alleles (Strittmatter et al. 1993). Thus, this theory allows incorporation of amyloid into the hypotheses about the effects of ApoE—that somehow the altered binding to the amyloid fragment that occurs with the E4 allele does not allow normal processing of the β-fragment and results in its accumulation. Still another therapy is that E4 itself can produce amyloid fibrils (Wisniewski et al. 1995). It is not known how the E2 allele might protect against AD. Knowledge of the mechanism by which this happens—both the protective effect of E2 and the susceptibility brought about by E4 (Corder et al. 1994), may lead to specific therapies directed against these effects, such as slowing the rate of production or altering the solubility characteristics of β-amyloid.

Developing Issues in the Biology of Alzheimer's Disease

Significant intellectual and financial resources are committed to understanding AD and its pathophysiology and to develop both palliative and curative therapies. The metabolism of amyloid will continue to be a major focus of such efforts, as will investigation of ways to enhance neurotransmission in degenerating neurotransmitter systems. Among several areas of research are investigation of the roles of free radicals in the neuronal death or pathophysiology of AD, the role of inflammation and anti-inflammatory therapy, the relation of estrogen treatment to AD, and the search for diagnostic tests.

The toxicity of β-amyloid may be mediated or increased by free radicals (Behl et al. 1994). Because there are treatments to suppress free radical formation, this area of inquiry may lead to both understanding of the pathophysiology and potential treatments.

NPs appear to contain an inflammatory reaction to the presence of β-amyloid (McGeer et al. 1989; Perlmutter et al. 1992; Styren et al. 1990). Elevation of cytokines such as IL-1β are found in NPs (Griffin et al. 1989). Populations of patients who have been on long-term anti-inflammatory agents that cross the blood-brain barrier, such as glucocorticoids (in rheumatoid arthritis) (McGeer et al. 1990) and dapsone (in leprosy), are reported to have lower prevalence of AD. Preliminary efforts have been to use anti-inflammatory medications to suppress the destructive process (Rogers et al. 1993). Further trials of such medications have been recommended (Aisen and Davis 1994) and are in process.

Some epidemiological studies suggest that women who have been on supplementary estrogen have lower prevalence of AD and that estrogen may protect against AD or its clinical manifestations (Henderson et al. 1993; Paganini-Hill and Henderson 1994). Estrogen has stimulatory effects on the cholinergic system and is a neurotrophic substance under some conditions. The mechanism by which estrogen may be protective is still under study.

The antemortem diagnosis of AD is a diagnosis of exclusion, and although accuracy rates of better than 90% are obtained by skilled clinicians, a diagnostic test would simplify the evaluation, eliminate uncertainty, and possibly identify presymptomatic cases. In autosomal-dominant FAD with mutations on chromosomes 14 or 21, both symptomatic and presymptomatic patients can be detected. Although patients homozygous for the E4 allele of ApoE have an eightfold chance of developing the disease, the presence of a single E4 allele does not predict the occurrence of disease in an individual patient (Roses et al. 1994).

There is not a great deal of accumulation of β-amyloid outside the brain. Detection of β-amyloid or other amyloidogenic fragments in the cerebrospinal fluid (CSF), however, has been an area of investigation. Although it is not known if the β-amyloid fragment is a pathological metabolite of APP metabolism, sensitive antibody assays have shown that it is produced in small amounts in normal humans (Haass et al. 1992; Seubert et al. 1992; Shoji et al. 1992). β-Amyloid is found in normal CSF, and the levels increase with increasing age (van Gool et al. 1994). Although there appears to be an inverse relationship between βamyloid concentration in CSF and dementia severity in AD (Nitsch et al. 1995), CSF β-amyloid levels do not differentiate AD patients from Parkinson's disease patients (van Gool et al. 1995). Differences in amounts of β-amyloid between AD CSF and normal age-matched patients may provide a diagnostic or confirmatory test. Soluble APP levels in CSF (whose formation makes it impossible to produce β-amyloid; see Figure 13–1) are reported to be decreased in AD as compared with control CSF (Van Nostrand et al. 1992). This suggests that lower levels of the major metabolite might also be used as a diagnostic test, especially because other non-AD dementias do not appear to have this change. There is a commercially available test for soluble APP, but there is little clinical experience with the test, and age-specific ranges of CSF levels in normal subjects have not been published. Thus, cutoff points for making the diagnosis are not available. Finally, the sensitivity of the test—how early in the course of disease it might reflect CNS changes—has not been defined. Although there are a number of ways that APP metabolism can be affected in AD, better antibodies and a fuller understanding of these metabolic pathways may enable a diagnostic test to be derived from some amyloid marker (Palmert et al. 1989).

Fibroblasts from skin biopsies have shown some differences in the potassium channel profile of AD patients as compared with control subjects, but this finding has not yet been applied to clinical testing (Etcheberrigaray et al. 1993). Epidermal growth factor receptor was found to be expressed in the capillaries of skin samples taken post mortem, as well as cerebral blood vessels in postmortem assessments of patients with AD and other dementias, whereas it is not present in the skin of normal aged control subjects (Styren et al. 1990). Such autopsy studies need confirmation in living patients, and these studies are under way.

Is AD one disease? The diverse clinical presentations have profound memory loss as a common feature, but there are widely varying rates of progression and specific cognitive, behavioral, and emotional disorders that are severe in some patients and mild in others. Similarly, some patients have parkinsonian features, whereas others never develop them. Pathologically, the absence of NFTs in some cases, the presence of cortical Lewy bodies in some cases, and the variable degree of subcortical neuronal loss suggest that different etiologies may produce similar pathological cascades. The common denominator of all of these cases is the presence of NPs. Understanding the pathoetiology of NPs and the role of β-amyloid will allow us to determine if there is a nosology of Alzheimer-type pathology.

Over the next several years, progress in the molecular neurobiology, epidemiology, and neuroimaging of AD are likely to provide us with significant information about the pathophysiology, diagnosis, and risk factors in this disease.

CHAPTER 14

Research in Treating Cognitive Impairment in Alzheimer's Disease

Robert G. Stern, M.D.
Kenneth L. Davis, M.D.

Progressive cognitive deterioration is the clinical hallmark of Alzheimer's disease (AD) and the main target of current therapeutic efforts. As for other diseases characterized by progressive deterioration, therapeutic goals can include alleviating symptoms, slowing or arresting the deterioration, or reversing the damage. The neurotransmitter-based approaches described in this chapter offer modest palliation by augmenting deficient neurotransmission. Many other empirically derived approaches have been assessed for potential palliative or deterioration-retarding properties in AD. Recent advances in understanding AD may permit the development of new strategies for retarding or halting the progression of the illness. These strategies, derived from various pathophysiological models of the illness, attempt to alter putative neurotoxic mechanisms such as glutamate's excitotoxic effects, free radical–mediated neuronal damage, chronic brain inflammation, amyloid production, aluminum accumulation, and others. Whereas development of neuroprotective strategies appear increasingly close, regenerative treatments that can restore damaged tissue are not yet in sight.

Cholinergic Hypothesis of AD and Cholinergic Enhancement Strategies

Several lines of evidence support the hypothesis that enhancing cholinergic neurotransmission will ameliorate cognitive dysfunction in patients with AD. Much of the evidence is reviewed in Chapters 6 and 13. Additional evidence comes from chemical, surgical, and pharmacological lesions of the cerebral cholinergic system, all of which impair learning and memory in animals. Such impairment is reversed by cholinomimetic agents (Bartus et al. 1985; Collerton 1986; Olton and Wenk 1987). Brains of AD patients exhibit consistent cholinergic cell loss in the septum and the nucleus basalis of Meynert. There is a decrease in the cholinergic markers choline acetyltransferase and acetylcholinesterase (AChE) and a correlation between these neurochemical changes and the degree of cognitive impairment (Davies and Maloney 1976; Perry et al. 1977, 1978).

Therapeutic trials in AD aimed at augmenting cerebral cholinergic neurotransmission have employed AChE inhibitors, cholinergic agonists, acetylcholine (ACh) precursors, ACh-releasing agents, and drugs with less well defined mechanisms. Despite the large number of known centrally active cholinomimetic agents, few are usable. Most such agents have a short biological half-life, poor blood-brain barrier penetration, instability in plasma, unpredictable absorption, frequent side effects, or a dangerously narrow therapeutic range. AChE inhibitors have been the most extensively studied drugs and have had the best clinical results.

Acetylcholinesterase Inhibitor Tetrahydroaminoacridine (Tacrine)

The synthetic aminoacridine 1,2,3,4,-tetrahydro-9-acridinamine, known as tacrine, was synthesized more than 40 years ago. Tacrine (Cognex) was approved by the Food and Drug Administration (FDA) in 1993 for the treatment of cognitive impairment in AD. Its administration, dosage, and side effects are discussed in Chapter 6. Tacrine monohydrochloride monohydrate is a reversible AChE inhibitor with a moderately long duration of action. Tacrine's AChE inhibitory activity is thought to be mediated by its binding to a hydrophobic area of the enzyme close to the active site. In addition to its AChE inhibitory activity, tacrine has multiple pharmacological effects that may contribute to its therapeutic effects in this illness. Tacrine binds to M_1 muscarinic and nicotinic receptor sites and two membrane sites whose pharmacological and clinical significance are unknown (Mena and Desai 1991). At therapeutic concentrations, tacrine is believed to produce a significant decrease in monoamine oxidase (MAO) activity, leading to enhanced monoaminergic activity. Furthermore, tacrine induces monoamine release and inhibits monoamine uptake, increasing several monoamine neurotransmitters, including dopamine, serotonin, and norepinephrine (Drukarch et al. 1987, 1988). Tacrine interacts with K^+, Na^+, and Ca^{++} channels. It appears to keep Na^+ channels open and K^+ channels closed (Adem 1992; Freeman and Dawson 1991; Nordberg et al. 1989). All these effects might be of therapeutic significance in AD.

Active tacrine metabolites include the 1-hydroxy metabolite velnacrine, an active but weaker AChE inhibitor. After chronic administration (several weeks at therapeutic dosage) tacrine plasma levels range from 10 to 100 ng/ml. Plasma levels are 50% higher in women than men. At steady state, mean maximum plasma concentrations are 5.1, 20.7, and 33.9 ng/ml following doses of 40, 80, and 120 mg qd, respectively (Cognex drug insert 1993 Cutler et al. 1990a, 1990b; Hartvig et al. 1990).

Clinical studies with tacrine in AD started in 1981 (Summers et al. 1981). Since then, eight large placebo-controlled studies have assessed the efficacy of tacrine with or without lecithin in larger samples of AD patients (Chatellier and Lacomblez 1990; K. L. Davis et al. 1992; Eagger et al. 1991; Farlow et al. 1992; Gauthier et al. 1990; Knapp et al. 1994; Maltby et al. 1994; Wilcock et al. 1993). Tacrine combined with lecithin resulted in significant improvement in two studies (Eagger et al. 1991; Gauthier et al. 1990) and in marginal or no improvement in two other studies (Chatellier and Lacomblez 1990; Maltby et al. 1994). A 6-week parallel trial using an enriched-population design (K. L. Davis et al. 1992) found that tacrine-treated patients had less decline in cognitive function than the placebo-treated group. In another study (Farlow et al. 1992), tacrine produced a significant dose-related cognitive improvement. Similar results were reported from a more recent 30-week study (Knapp et al. 1994). Two other studies—one with a crossover design (Wilcock et al. 1993) and one with a parallel design (Maltby et al. 1994)—failed to find statistically significant differences between tacrine and placebo.

The studies reviewed here suggest that lecithin is not essential and probably not contributory to the therapeutic effect. Furthermore, these studies suggest that tacrine administered for at least 2 weeks in doses of 80–160 mg po qd produces significant improvements that can be ascertained on cognitive performance tests, such as the Alzheimer's Disease Assessment Scale (see Chapter 1 and Appendix 8), and on global clinical measures. The effect of tacrine was equivalent to slowing cognitive deterioration by 6–12 months. The crossover design trials studied smaller groups and were therefore less likely to identify tacrine's therapeutic effects. It is possible that low tacrine dosage, the crossover design, and lower power to detect change due to smaller sample sizes are responsible for the apparent lack of efficacy reported in some studies.

The response to tacrine is as heterogeneous as the clinical and histopathological presentation of the illness itself. Whereas 10% of patients showed large benefit, 20% demonstrated more modest benefits and 20% smaller but statistically significant improvement in cognitive performance or clinical status. The remaining patients showed no short-term benefits. Although the amelioration achieved with tacrine is limited, these results are encouraging as they represent the first successful attempt to improve cognitive performance and functional ability in AD.

Investigational Tacrine Derivatives

Velnacrine maleate (HP-029, 9-amino-1,2,3,4,-tetrahydro-1-acridinol maleate), is the main tacrine metabolite in man. It is a reversible AChE inhibitor with a shorter half-life than tacrine. Velnacrine is a less-potent AChE inhibitor on a weight basis but induces the same degree of AChE inhibition as tacrine (Shutske et al. 1988). Initial studies showed velnacrine to be safe in healthy young volunteers (Puri et al. 1989) and in elderly volunteers (Fielding et al. 1989). More recently, a 28-day course of 300 mg velnacrine po qd was tolerated well by elderly (60- to 74-year-old) volunteers but not by patients with AD. In the AD group, doses greater than 225 mg qd were associated with dizziness, fainting, nausea, vomiting, headache, and severe diarrhea (Cutler et al. 1992a, 1992b). Velnacrine is rapidly absorbed after oral administration, reaching peak plasma levels after 0.75–1.20 hours. The mean plasma half-life is approximately 2 hours. There seems to be marked intersubject variability in tolerance to the drug (Cutler et al. 1990b). Preliminary results suggest that one-third of the patients benefit from the drug (Murphy et al. 1991) and that cognitive performance improved significantly (Schneider 1993). However, hepatotoxic effects have been reported, and the drug will probably not be further developed.

The agent **suronacrine maleate** (HP-128, 9-[benzylamino]-1,2,3,4-tetrahydro-1-acridinol maleate), is another tacrine derivative. Suronacrine inhibits AChE in vitro and improves memory in an animal model of AD. Suronacrine is a weaker AChE inhibitor than tacrine or velnacrine. The latter is one of suronacrine's main metabolites. The drug inhibits the uptake of norepinephrine and dopamine in vitro and has blocking effects on cholinergic receptors and certain ion channels (Braga et al. 1991; Shutske et al. 1989). Suronacrine reaches peak plasma levels 1.4–5.0 hours after oral administration and has a plasma half-life of 1.5–8.6 hours. Suronacrine

200 mg po qd is well tolerated and safe in patients with AD, but its therapeutic efficacy is unclear (Huff et al. 1991).

Methoxytacrine (7-methoxy-1,2,3,4-tetrahydroaminoacridine), is a reversible cholinesterase inhibitor developed in Czechoslovakia. Animal studies suggested that methoxytacrine might have cholinomimetic properties consistent with a therapeutic effect in AD (Dolezal and Tucek 1991; Musilkova and Tucek 1991; Svejdova et al. 1990; Tucek and Dolezal 1991). Initial safety trials in healthy volunteers have shown methoxytacrine up to 8 mg/kg body weight po to be well tolerated. Peak plasma levels were reached 4 hours after oral administration and $T_{1/2}$ was 8.73.9 hours (Filip et al. 1991). Data on the agent's therapeutic effects are pending.

SM-10888 (9-amino-8-fluoro-1,2,3,4-tetrahydro-2,4-methanoacridine) is thought to be a potent AChE inhibitor with a high brain-periphery partition coefficient and fewer peripheral cholinergic side effects than tacrine, velnacrine, or physostigmine (PHS) (see following section). Consistent with its postulated selectivity for the central nervous system (CNS), SM-10888 enhanced learning in animal models at much lower doses than tacrine (Natori et al. 1990; Okazaki et al. 1990).

Other Experimental AChE Inhibitors

Various other compounds with AChE-inhibitory activity are being considered for their therapeutic potential in AD. Bioavailability, pharmacokinetic properties, and brain-plasma partition pattern are some of the major properties affecting the therapeutic potential of various AChE inhibitors in AD. A compound's relative affinity for AChE and butyrylcholinesterase (BuChE) may affect its therapeutic potential as well. Because inactivated BuChE, the precursor of AChE, does not contribute to the pool of AChE, AChE inhibitors with higher BuChE-AChE affinity ratio may have a detrimental effect on the cholinergic neurotransmission. The administration of an AChE inhibitor with a high affinity for BuChE might produce a prolonged drop in the precursor level and ultimately decrease AChE level (Koelle et al. 1977, 1987).

Physostigmine (PHS) is a natural alkaloid, first isolated in 1864. PHS is a lipid-soluble tertiary amine readily absorbed from the gastrointestinal tract, subcutaneous tissue, and mucous membranes and is able to cross the blood-brain barrier. It reaches maximal levels in a short time. It is hydrolyzed and inactivated within 2 hours. Orally administered PHS has been used in the treatment of exophthalmos, gastric atony, tachycardia, inherited ataxias, and myasthenia gravis.

PHS was one of the first AChE inhibitors to be assessed in the treatment of AD. Of the 11 studies of PHS in AD reviewed by Mohs and Davis (1987), all five studies using parenterally administered PHS, and four of the six using orally administered PHS found some improvement in at least a subpopulation of the patients studied. Two recent studies confirmed the beneficial effect of oral PHS on an auditory verbal learning test (Sevush et al. 1991) and on a selective reminding test in outpatients with AD (Sano et al. 1992). The effects of intracerebroventricular (ICV) administration of PHS in AD patients have also been evaluated (Becker et al. 1988). ICV administration of PHS was not associated with peripheral side effects; however, the drug caused increased irritability and sleepiness. It produced no clinically meaningful effects, despite some improvement of performance in a word-recognition test.

Results from a few uncontrolled studies suggest that long-term PHS administration might delay or prevent cognitive deterioration in AD patients (Beller et al. 1988; Jenike et al. 1990). A 1-year controlled study with up to 15 mg qd of oral PHS in outpatients with AD appears to support the notion that long-term PHS treatment improves or stabilizes neuropsychological function (Storey et al. 1993).

Heptylphysostigmine, which is a carbamate derivative of PHS, is more lipophilic, produces longer inhibition of brain cholinesterase than PHS, and has fewer peripheral side effects than PHS (Brufani et al. 1986; DeSarno et al. 1989). Despite initially promising results in clinical trials, heptylphysostigmine trials in humans have been abandoned because of drug-induced neutropenia. Other PHS analogues similar to heptylphysostigmine are being assessed as well. **Heptastigmine** has a longer half-life, a more favorable brain-plasma partition pattern, and possibly less peripheral toxicity than PHS (Segre et al. 1992). **Eptastigmine,** a long-acting cholinesterase inhibitor, was shown to have a strong cholinomimetic effect (Cella et al. 1993). Eptastigmine was shown to produce prolonged changes in regional cerebral blood flow studies in rats (Scremin et al. 1993). Further preclinical evaluation of these agents is needed before their clinical efficacy can be tested.

Galanthamine is a tertiary amine alkaloid. It is a competitive inhibitor of cholinesterase activity. Administration of this medication resulted in cerebral concentrations three times higher than its plasma level. Galanthamine's 7-hour half-life is longer than that of tacrine or PHS. Administration of galanthamine 30 mg po qd in divided doses over 2 months to 9 AD patients appeared to have beneficial effects and was well tolerated (Rainer et al. 1989). In an open trial, galanthamine produced no significant changes on neuropsychological tests in 18 patients treated with 30 mg po qd for 2 months (Dal-Bianco et al. 1991). Research on this drug has been discontinued.

Metrifonate is an organophosphorus compound that has been employed as an insecticide and as a treatment for human infections with the parasite *Schistosoma haematobium*. Metrifonate is transformed nonenzymatically into dichlorvos, an AChE inhibitor with a half-life longer than PHS. Although toxic reactions in humans have been reported, orally administered metrifonate in doses of 7.5–10.0 mg/kg body weight seem to be safe. Metrifonate has been shown to induce AChE inhibition in the CNS after intramuscular and intraperitoneal administration in rodents (Nordgren and Holmstedt 1988). The drug has also been shown to inhibit plasma and red blood cell AChE activity in humans after oral administration (Hallak and Giacobini 1987).

Huperzine-A and -B are two natural alkaloids isolated by Chinese scientists from the plant *Huperzia serrata*. Huperzine-A is a reversible AChE inhibitor that is more selective and more potent than PHS (Wang et al. 1986). A double-blind, placebo-controlled study with 0.05 mg im bid or 0.03 mg im tid huperzine-A reported positive effects in patients with multi-infarct dementia and presenile or senile-onset AD (Zhang et al. 1991).

SDZ ENA-713 has been shown to have neuroprotective effects in a gerbil brain ischemia model of dementia (K. Tanaka et al. 1993). In humans, SDZ ENA-713 was shown to be safe in doses up to 4.6 mg po (Enz et al. 1991).

E-2020 (1-benzyl-4-((5,6-dimethoxy-1-indanon)-2-yl)-methyl-piperidine hydrochloride) is an AChE inhibitor under development for the treatment of AD in Japan and the United States. The drug is 92.6% protein bound in serum, is secreted in the urine, and has an exceptionally long plasma half-life of 50 hours. Plasma steady-state was achieved after approximately 2 weeks of daily dosing (Mihara et al. 1993).

NIK-247 (9-amino-2,3,5,6,7,8-hexahydro-1*H*-cyclopenta-(b)-quinoline monohydrate hydrochloride) is an AChE inhibitor under development in Japan with central cholinomimetic effects (Yamamoto et al. 1993a) and improves experimentally induced deficits in working memory (Yamamoto et al. 1993b).

Cholinergic Agonists and Antagonists

Although the administration of cholinergic agonists provides a nonphysiological, tonic stimulation at the postsynaptic receptor, this approach had beneficial effects on memory and learning in animals with experimentally induced hypocholinergic states (Haroutunian et al. 1985). Most of the cholinergic agonists that have been evaluated in AD are choline derivatives, natural alkaloids, or synthetic analogues. The initial results from trials with cholinergic agonists in AD were modest at best. Since the discovery of muscarinic receptor subtypes (M_1–M_5), receptor-subtype-selective cholinergic agents have been developed (Davis et al. 1993a). It is believed that such selective agents could enhance cholinergic neurotransmission by blocking presynaptic cholinergic autoreceptors and activating postsynaptic muscarinic receptors. The blockade of presynaptic autoreceptors is believed to enhance neurotransmission by reducing or abolishing feedback inhibition.

RS-86 (2-ethyl-8-methyl-2,8-diazospiro-4,5-decan-1,3-dionhydrobromide), a long-acting cholinergic agonist with good CNS permeability, has not been found to produce significant improvements in AD (Bruno et al. 1985; Hollander et al. 1987; Mouradian et al. 1988; Wettstein and Spiegal 1984). **Oxotremorine,** another synthetic cholinergic agonist with a half-life of several hours, had no beneficial effect in AD (Davis et al. 1987).

Bethanechol, a synthetic ACh analogue, is a relatively short acting muscarinic agonist that does not cross the blood-brain barrier. Bethanechol was the first drug to be administered by the ICV route to AD patients but had no significant therapeutic effects (Harbaugh 1987; Penn et al. 1988b). Moreover, the ICV route of administration carried considerable risks related to anesthesia, surgery, infection, and hemorrhage. Reported complications include pneumocephalus and seizures (Gauthier et al. 1986) and hemiparesis accompanied by dysphasia and chronic subdural hematoma (Penn et al. 1988a).

Arecoline, a natural alkaloid with muscarinic and nicotinic agonistic properties, was one of the first cholinergic agonists to be evaluated in AD. Two studies found no significant effects with intravenously administered arecoline in AD patients (Christie et al. 1981; Tariot et al. 1988a). More recently, arecoline administered as an intravenous continuous infusion for 5 days in a placebo-controlled trial produced significant improvement on a verbal memory test (Raffaele et al. 1991a). No significant group mean changes were observed in a related study upon acute arecoline infusion (Raffaele et al. 1991b).

Nicotine administered intravenously had significant effects on mood and cognitive performance in patients with AD (Newhouse et al. 1988; Sunderland et al. 1988). Although higher doses produced anxiety and mood changes, these studies and other animal and human experi-

mental data point to the possible involvement of central nicotinic cholinergic neurotransmission in some cognitive processes. Further studies of
nicotinic cholinergic mechanisms in AD are warranted, but careful attention must be paid to toxicity.

New Cholinergic Agonists

Several new cholinergic agonists are being developed. Animal experiments suggest that some of these agents might produce better therapeutic effects in AD with fewer side effects than the agents assessed in the
past (Doods et al. 1993).

AF-102B (*cis*-2-methylspiro-(1,3-oxathiolane-5,3')quinuclidine) is an
M_1-selective agonist that crosses the blood-brain barrier (Ono et al. 1988)
and is considered for cholinergic enhancement in AD (Nakahara et al.
1988). The related agents AF-150 and AF-151 are also selective for brain-
M_1 receptors (L. J. Fisher et al. 1993a).

L-689,660 is an arecoline derivative and a muscarinic agonist that pene-
trates freely into the CNS and exhibits functional selectivity. L-689,660 is a
potent partial agonist at M_1 and M_3 receptors and acts as an antagonist at
M_2 receptors (Iversen 1993).

PD-142505 and **CI-979** are two other novel cholinergic muscarinic
agonists thought to have a more advantageous receptor-binding profile.
In particular, PD-142505 appears to have a selectively higher affinity for
M_1 than M_2 receptors. In addition, it has been suggested that PD-142505
acts as a partial agonist/antagonist at some muscarinic receptor sites
(Davis et al. 1993b).

The list of new M_1 or brain selective muscarinic agonists such as SR-
95639 (Boast et al. 1991), SDZ ENS 163 (Enz et al. 1992, 1993), and WAL-
2014 (Ensinger et al. 1993) is continuously growing. Some of these
agonists are selective M_1 partial agonists and M_2 partial antagonists.
Such compounds might alleviate central cholinergic deficits in AD with
fewer peripheral side effects. For maximal effects, both muscarinic and
nicotinic stimulation may be required.

Acetylcholine Precursors

An early strategy to enhance central cholinergic transmission was the
administration of ACh precursors, mainly choline and lecithin, in the
hope of increasing ACh synthesis and cholinergic transmission. The rate
of ACh release is ultimately dependent on its rate of synthesis, which, in
turn, appears to depend on the rate of choline uptake into the choliner-

gic neuron by the high-affinity choline-uptake system. Under normal conditions, this system is saturated, and an increase in the availability of extracellular choline does not increase synthesis or release of ACh. However, during intense cholinergic activity and greater demand for additional precursor, the increased extracellular concentration of choline might be beneficial. Furthermore, choline itself might have cholinomimetic properties. Thus, ACh precursor therapy might slightly improve cognitive performance in AD under normal conditions by increasing the cholinergic tonus, with more significant improvement under conditions of increased cholinergic demand, when ordinarily the rate of ACh synthesis would be limited by insufficient extracellular choline. A review of 17 studies performed between 1977 and 1982 provided little or no evidence for the efficacy of this approach (Bartus and Dean 1982). Other studies have examined the ability of ACh precursors to delay or prevent cognitive deterioration in AD patients.

A 1-year study with lecithin in AD patients found no significant effects (Levy et al. 1983), whereas two other long-term studies suggested a beneficial preventive effect (Christie et al. 1979; Little et al. 1985). Whether this approach provides consistent benefit in preventing or slowing the progression of the disease requires further study. ACh precursors other than choline and lecithin have also been assessed.

Phosphatidylserine (PS) is a phospholipid component of the cell membrane. The therapeutic effects of PS in AD have been studied since the mid-1980s. Two controlled studies with PS in AD (Amaducci and the SMID group 1988; Crook et al. 1992) suggested that PS in doses of 200 mg po qd and 300 mg po qd is superior to placebo, particularly in more severely affected AD patients. Treatment with PS in combination with cognitive training was superior to cognitive training alone (Heiss et al. 1993). Although PS administration over a period of 3–6 months seemed to produce small improvements on specific cognitive tests, the overall clinical relevance of these effects is questionable.

L-α-Glyceryl-phosphorylcholine (LAGPC), a lecithin derivative, is an ACh precursor believed to have cholinomimetic and cognition-enhancing properties. After absorption, this compound is converted to phosphorylcholine, the metabolically active form of choline (Gatti et al. 1992). In 65 patients with AD who received LAGPC 800 mg po qid for 6 months in an open study, there was progressive amelioration on Mini-Mental State scores and on immediate and delayed recall tests (Parnetti et al. 1993). **Cytidine diphosphate choline** (CDP-choline), another ACh precursor, has been assessed for its therapeutic potential in dementia. Clinical trials have repeatedly shown positive effects of CDP-choline in demented patients (de la Morena 1993). A recent study in patients with AD found that the majority of patients benefited from a 3-month course of CDP-choline 1,000 mg po qd (Cacabelos et al. 1993).

ACh-Release-Enhancing Agents

The use of ACh releasers is based on their ability to enhance stimulus-induced ACh delivery into the synapse. Such an action could improve the signal-to-noise ratio during neuronal transmission without the toxicity of cholinesterase inhibitors or the distorted temporal pattern of neurotransmission observed with cholinergic agonists.

4-Aminopyridine (4-AP) increases the amount of ACh released into the synaptic space with each activation of the synapse. Some improvement in cognitive functions was found in a study with 4-AP in AD patients (Wesseling et al. 1984). In contrast, no significant effect of 4-AP on cognitive performance was found in a more recent study employing a best-dose finding phase in 14 AD patients (Davidson et al. 1988). The different results in these two studies may relate to differences in the characteristics of the two populations studied (i.e., age and severity of the disease) and length of treatment (6 weeks in the former, 4 days in the latter). Study results suggest that after an initial phase of increased release 4-AP may deplete ACh storages and that the combined administration of 4-AP with an ACh precursor might be more efficient (Branconnier 1983b).

Linopirdine (DuP 996) (1-phenyl-3,3-bis[4-pyridinylmethyl]-2-phenylindolinone) is a compound with properties similar to 4-AP. DuP 996 enhances the stimulus-induced release of ACh as well as other neurotransmitters such as dopamine and serotonin. The drug has been found to improve learning performance in various models in mice, rats, and monkeys (Cook 1988; Cook et al. 1990; Nicholson et al. 1990), but it has been abandoned by the manufacturer.

HP 749 *(N-(n-propyl)-N-(4-pyridinyl)-1H-indol-1-amine)* is an indole-substituted analogue of 4-AP that is well absorbed after oral administration (Hsu et al. 1991). In preclinical studies, HP 749 reversed the passive avoidance deficit produced by nucleus basalis lesions in rodents (Cornfeldt et al. 1990). Data from clinical trials have not been published.

Limitations to the Cholinomimetic Approach

Adverse effects of AChE inhibitors and muscarinic agonists are primarily due to the enhancement of peripheral cholinergic tonus. Cholinergic toxicity is often manifested by gastrointestinal symptoms (nausea, vomiting, abdominal cramping, and diarrhea), diaphoresis, light-headedness, and occasionally by cardiovascular symptoms such as bradycardia and hypotension. Depression and agitation have also been encountered. Individual susceptibility to such side effects varies widely. Considering the inverted U-shape form of the dose-response curve to cholinergic enhancement in AD, drug plasma levels that are too high or too low may easily interfere with optimal therapeutic efficacy. Nonoptimal levels may easily occur, with fluctuations in drug levels caused by poor or unreliable CNS availability of the drug. Under such circumstances, fixed-dose treatment studies are of limited benefit. Thus, newer studies have included individual best-dose trials, plasma level assays, and confirmation of CNS penetration by various means. It is also important to recognize that some patients may present with such a severe degree of presynaptic cholinergic cell loss that any cholinomimetic agent active at the presynaptic site would fail to induce a clinically effective enhancement of the cholinergic transmission.

There are limitations to the postsynaptic agonistic strategy as well. Postsynaptic muscarinic agonists provide a nonphysiological tonic stimulation, whereas the physiological state is characterized by phasic processes. Also, it appears that the CNS contains spare cholinergic receptor sites that have lost functional innervation during development and maturation. The stimulation of such "spare" receptors and the resulting untoward effects might present one of the more significant impediments to the agonist approach. The therapeutic efficacy of cholinergic agonists could possibly be further enhanced by augmenting both muscarinic and nicotinic cholinergic transmission at hypothesized specific nicotinic receptor subtypes. This possibility is supported by the finding that scopolamine administration in young volunteers produces a single photon emission computed tomography (SPECT) brain scan pattern of predominantly frontal flow reduction (Honer et al. 1989), unlike the pattern found in AD patients, which is characterized by temporoparietal flow reduction. The difference in these two patterns could be explained by the fact that scopolamine primarily induces a central cholinergic muscarinic blockade, whereas the AD pattern might be produced by additional deficits such as cholinergic nicotinic or other noncholinergic deficits.

The pharmacology of the cholinergic system is far from being fully understood. Yet unrecognized variables may still emerge, and the clinical implications of the various parameters need more accurate assessment.

Noncholinergic Neurotransmitter Replacement Strategies

AD is characterized by a marked noradrenergic (Bondareff et al. 1982; Rossor and Iversen 1986) and serotonergic (Bowen et al. 1983; Cross et al. 1986; Yamamoto and Hirano 1985) deficit. In addition, deficits in neuropeptidergic neurotransmission have been found (somatostatin in particular) (reviewed in Husain and Nemeroff 1990). Based on these findings and on encouraging experimental results, investigators have attempted to manipulate these neurotransmitter systems.

Monoaminergic Drugs

Selegiline or L-deprenyl (Eldepryl) is an MAO-B inhibitor, first synthesized in 1972, with good brain permeability that is used in the treatment of Parkinson's disease (Knoll 1992). Selegiline has been evaluated in several studies with AD patients. Double-blind, placebo-controlled trials with small patient samples suggest that subchronic treatment at 10 mg qd improves performance on attention, memory, and learning tasks (Martignoni et al. 1991; Piccinin et al. 1990; Tariot et al. 1987a, 1987b). Higher doses were not as efficacious and were associated with more side effects (Tariot et al. 1987b). The beneficial effects of selegiline do not appear to be due its antidepressant action, because the MAO-A inhibitor tranylcypromine did not improve cognitive performance and produced significant side effects (Tariot et al. 1988b). A large multicenter study of selegiline is currently under way in the United States.

Clonidine, a centrally active α_2-adrenoreceptor agonist, has been assessed for its therapeutic potential in AD. In a double-blind, placebo-controlled trial, eight AD patients received 0.1–0.4 mg clonidine qd and one patient received up to 1.2 mg po qd. This study found no beneficial effect of acute clonidine administration on cognition in AD (Mohr et al. 1989).

Guanfacine is another centrally active α_2-adrenoreceptor agonist that has been assessed in AD. After an initial open-drug titration and best-dose finding phase, 5 AD patients and 5 age-matched healthy control subjects entered a double-blind, placebo-controlled study. Neuropsychological tests did not identify a best dose, and the highest tolerated dose of guanfacine (mean, 0.7 mg; range, 0.5–1.0 mg po) did not produce a significant effect on cognitive functions, except for a small improvement in mood (Schlegel et al. 1989). In another double-blind, placebo-controlled study (Crook et al. 1992), 15 AD patients received 0.5 mg guanfacine po qd, whereas 14 patients received placebo. Guanfacine produced no significant improvement. These negative results do not mean that adrenergic enhancement is ineffective in AD or that it might not be a critical complement to a cholinergic therapy. It is possible that agonists have a significant activity at presynaptic receptors and inhibit transmitter release to an extent that yields a net diminution in noradrenergic activity. Therefore, an alternative strategy could employ an α_2-adrenoreceptor antagonist, selectively active at the presynaptic receptor, which would interrupt the feedback inhibition path and could lead to increased norepinephrine release. Both agonists and antagonists require further investigation.

Cholinergic-Monoaminergic Combinations

Animal experiments have demonstrated that noradrenergic brain lesions block cholinomimetic enhancement of memory and that the efficacy of cholinomimetic treatment can be restored by administration of clonidine (Davis et al. 1987; Haroutunian et al. 1990). Similarly, the combined administration of clonidine and PHS was found to enhance memory performance in primates beyond the improvement observed after the administration of either drug alone (Buccafusco et al. 1992). Taken together, these data suggest that simultaneous enhancement of the cholinergic and noradrenergic systems is feasible, may be necessary, and could render results superior to the isolated neurotransmitter systems enhancement approaches.

A pilot study of clonidine combined with PHS in nine AD patients confirmed the safety of this combined treatment (Davidson et al. 1989), whereas another study found that the combination of PHS with yohimbine may have significant cardiovascular side effects in AD (Bierer et al. 1993). One double-blind, placebo-controlled study suggested that L-deprenyl combined with either tacrine or PHS may improve cognitive functions (Schneider et al. 1993). However, another double-blind, placebo-controlled study found no significant improvement with the combination of physostigmine and L-deprenyl (Sunderland et al. 1992). Further studies are needed to clarify the potential efficacy of combination treatments.

Neuropeptides

Over the last 20 years, animal experiments have generated convincing evidence for the involvement of adrenocorticotrophic hormone (ACTH) and vasopressin (VP) in learning and memory (De Wied 1984). Studies in animals with the ACTH and VP analogues $ACTH_{4-10}$, $ACTH_{4-9}$ (Org 2766), arginine VP, 1-desamino-8-D-arginine VP, and *des*-9-glycinamide-arginine VP (Org 5667), and studies in normal volunteers and various patient groups have reported positive effects on attention. In analyzing the clinical studies with ACTH and VP analogues in AD, several reviews (Jolles 1986; Kopelman and Lishman 1986; Kragh-Sorensen and Lolk 1987) as well as one recent high-dose trial (Miller et al. 1993) concluded that there is no evidence for a beneficial effect of these peptides on cognition in this patient population. Another ACTH analogue, HOE 427 (ebiratide), showed poor results in patients with AD (Siegfried 1991).

One trial with the somatostatin analogue L-363,586, MSD in 10 AD patients failed to demonstrate any significant effects, and the drug could not be detected in the cerebrospinal fluid (CSF) (Cutler et al. 1985). In a subsequent trial in 14 AD patients, the somatostatin analogue octreotide (sandostatin or SMS 201-995) appeared to have CNS effects but failed to improve cognitive functions (Mouradian et al. 1991).

Preclinical studies with the cholecystokinin-8 analogue SUT-8701 seem promising. The drug has been shown to have neuroprotective effects and to enhance learning in aged and nucleus basalis-lesioned rats (Sugaya et al. 1993).

Glutamatergic Drugs

Experimental data indicate that excitatory amino acid (EAA)-mediated toxicity may produce lesions similar to the neurofibrillary tangles of AD. Furthermore, the glutamatergic system has been implicated in learning and memory. Blockade of *N*-methyl-D-aspartic acid (NMDA) receptors disrupts spatial learning and prevents long-term potentiation (LTP), which is thought to be the physiological basis of memory (Brown et al. 1988; Squire 1987).

NMDA-receptor blockers have been shown to provide significant protection against ischemic and EAA-mediated cortical insults (Greenamyre and Young 1989; Palmer 1991). Glycine, an NMDA-receptor modulator, is thought to enhance glutamate's effects at the NMDA-receptor site and thus to augment LTP processes and memory. It appears that the blockade of certain glutamate-receptor subtypes may protect against EAA-excitotoxicity, whereas activation of other subtypes may enhance cognitive functions in AD.

Milacemide, a glycine prodrug, enhances learning in normal and amnestic rodents. In addition, milacemide enhanced performance on certain neuropsychological tests in young healthy volunteers. However, in two large double-blind, placebo-controlled trials in AD, milacemide did not enhance cognition and was accompanied by significant liver toxicity (Dysken et al. 1992; Herting et al. 1991).

D-Cycloserine, a partial glycine agonist, enhances learning in rodents. In human volunteers, D-cycloserine was shown to ameliorate scopolamine induced cognitive impairment (Jones et al. 1991). However, preliminary reports suggest that little benefit was achieved by AD patients treated with D-cycloserine for 26 weeks (Mohr et al. 1993). Glutamatergic modulating agents require further studies. The pharmacology of the EAA is a rapidly developing field. New NMDA-receptor blockers as well as possible EAA-receptor subtype-specific partial agonists may open new avenues in the treatment of AD.

Miscellaneous

Classic Nootropics

Piracetam, the prototype nootropic, is mentioned in Chapter 6. A recent study (Croisile et al. 1993) with this agent suggested that long-term administration of high doses might slow the rate of cognitive deterioration in patients with AD. Studies of piracetam combined with the cholinergic precursors lecithin or choline showed no significant effects on cognition in AD (Davidson et al. 1987; Friedman et al. 1981; Growdon et al. 1986; R. C. Smith et al. 1984).

Other piracetam-like compounds have also been evaluated in clinical studies. Studies with pramiracetam (Branconnier et al. 1983; Claus et al. 1991) and oxiracetam (Green et al. 1992) were not successful in improving cognitive function in AD patients. Data on aniracetam (Ro 13-5057) in AD is inconclusive. Although a preliminary report from Japan seemed favorable (Mizuki 1984), a subsequent study failed to show aniracetam to be superior to placebo (Sourander et al. 1987). More recently, a controlled multicenter clinical study showed aniracetam to be superior to placebo (Senin et al. 1991).

Acetyl-L-carnitine (ALC), also discussed in Chapter 6, is a naturally occurring substance involved in mitochondrial energy processing. ALC may have multiple effects at the cellular level that might be consistent with a therapeutic potential in AD. ALC is thought to have antioxidant neuroprotective properties and is believed to enhance cellular energy supply, membrane stability, and cholinergic neurotransmission. Double-blind, placebo-controlled studies conducted in Europe and the United States suggest that 2–3 g ALC po qd administered for 6–12 months may improve cognitive performance and slow the rate of progression of AD (Carta and Calvani 1991). Further trials are necessary to prove ALC's effects conclusively.

Antioxidants

Aging and AD may be associated with increased free radical production (Papolla et al. 1992). Increased superoxide dismutase-derived hydrogen peroxide fluxes, metal ions, and damaged mitochondria can contribute to cell damage mediated by free radicals (Gutteridge et al. 1986). Free radical production in AD may also be caused by amyloid beta protein and glutamate (Behl et al. 1992). Therefore, it has been hypothesized that antioxidant agents could have beneficial effects in AD by reducing free radical production and preventing subsequent cell injury.

Selegiline is thought to have neuroprotective effects in AD as well as in Parkinson's disease by acting as a scavenger of free radicals (Knoll 1992). Vitamin E and idebenone are also potential antioxidant treatments for AD because they prevent cell death caused by glutamate and amyloid beta protein (Behl et al. 1992; Oka et al. 1993). A clinical trial with selegiline and vitamin E is currently evaluating their ability to slow the progression of AD.

Chelating Agents

An association between aluminum and AD has been suspected for more than a decade. Epidemiological studies have reported an association between the aluminum concentration in drinking water and the occurrence of AD (Martyn et al. 1989; Perl and Brody 1980). In addition, aluminum is toxic to the cholinergic system (Clayton et al. 1992). These findings have led to clinical trials in AD of desferrioxamine mesylate, which has a particularly high affinity for aluminum and has been used to treat iron and aluminum overload (Chang et al. 1983; Propper et al. 1977). In a 2-year, double-blind controlled trial with intramuscular desferrioxamine, patients who received desferrioxamine treatment showed less decline in daily living skills than the placebo group (Crapper McLachlan et al. 1991). The therapeutic effects observed with this agent may not be due to its chelating action because it has been shown to inhibit free radical formation and inflammation as well (Crapper et al.

1991). The required intramuscular administration and toxic side effects of this compound might limit its clinical utility. Replication studies are necessary to confirm the efficacy of this approach.

Vitamins

Pyritinol (Encephabol), a pyridoxine (vitamin B_6) derivative, was administered in doses of 600 mg po qd to 100 AD patients in a 12-week, double-blind, placebo-controlled parallel study (Fischhof et al. 1992). Although pyritinol appeared to be superior to placebo, the differences between placebo and the active agent were not significant.

Mecobalamin (vitamin B_{12}) (0.5 mg iv qod) was given to 10 AD patients for 8 weeks. The results suggest that cognitive functions and communication abilities improved and that the improvements correlated with high levels of B_{12} in CSF (Ikeda et al. 1992).

New Outlooks

Nerve Growth Factor

Another potential therapeutic approach for AD is based on the administration of neurotrophic factors. Nerve growth factor (NGF) is a 118-amino acid polypeptide that does not cross the blood-brain barrier. Other substances with neurotrophic activity, such as epidermal growth factor, brain-derived neurotrophic factor, gangliosides, and the β1–28 peptide of the β-amyloid protein (Whitson et al. 1989), might have a therapeutic potential as well. ICV administration of NGF partially reverses lesion-induced deficits of cortical AChE and choline acetyltransferase (CHAT) activities (Haroutounian et al. 1985), promotes survival of septal cholinergic neurons after fimbrial transection in adult rats (Hefti 1986), and reverses behavioral deterioration in rats with such lesions (Will and Hefti 1985).

Human NGF (hNGF) has been produced by recombinant techniques (Bruce and Heinrich 1989), and in the near future, sufficient amounts of pure hNGF may be available for experimental assessment and therapeutic trials in AD. There are promising pharmacological strategies, such as the synthesis of liposomes, drug lipidization, development of lipid-soluble prodrugs, and chimeric nutrients or peptides, that might provide ways for improved noninvasive drug delivery to the CNS (reviewed in Brewster 1989; Pardridge 1989).

Other routes of administration could also be considered. NGF has already been administered to Parkinson's patients surgically by intraputaminal infusion (Olson and Hoffer 1992). Genetically modified NGF-secreting fibroblasts grafts have been shown to prevent degeneration of cholinergic neurons after surgical lesions of the fimbria-fornix in rats (Rosenberg et al. 1988). This opens the possibility of infusing or grafting genetically engineered cells that would secret in situ the factor or neurotransmitter required (Olson and Hoffer 1993). For example, a fibroblast cell line was genetically modified to express choline acetyltransferase. The altered cells produced and released ACh in vitro and in vivo after grafting into rat hippocampus. Thus, specially designed fibroblasts could provide a vehicle for delivering various substances to the brain. This strategy may be a useful approach for AD (Fisher et al. 1993b). It is conceivable that in the future neuronal stem cells or neurotransmitter secreting cell implants will become available for clinical trials in the treatment of AD. Most recently, NGF conjugated to an antibody to the transferrin receptor was shown to cross the blood-brain barrier and to increase the survival of cholinergic and noncholinergic neurons after peripheral injection in rats (Frieden et al. 1993).

Anti-Inflammatory Agents

The involvement of the immune system and of inflammation in the pathophysiology of AD has been suggested by a number of investigators and reviewed by McGeer et al. (1994). Findings include the presence of acute-phase reactants in CSF (Brugge et al. 1992), along with elevated levels of various cytokines including tumor necrosis factor in serum (Fillit et al. 1991) and interleukins 1 and 6 in brain (Bauer et al. 1991; Griffin et al. 1989). Cellular immune responses include T4 and T8 lymphocytes and microglia (Rogers et al. 1992a) and the production of complement (McGeer and McGeer 1992). The use of anti-inflammatory agents in the treatment of AD is further supported by the low prevalence of AD in patients with rheumatoid arthritis (McGeer et al. 1990), a finding that could be explained by the long-standing exposure of these patients to anti-inflammatory therapy. Furthermore, preliminary observations suggest that steroids and nonsteroidal anti-inflammatory drugs such as indomethacin and aspirin may have protective effects against AD (Breitner et al. 1994). In a 6-month, double-blind, placebo-controlled study of AD, indomethacin 100–150 mg po qd was found to improve cognitive function and to delay further deterioration. These results are promising, but indomethacin's toxicity might limit its use (Rogers et al. 1993).

Corticosteroid use is another possible anti-inflammatory strategy for AD (Aisen and Davis 1994). These agents are widely used for the treatment of CNS inflammatory diseases, including lupus cerebritis and multiple sclerosis. Unfortunately, the systemic toxicity of steroids limit the dosage and length of treatment with these agents. Colchicine is another possible anti-inflammatory candidate for the treatment of AD. This drug effectively treats familial Mediterranean fever, a condition in which recurrent inflammation and amyloidosis occur. Although the amyloid constituents in familial Mediterranean fever and AD differ, both illnesses involve chronic inflammation, elevated acute-phase proteins, and abnormal processing of a precursor protein leading to deposition of insoluble amyloid fragments. Hydroxychloroquine, an antimalarial agent and an effective second-line drug for the treatment of rheumatoid arthritis and lupus erythematosus, is thought to affect the immune response by interacting with lysosomal functioning. This agent suppresses cytokine and acute-phase reactant levels (Ertel et al. 1991). The drug is relatively safe when administered chronically for the treatment of rheumatoid arthritis and could be a candidate for treating AD.

Anti-Amyloidogenesis Agents

Extracellular deposits of β-amyloid protein in plaques may be toxic and may cause cell death and neurofibrillary tangle formation (Hardy and Higgins 1992; Higgins et al. 1995). β-Amyloid protein is derived from the processing of the amyloid precursor protein (APP), but, as indicated in Chapter 13, normal APP processing does not result in β-amyloid secretion (Gandy et al. 1988; Suzuki et al. 1992). Aberrant lysosomal processing of APP may generate amyloidogenic fragments (Estus et al. 1992). Thus, agents that interfere with β-amyloid production may represent an alternative strategy to alter the course of AD. The effects of colchicine and hydroxychloroquine on lysosomal processing suggest that these agents could have beneficial effects in AD by interfering with the amyloidogenic pathway. Although colchicine is used as a neurotoxin in laboratory studies, no significant CNS toxicity has been reported with clinical use of this agent. Other such substances are small-molecule anionic sulphonates or sulphates (Kisilevsky et al. 1995). If amyloidogenesis results from inadequacy of normal sequestering substances such as transthyretin (Schwarzman et al. 1995), analogues of this substance might be devised.

Recent data suggest that cholinergic receptors may influence intracellular APP concentrations and processing. Cholinergic agonists were shown to alter the processing of the β-amyloid precursor protein by increasing the secretory cleavage pathway of the protein (see Figure 13–1). The cholinergic agonist carbachol increases the rate of APP secretion in transfected human embryonic kidney cell lines by stimulating M_1 and M_3 receptors. This increase is probably mediated by the activation of protein kinases (Buxbaum et al. 1992; Nitsch et al. 1992). These data suggest that cholinergic receptors may modulate intracellular APP processing and secretion and may thereby affect extracellular senile plaque formation.

Apolipoprotein E

There is a threefold higher prevalence of apolipoprotein E4 (ApoE4) allele in patients with late-onset familial AD than in control subjects. ApoE is present in senile plaques, vascular amyloid, and neurofibrillary tangles of AD. Based on experimental data, it has been suggested that the protein generated by the ApoE4 allele (unlike the proteins generated by the alleles ApoE3 or ApoE2) lacks microtubule-protective properties. Thus, the absence of the alternative alleles ApoE3 or ApoE2 may be amyloidogenic and associated with an increased risk for AD (Strittmatter et al. 1994). This hypothesis suggests that new pharmacological strategies in AD could consist of agents with ApoE3- or ApoE2-like microtubule-stabilizing properties or of compounds that alter the expression of the ApoE gene.

Transplants

Autologous neuronal tissue from the adrenal medulla has been grafted successfully into the caudate nucleus in Parkinson's disease patients (Madrazzo et al. 1987), as have transplants of adrenal medulla (Penn et al. 1988a) and ventral mesencephalic tissue from aborted human fetuses (Lindvall et al. 1989). Cholinergic neuronal tissue transplanted into brains of animals with cholinergic lesions partially reversed neurochemical and behavioral deficits produced by the lesions (Fine et al. 1985). Recently, a fibroblast cell line was genetically modified to express choline acetyltransferase. The altered cells produced and released acetylcholine in vitro and after grafting into rat hippocampus. Thus, genetically modified fibroblasts could provide a vehicle for delivering various substances to the brain. This strategy may represent a most promising approach for the amelioration of cognitive impairment in AD (Fisher et al. 1993b). Considering these results and other comparably promising reports with implants of NGF-secreting cells (Rosenberg et al. 1988), it is conceivable that neuronal stem cells or neurotransmitter-secreting cell implants will become available for clinical trials in the treatment of AD.

Genetics and Prevention

Epidemiological studies have identified no other strongly consistent risk factors for AD except advanced age, a history of AD in a first-degree relative, and the ApoE4 allele. Mutations of the APP gene on chromosomes 21 and unidentified mutations at other loci on chromosome 21, 19, and 14 are thought to be associated with an increased risk for the disease (for review see Clark and Goate 1993). Although most AD cases are probably not linked to those loci, they may still retain an important genetic influence. Given the heterogeneity in age at onset, rate of progression, and clinical characteristics of the disease, it must be assumed that the phenotypic expression is modulated by a complex interaction between the genetic vulnerability, the aging process, and some yet-unidentified environmental factors.

Neurochemical, neuroendocrinological, and brain imaging studies so far have not identified any reliable in vivo biological marker for AD. Currently available diagnostic criteria allow the recognition of the disease at a stage when the degenerative process may have advanced well beyond the compensatory reserves of the CNS. Thus, present therapeutic attempts act on a severely compromised system. The identification of a reliable early marker for AD would allow for the development of treatments to be administered to the population at risk for AD long before the disease manifests. It has been suggested that delaying the age at onset by 5 years would cut AD morbidity in half (Breitner et al. 1989). The identification of an early AD marker could be the first step toward the treatment of the disease by manipulations of the pathogenetic mechanisms or even the eradication of the disease by means of genetic engineering.

Summary and Conclusions

Multiple empirical pharmacological strategies have failed in AD. The neurotransmission-enhancing strategies and in particular the cholinomimetic strategies have shown some promise. The AChE inhibitor tacrine has been approved by the FDA for the treatment of cognitive impairment in AD, and a second generation of cholinesterase inhibitors is on the horizon. Combined neurotransmission-enhancing therapies might prove superior to the isolated cholinomimetic augmentation. Newer strategies are based on an increasing understanding of the pathophysiological processes involved in this illness. Strategies aimed at slowing or arresting the progression of the illness are beginning to be explored and will undoubtedly lead to therapeutic breakthroughs in the near future.

Dementia Questionnaire

Patient Name _____ Age _____ Date _____

Informant _____

Relation to patient _____

MEMORY

Does_____

have any problem with:

	Yes	No	Don't know	Date
1) Memory	____	____	____	____
2) Remembering people's names	____	____	____	____
3) Recognizing familiar faces	____	____	____	____
4) Finding way about indoors	____	____	____	____
5) Finding way on familiar streets	____	____	____	____
6) Remembering a short list of items	____	____	____	____
7) Did trouble with memory begin suddenly	____	or slowly	____	
8) Has the course of the memory problems been a steady downhill progression or have there been abrupt declines	____	____	____	

EXPRESSION

	Yes	No	Don't know	Date
9) Ever have trouble finding the right word or expressing self	____	____	____	____
10) Talking become less over time	____	____	____	____
11) Tendency to dwell in the past	____	____	____	____

DAILY FUNCTIONING

	Yes	No	Don't know	Date
12) Trouble with household tasks	____	____	____	____
13) Trouble handling money	____	____	____	____

		Yes	No	Don't know	Date
14)	Trouble grasping situations or explanations	___	___	___	___
15)	Difficulty at work (check if N/A___)	___	___	___	___
16)	Trouble dressing or caring for self	___	___	___	___
17)	Trouble feeding self	___	___	___	___
18)	Trouble controlling bladder and bowels	___	___	___	___
19)	Agitation and nervousness	___	___	___	___

OTHER PROBLEMS

		Yes	No	Don't know	Date
20)	High blood pressure	___	___	___	___
21)	Stroke	___	___	___	___
22)	More than 1 stroke	___	___	___	___
23)	Is one side of the body weaker than other side	___	___	___	___
24)	Parkinson's disease (tremors, shuffling gait, rigidity of limbs)	___	___	___	___
25)	Injury to the head resulting in a loss of consciousness for more than a second or two	___	___	___	___
26)	Seizure or fits	___	___	___	___
27)	Syphilis	___	___	___	___
28)	Diabetes	___	___	___	___
29)	Drinking problem (describe type and amount consumed per day, duration, blackouts, DTs)_____				
30)	Did memory problems coincide with drinking	___	___	___	___
31)	Ever depressed or sad for two weeks or more	___	___	___	___
32)	If yes, ever seek treatment	___	___	___	___
33)	Ever very high, euphoric, top of the world	___	___	___	___
34)	If yes, ever seek treatment	___	___	___	___
35)	Ever seek psychiatric or psychological help for any reason	___	___	___	___
36)	If yes, ever hospitalized for psychiatric illness	___	___	___	___
	Where? _____				

	Yes	No	Don't know	Date
37) Down's syndrome (subject or family member)	____	____	____	____
38) Other medical problems we have not talked about_____				

MEDICAL CONTACTS

39) Name and address of doctors seen for memory or related problems:

_____

_____

_____

	Yes	No	Don't know	Date
40) Ever receive medications	____	____	____	____
41) A neurological exam or a psychiatric exam	____	____	____	____
42) CAT scan	____	____	____	____
43) What was diagnosis given for problems_____				

RECOGNITION OF PROBLEM

44) Who was the first person to notice something wrong _____

45) What was noticed_____

46) When was the last time (the subject seemed to be really well, or his old self)_____

_____

MEDICATIONS

47) What medications are currently being taken_____

FAMILY HISTORY

48) Anyone else in the family with similar problems _____Yes _____No. If yes, what is the name of the person _____; relationship _____; age _____. How can we obtain history about that person _____

_____

Source.   Modified with permission from Breitner and Folstein 1984.

Mental Status Examination

Patient name_____ Date:__/__/__
Handedness__R__L Age____ Sex___ Marital status_____
Years of education_____   Occupation_____

	NORM	ABN	UNK
1. APPEARANCE AND BEHAVIOR			
Grooming and dress (circle one):	0	1	9
Hearing _____	0	1	9
Eyesight _____	0	1	9
2. BEHAVIORAL HISTORY OR OBSERVATION			
Wandering _____	0	1	9
Verbal aggression _____	0	1	9
Physical aggression _____	0	1	9
Apathy _____	0	1	9
Sundowning _____	0	1	9
Crying _____	0	1	9
3. ORIENTATION	0	1	9

Time __ day __ date __ month __ year
Place __ city __ hospital __ home address
Person __ name __ age __ birth date

	NORM	ABN	UNK
4. EMOTION (AFFECT)			
Blunted _____	0	1	9
Shallow _____	0	1	9
Labile _____	0	1	9
Appropriateness _____	0	1	9
Other _____	0	1	9
5. MOOD			
Depressed _____	0	1	9
Euphoric _____	0	1	9
Other _____	0	1	9

6. THOUGHT PROCESS	NORM	ABN	UNK

Associations

Loose _____	0	1	9
Klang _____	0	1	9
Other _____	0	1	9

Flow

Tangential _____	0	1	9
Circumstantial _____	0	1	9
Flight of ideas _____	0	1	9
Blockage _____	0	1	9
Derailment _____	0	1	9
Perseveration _____	0	1	9
Other _____	0	1	9

7.   THOUGHT CONTENT

Delusions _____	0	1	9
Hallucinations _____	0	1	9
Illusions _____	0	1	9
Suspicions _____	0	1	9
Misidentification syndrome _____	0	1	9

8.   ATTENTION

3-7
2-4-9   Digits forward: 0   1   9
8-5-2-7
2-9-6-8-3   Digits reversed: 0   1   9
5-7-1-9-4-6
8-1-5-9-3-6-2
3-9-8-2-5-1-4-7

CONCENTRATION—serial subtraction of 3s or 7s

Subtraction of 3s (20, 17, 14, 11, 8, 5, 2, -1)	0	1	9
Subtraction of 7s (100, 93, 86, 79, 72, 65, 58, 51)	0	1	9

9.   LANGUAGE

Articulation _____	0	1	9
Fluency overall _____	0	1	9

__ increase   __ decrease   __ delayed word finding
__ neologisms   __ paraphasias
__ other _____

10.   Name as many animals as you can in 1 minute: 0   1   9
(normal = 18: plus or minus 6)

		MILD—		
11. EXPRESSIVE LANGUAGE	**NONE**	**MOD**	**SEV**	**UNK**

Word finding difficulty in
spontaneous speech: _____ 0   1   2   9

Global rating of amount of spoken
language: _____ 0   1   2   9

	NORM	**ABN**	**UNK**
12. COMPREHENSION	**0**	**1**	**9**

__ Point to floor   __ ceiling   __ desk, chair, door
__ Are you 150 years old?   __ Is the sky green?
__ Do you put on your coat before or after your shirt/blouse?
__ If you cross from the north to the south side of the street, which side are
   you on?
__ Is my cousin's mother a man or a woman?

13. REPETITION   0   1   9

__ walk   __ hospital   __ Mississippi river
__ the little boy next door
__ I saw the train arrive yesterday

14. NAMING   0   1   9

__ watch   __ back   __ crystal   __ band   __ stem

15. READING ALOUD (see p. 364)

P   G   R   0   1   9
I am going to a movie   0   1   9
It is a thriller and bound to be scary   0   1   9

16. WRITING (see p. 366)

Dictated sentence   0   1   9
Spontaneous sentence   0   1   9

17. MEMORY

Remote: __ name four presidents during your lifetime   0   1   9
Recent: **unrelated words**   **5 minutes**   **cued**
                  book   _____   _____   0   1   9
                  chair   _____   _____   0   1   9
                  green   _____   _____   0   1   9

18. PRAXIS	NORM	ABN	UNK
Imitation	0	1	9
Ideomotor:			
salute flag	0	1	9
comb hair	0	1	9
Blow out match	0	1	9
Construction (see p. 365):	0	1	9
__ intersecting rectangles	0	1	9
__ Greek cross	0	1	9
__ cube	0	1	9

19.   HIGHER COGNITIVE FUNCTION

Fund of information	0	1	9

__ How many weeks in a year?
__ Why do people have lungs?
__ Name four states
__ Where is Denmark?
__ How far is it from New
    York to Los Angeles?
__ Who wrote the Odyssey?

__ Why are light colored clothes
    cooler in the summer than dark
    colored clothes?
__ Who was president during the
    American Civil War?
__ What causes rust?
__ What is the Koran?

20.   CALCULATION

$2 \times 2 = 4, 2 \times 4 = 8, 2 \times 8 = 16, \ldots$ (through 1,024)	0	1	9

21.   PROVERBS: What do people mean when they say . . .

	NORM	ABN	UNK
Don't cry over spilled milk.	0	1	9
The grass is always greener on the other side of the street.	0	1	9
People who live in glass houses shouldn't throw stones.	0	1	9
Overall rating	0	1	9

22.   SIMILARITIES: An apple and a banana are similar in that they are fruits. What is the similarity between . . .

potato	—	carrot _____	0	1	9
cat	—	rabbit _____	0	1	9
airplane	—	motorcycle _____	0	1	9
dancing	—	swiming _____	0	1	9
hot	—	cold _____	0	1	9
nose	—	tongue _____	0	1	9
Overall rating		_____	0	1	9

23.   JUDGMENT—What would you do if . . .

	NORM	ABN	UNK
You found a sealed, addressed, stamped envelope on the street?	0	1	9
You were in a crowded theater when a fire broke out?	0	1	9
A check you wrote bounced?	0	1	9
Overall assessment	0	1	9

24. INSIGHT: 0 = normal; total insight into illness and implications
                     1 = partial awareness of disease or implications
                     2 = unaware of or denial of symptoms or illness
                     3 = uncertain or irrelevant response or not applicable

DIAGNOSIS (DSM-IV)

Axis I: Clinical syndromes or conditions that are the focus of treatment: ___

_____

_____

_____

Axis II: Personality or specific developmental disorders: _____

_____

_____

Axis III: Physical disorders and conditions: _____

_____

_____

P   G   R

I AM GOING TO A MOVIE

*IT IS A THRILLER AND BOUND
TO BE SCARY*

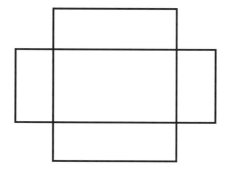

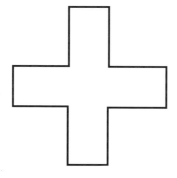

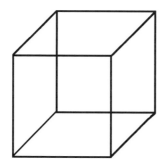

Dictated sentence:

_____

Spontaneous sentence:

_____

Draw figures below:

Neurological Examination

Patient _____   Date ___/___/___
Handedness: R   L
Age _____   Sex _____

CRANIAL NERVES	NORMAL	ABNORMAL	N/A
1. Olfaction _____	0	1	9
2. Visual acuity _____	0	1	9
3. Pupils (ERRLA) _____	0	N = neurologic P = physical	9
4. Visual fields _____	0	1	9
5. Fundi _____	0	1	9
6. EOMs _____	0	1	9
7. Facial sensation _____	0	1	9
8. Muscles of mastication _____	0	1	9
9. Jaw jerk _____	0	1	9
10. Facial muscles _____	0	N = neurologic P = physical	9
11. Auditory activity _____	0	1 = unilateral 2 = bilateral	9
12. Palate elevation _____	0	N = neurologic P = physical	9
13. Cough, gag, swallow _____	0	1	9
14. Traps and SCM (CNXI) _____	0	1	9
15. Tongue _____	0	1	9
16. Bulk _____	0	F = foc D = diff	9
17. Spasticity (tone) _____	0	F = foc D = diff	9

18. "Lead pipe" rigidity   None   Mild   Moderate Severe N/A
    a) Right extremities   0   1   2   3   9
    b) Left extremities   0   1   2   3   9
    Note. Do not consider cog-wheel rigidity here.

19. Strength (circle one)
    5 = normal   2 = unable to overcome gravity
    4 = reduced strength   1 = trace of movement only
    3 = unable to overcome resistance 0 = no strength
              9 = N/A

20. Muscle stretch refelxes (circle one for each side)

a) Right		b) Left
0	absent reflexes	0
1	reflexes reduced but not present	1
2	normal	2
3	increased reflexes	3
4	nonsustained clonus	4
5	sustained clonus	5
9	N/A	9

                                    NORMAL ABNORMAL   N/A

21. Primitive reflexes (check all that apply)   0   1   9

    ____Palmomental
    ____Grasp
    ____Snout
    ____Suck

22. Extensor plantar response _____   0   L = left   9
                                         R = right
                                         B = bilateral

23. Finger-nose-finger _____   0   1   9

24. Heel-knee-shin _____   0   1   9

25. Rapid alternating movements (RAMs)

		Right Impairment						Left Impairment			
		Norm	Mild	Mod	Severe	N/A		Norm	Mild	Mod	Severe	N/A
a)	Finger or hand clasps	0	1	2	3	9	d)	0	1	2	3	9
b)	Heel taps	0	1	2	3	9	e)	0	1	2	3	9
c)	Prone/supine	0	1	2	3	9	f)	0	1	2	3	9

		Normal	Abnormal	N/A

26. Abnormal movements

		Normal	Abnormal	N/A
a)	Benign essential tremor _____	0	1	9
b)	Myoclonus _____	0	1	9
c)	Dyskinesia _____	0	1	9
d)	Rest tremor—right extremities _____	0	1	9
e)	Rest tremor—left extremities _____	0	1	9
f)	Action tremor—right extremities _____	0	1	9
g)	Action tremor— left extremities _____	0	1	9

27. Sensation (decreased) overall _____   0   F = focal   9
                                                       D = diffuse

     _____ Light touch
     _____ Vibration
     _____ Joint position sense
     _____ Cold
     _____ Pinprick

28. Gait and station
     Gait and posture _____   0   1   9

29. Other extrapyramidal symptoms

		Normal	Abnormal	N/A
a)	Body bradykinesia _____	0	1	9
b)	Postural stability _____	0	1	9
c)	Arising from a chair _____	0	1	9
d)	Voice (hypovocalization) _____	0	1	9
e)	Facial movement (hypomania) _____	0	1	9
f)	Turning en bloc _____	0	1	9
g)	Cogwheel rigidity _____	0	1	9

30. Patient cooperativeness (circle one)
     0 = fully coperative
     1 = mildly to moderately cooperative
     2 = very uncooperative
     9 = couldn't examine/don't know

31. Overall neurological assessment   0   1   9
        (excluding mental status)

32. Overall mental status _____   0   1   9

Notes:

_____

_____

_____

_____

_____

_____

_____

Blessed Dementia Rating Scale (BDRS)

1) Memory and performance of everyday activities

Loss of ability	NONE	SOME	SEVERE
(Score: 0 = none; 0.5 = sometimes; 1 = frequently)			
A. Ability to perform household tasks	0	0.5	1
B. Ability to cope with small sums of money	0	0.5	1
C. Ability to remember a short list of items (e.g., shopping list)	0	0.5	1
D. Ability to find way about indoors (patient's home or other familiar locations)	0	0.5	1
E. Ability to find way around familiar streets	0	0.5	1
F. Ability to grasp situations or explanations	0	0.5	1
G. Ability to recall recent events	0	0.5	1
H. Tendency to dwell in the past	0	0.5	1

2) Habits
A. Eating
    0 = Feeds self without assistance
    1 = Feeds self with minor assistance
    2 = Feeds self with much assistance
    3 = Has to be fed

B. Dressing
    0 = Unaided
    1 = Occasionally misplaces buttons, etc., requires minor help
    2 = Wrong sequence, forgets items, requires much assistance
    3 = Unable to dress

C. Toilet
    0 = Clean, cares for self at toilet
    1 = Occasional incontinence, or needs to be reminded
    2 = Frequent incontinence, or much assistance
    3 = No control

3) TOTAL SCORE OF ALL ITEMS (maximum score 17) _____

Source. Modified with permission from Blessed et al. 1968.

Washington University Clinical Dementia Rating (CDR) Scale

	Healthy CDR 0	Questionable dementia CDR 0.5
Memory	No memory loss or slight inconsistent forgetfulness	Mild consistent forgetfulness, partial recollection of events; "benign" forgetfulness
Orientation	Fully oriented	
Judgment—problem solving	Solves everyday problems well; judgment good in relation to past performance	Only doubtful impairment in solving problems, similarities, differences
Community affairs	Independent function at usual level in job, shopping, business, and financial affairs, volunteer and social groups	Only doubtful or mild impairment in these activities
Home—hobbies	Life at home, hobbies, intellectual interests well maintained	Life at home, hobbies, intellectual interests slightly impaired
Personal care	Fully capable of self-care	

Score only impairment due to cognitive loss, not impairment due to other factors.

Source. Reprinted with permission from Hughes CP, Berg L, Danziger WL: "A New Clinical Scale for the Staging of Dementia." *British Journal of Psychiatry* 140:566–572, 1982.

Mild dementia CDR 1	Moderate dementia CDR 2	Severe dementia CDR 3
Moderate memory loss more marked for recent events; defect interferes with everyday activities	Severe memory loss: only highly learned material retained; new material rapidly lost	Severe memory loss: only fragments remain
Some difficulty with time relationships: oriented for place and person at examination but may have geographic disorientation	Usually disoriented in time, often to place	Orientation to person only
Moderate difficulty in handling complex problems; social judgment usually maintained	Severely impaired in handling problems, similarities, differences; social judgment usually impaired	Unable to make judgments or solve problems
Unable to function independently at these activities though may still be engaged in some; may still appear normal to casual inspection	No pretense of independent function outside home	
	Appears well enough to be taken to functions outside a family home	Appears too ill to be taken to functions outside a family home
Mild but definite impairment of function at home; more difficult chores abandoned; more complicated hobbies and interests abandoned	Only simple chores preserved; very restricted interests, poorly sustained	No significant function in home outside of own room
Needs prompting	Requires assistance in dressing, hygiene, keeping of personal effects	Requires much help with personal care; often incontinent

The Mini-Mental State Exam (MMSE)

		Score	Points
Orientation			
1. What is the	Year?		1
	Season?		1
	Date?		1
	Day?		1
	Month?		1
2. Where are we?	State?		1
	County?		1
	Town or city?		1
	Hospital?		1
	Floor?		1

Registration

3. Name three objects, taking one second to say each.
   Then ask the patient all three after you have said
   them. Give one point for each correct answer.
   Repeat the answers until the patient learns all three.   3

Attention and Calculation

4. Serial 7s. Given one point for each correct answer.
   Stop after five answers. *Alternative:* Spell WORLD
   backwards.   5

Recall

5. Ask for names of three objects learned in
   Question 3. Give one point for each correct answer.   3

Language

6. Point to a pencil and a watch. Have the patient name
   them as you point.   2

7. Have the patient repeat "No ifs, ands, or buts."   1

8. Have the patient follow a three-stage command:
   "Take the paper in your right hand. Fold the paper
   in half. Put the paper on the floor."   3

Language *(continued)*   *Score   Points*

9. Have the patient read and obey the following:
    "CLOSE YOUR EYES." (Write it in large letters.)   1

10. Have the patient write a sentence of his or her
    own choice. (The sentence should contain a subject
    and an object and should make sense. Ignore spelling
    errors when scoring.)   1

11. Enlarge the design printed below to 1 to 5 cm per side
    and have the patient copy it. (Give one point if all sides
    and angles are preserved and if the intersecting sides
    form a quadrangle.)   1

                                              _____ = Total 30

Source.   Reprinted with permission from Folstein MF, Folstein SE, McHugh PR: "Mini-Mental State: A Practical Method for Grading the Cognitive State of Patients for the Clinician." *Journal of Psychiatric Research* 12:189–198, 1975.

Alzheimer's Disease Assessment Scale (ADAS)

The examiner is seated facing the subject across a small table. The word recall task is administered first and is followed by the remaining cognitive tasks. Some time (as long as 10 minutes) is spent in open-ended conversation to assess various aspects of expressive speech. Noncognitive behaviors are evaluated from reports of the patient and/or reliable informants and from observations made during the interview. It is best, but not absolutely necessary, to interview subject or informant separately.

The rating scale of 0–5 indicates the severity of dysfunction.

0 = no impairment on a task or absence of a particular behavior
1 = very mild
2 = mild
3 = moderate
4 = moderately severe
5 = the most severe degree of impairment or a very high frequency of a behavior

Ratings of many cognitive behaviors correspond to specific levels of performance on tasks.

COGNITIVE BEHAVIORS

1. WORD RECALL TASK. The subject reads 10 high-imagery words exposed for two seconds each. Each word is printed in 5/8" (16-mm) letters on a separate 4" × 6" card. The subject is asked to recall the words aloud. The cards are then shuffled and re-presented. Three trials of reading and recall are given. The score equals the mean number of words NOT recalled on three trials (maximum = 10). If subject is unable to comprehend or perform task, the score is 10.

Note: Language abilities are evaluated throughout the interview and on specific tests. Questions eliciting "yes" and "no" answers assess

basic comprehension. Other questions should require specific information and well-developed communication skills commensurate with educational level or estimated premorbid intelligence level. Do NOT rate
word finding here.

2. SPOKEN LANGUAGE ABILITY.   This is a global rating of speech
quality such as clarity and ability to make oneself understood. Do NOT
rate quantity of speech or word-finding difficulty here.

    0 = no difficulty
    1 = one instance of lack of understanding
    2 = subject understandable > 75% of the time
    3 = subject understandable 50%–75% of the time
    4 = subject NOT understandable 50% of the time
    5 = one or two word utterances; fluent but empty speech; mute

3. COMPREHENSION.   Evaluate the subject's ability to understand
speech. Do not include responses to commands.

    0 = no misunderstandings
    1 = one instance of misunderstanding
    2 = 3–5 instances of misunderstanding
    3 = requires several repetitions and rephrasing
    4 = occasional correct response, such as yes-no questions
    5 = rarely responds to questions appropriately, not due to poverty
        of speech

4. REMEMBERING TEST INSTRUCTIONS.   The subject's ability to
remember the requirements of the recognition task is evaluated. On each
recognition trial, the subject is asked prior to presenting the first two
words, "Did you see this word before or is it a new word?" For the third
word, the subject is asked, "How about this one?" If subject responds
appropriately, i.e., "yes" or "no," recall of instructions is accurate. Failure
to respond indicates that instructions have been forgotten. The instruction is then repeated. The procedure for the third word is repeated for
words 4–24; each instance of recall failure is noted.

    0 = remembers well
    1 = forgets once
    2 = must be reminded twice
    3 = must be reminded 3–4 times

4 = must be reminded 5–6 times
5 = must be reminded 7 or more times

5. WORD-FINDING DIFFICULTY IN SPONTANEOUS SPEECH.
Subjects have difficulty finding the desired word in spontaneous speech.
They may deal with this by circumlocution or giving explanatory
phrases or nearly satisfactory synonyms. Do NOT include finger and
object naming in this rating.

0 = none
1 = 1–2 instances
2 = noticeable circumlocution or word substitution
    3 = occasional loss of words without compensation
4 = frequent loss of words without compensation
5 = nearly total loss of content words; speech sounds empty; 1- to
    2-word utterances

6. COMMANDS.   Receptive speech is also assessed by subject's ability
to carry out 1- to 5-step commands.

1 = Make a FIST.
2 = Point to the CEILING and then to the FLOOR.

Line up a pencil, watch and 4" × 6" card, in that order, on the table in front
of the patient.

3 = Put the PENCIL ON TOP OF THE CARD and then PUT IT
    BACK.
4 = Put the WATCH on the OTHER SIDE OF THE PENCIL and
    then TURN OVER THE CARD.
5 = Tap EACH SHOULDER TWICE, WITH TWO FINGERS,
    KEEPING YOUR EYES SHUT.

Each capitalized element is a single step. The command may be repeated
once in its entirety. Each command is scored as a whole. The rating is the
number of commands performed correctly.

0 = accomplishes 5-step command
1 = accomplishes 4-step command
2 = accomplishes 3-step command
3 = accomplishes 2-step command

4 = accomplishes 1-step command
5 = cannot follow 1-step command

7. NAMING OBJECTS AND FINGERS.   The subject is asked to name 12 randomly presented real objects whose frequency values (2) are high, medium and low. Then, subjects are asked to place the dominant hand on the table and to name the fingers: thumb, index (pointer, first finger forefinger), middle, ring, and little (pinky) or other culturally acceptable name. Standard clues may be used to assist subjects having difficulty. The objects, their frequency, and the clues are:

High Frequency:
    Flower (plastic): grows in the garden
    Bed (dollhouse furniture): used for sleeping
    Whistle: makes sound when blown
    Pencil: used for writing

Medium Frequency:
    Rattle: a baby's toy
    Mask: hides your face
    Scissors: cuts paper
    Comb: used on hair

Low Frequency:
    Wallet: holds your money
    Harmonica: a musical instrument
    Stethoscope: doctor uses it to listen to your heart
    Tongs: picks up food

0 = 0–2 objects named incorrectly (objects + fingers named)
1 = 3–5 objects named incorrectly
2 = 6–8 objects named incorrectly
3 = 9–11 objects named incorrectly
4 = 12–14 objects named incorrectly
5 = 15–17 objects named incorrectly

8. CONSTRUCTIONAL PRAXIS. The ability to copy four geometric forms is assessed. These forms, in order of presentation, are:

1. Circle, approximately 20 cm in diameter.
2. Two overlapping rectangles forming a cross. The vertical rectangle is 20 × 25 cm; the horizontal, 10 × 35 cm.
3. Rhombus, each side 20 cm, acute ≤ 50 deg, obtuse ≤ 130 deg.
4. Cube, each side = 20 cm, with internal lines present.

Each form is located in the upper middle of a 5 ½" × 8 ½" sheet of white paper. The subject is asked, "Do you see this figure," and then told, "Make one that looks like this anywhere on the paper." Two attempts are permitted.

Scoring criteria are:
1. Circle. A closed, curved figure.
2. Two overlapping rectangles. Figures must be four-sided and overlap similar to presented form. Do NOT score for size.
3. Rhombus. Figure must be four-sided, obliquely oriented and the sides of approximately equal length. Four measurements are taken: ac, a'c, bc, b'c. The ratio of ac/a'c ranges from 0.75 to 1.0. The ratio of bc/b'c ranges from 0.6 to 1.0. The ratio bb'/aa' ranges from 3 to 0.75. Figure is incorrect if any ratio is outside these ranges.
4. Cube. The form is three-dimensional with front face in the correct orientation, internal lines drawn correctly between corners. Opposite sides of faces not parallel by more than 10 deg is incorrect.

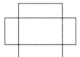   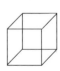

9. IDEATIONAL PRAXIS. The subject is given an 8 ½" × 11" sheet of paper and a long envelope. Subjects are instructed to pretend to send the letter to themselves. Subjects are told to fold the paper, put the paper in the envelope, seal it, address it to themselves and to indicate where the stamp goes. If subject forgets part of the task or has difficulty, reinstruction is given. Impairment on this task should reflect dysfunction in executing an overlearned task and NOT recall difficulty. Task components are: 1) fold letter, 2) put letter in envelope, 3) seal envelope, 4) address envelope, and 5) mark where stamp goes. Any address containing name, street, city and state (ZIP code is optional).

```
0 = performs all components
1 = failure to perform 1 component
2 = failure to perform 2 components
3 = failure to perform 3 components
4 = failure to perform 4 components
5 = failure to perform 5 components
```

10. ORIENTATION.   The components of orientation are date, month, year, day of the week, season, time of day, place, and person. One point is given for each INCORRECT response (maximum = 8). Acceptable answers include ±1 for the date, ±1 for the hour, partial name for place, naming of upcoming season within one week of its beginning and name of previous season for 2 weeks after its end.

11. WORD RECOGNITION TASK.   The subject reads aloud 12 high-imagery words printed in 16-mm letters on 4" × 6" cards. These cards are then randomly mixed with 12 words the subject has not seen. The subject indicates whether the word was shown previously. Then two more trials of reading the original words and of recognition are given. The score is the mean number of incorrect responses for the three trials (maximum = 12). If subject is unable to perform the task, a score of 12 is given.

NONCOGNITIVE BEHAVIORS

12. TREMORS.   Subject extends both hands in front of body and extends the fingers, holding this position for approximately 10 seconds.

```
0 = none
1 = very slight tremor, barely noticeable
2 = noticeable tremor that does not interfere with activities
3 = tremor that interferes with activities such as holding pencil or
    buttoning shirt
4 = tremor that interferes with gross activities such as holding a
    glass of water
5 = very rapid movements with sizable displacement
```

13. TEARFUL.   Subject/informant is asked about the frequency of tearfulness in the prior week.

0 = no tears or crying
1 = occurs one time during week or testing session
2 = occurs 2–3 times during the week
3 = occasional outbursts of short duration
4 = frequent crying spells nearly every day
5 = frequent and prolonged crying spells every day

14. DEPRESSION.   Subject/informant is asked about sadness, discouragement, being down. If response is positive, inquire as to severity and pervasiveness of mood, loss of interest or pleasure in activities, and reactivity to environmental events. Interviewer notes presence of depressed faces and ability to respond to encouragement and jokes. Include past week.

0 = feels good
1 = feels slightly dysphoric
2 = appears and reports mild dysphoric mood, reactivity present, some loss of interest
3 = feels moderately dysphoric often
4 = feels dysphoric almost all the time with considerable loss of reactivity and interest
5 = pervasive and severe dysphoric mood; total lack of reactivity; pervasive loss of interest and/or pleasure

15. CONCENTRATION/DISTRACTIBILITY.   Rate the frequency with which subject is distracted by irrelevant stimuli and/or must be reoriented to the ongoing task. Information from informant may also be used, for example, ability to watch TV, finish meals, have conversations. A score of 1 may be given subjects who are reported by the informant as distractible but do not exhibit this behavior during the interview.

0 = concentrates well
1 = one instance of poor concentration
2 = 2–3 instances of poor concentration/distractibility
3 = 4–5 instances during interview; frequent episodes at home
4 = poor concentration; highly distractible throughout much of the interview and at home
5 = extreme difficulty in concentration; extremely distractible, unable to complete tasks

16. UNCOOPERATIVE TO TESTING.   Rate the amount of subject's resistance to various aspects of the interview.

   0 = no instance of uncooperativeness
   1 = one instance of uncooperativeness
   2 = few instances of uncooperativeness; readily complies if asked
        to continue
   3 = several instances of uncooperativeness
   4 = needs constant cajoling to complete interview
   5 = refuses to complete interview

17. DELUSIONS.   Rate the subject's belief in ideas that appear untrue, for example, persons entering house, stealing possessions. In rating severity consider conviction in delusions, preoccupation and effect on subject's actions. Include prior week's observations.

   0 = none
   1 = one transient delusional belief
   2 = delusion present, but subject questions own belief
   3 = patient convinced of delusion, but belief doesn't affect behavior
   4 = delusion affects behavior
   5 = significant actions based on delusions

18. HALLUCINATIONS.   Inquiry about visual, auditory, and tactile hallucinations. The frequency and degree of disruptiveness of hallucinations are rated.

   0 = none
   1 = very mild; hears voice saying one word; visual hallucination
        once
   2 = mild
   3 = moderate; hallucinates numerous times during day, which
        interferes with normal functioning
   4 = moderately severe
   5 = severe; nearly constant hallucinating, which totally disrupts
        normal functioning

19. PACING.   Distinguish between normal physical activity and excessive walking back and forth. Include the prior week.

    0 = none
    1 = very rare occurrence
    2 = paces for short intervals at certain times of the day
    3 = paces frequently each day
    4 = paces for the greater portion of the day, but can stop for
        activities such as meals
    5 = cannot sit still and paces excessively

20. INCREASED MOTOR ACTIVITY.   Rate in relation to the subject's normal level of motor activity or a previously obtained baseline. Include the prior week. A score of 1–2 is permissible if increased motor activity is reported by the informant but does not occur during the interview.

    0 = none
    1 = very slight increase
    2 = noticeable fidgeting and restlessness
    3 = moves frequently; fidgets very often
    4 = significant increase in movement that interferes with other
        activity
    5 = must be moving constantly; rarely sits still

21. INCREASED/DECREASED APPETITE.   Rate relative to subject's normal appetite or previously obtained baseline. Include prior week.

    0 = none
    1 = slight appetite change without weight change
    2 = appetite change with weight change, but eats without en-
        couragement
    3 = appetite and weight change with encouragement needed to eat
        OR asks for more food
    4 = moderately severe
    5 = will not eat/requires forced feeding OR complains of constant
        hunger despite adequate food intake

ALZHEIMER'S DISEASE ASSESSMENT SCALE SCORING

Subject _____   Rater _____   Date _____

COGNITIVE BEHAVIORS
1. Word recall _____   Avg. Error Score____
2. Spoken language ability _____
3. Comprehension spoken language _____
4. Recall test instructions _____
5. Word finding difficulty _____
6. Commands: 1 2 3 4 5 _____
7. Naming _____
    H: 1 2 3 4 Fingers:
    M: 1 2 3 4 T I M R P
    L: 1 2 3 4
8. Constructions   Figures: 0 1 2 3 4
9. Ideational praxis   Steps: 0 1 2 3 4 5
10. Orientation
    Day _____ Year _____ Person _____ Time of Day _____
    Date _____ Month _____ Season _____ Place _____
11. Word recognition . . . . Avg. Error Score _____

NONCOGNITIVE BEHAVIORS
12. Tremor _____   17. Delusions _____
13. Tearful _____   18. Hallucinations _____
14. Depresed mood _____   19. Pacing _____
15. Concentation _____   20. Inc motor activity _____
16. Uncooperative to testing _____   21. Inc/dec appetite _____

TOTAL SCORES
Word Recall (Item 1) . . . . _____
Word Recognition (Item 11) . . . . _____
Total Cognitive Behaviors . . . . _____
Other Cognitive Behaviors (Items 2–10) . . . . . _____
Noncognitive Behaviors (Items 12–21) . . . . . . _____
Total . . . . _____

Source. Reprinted with permission from Rosen WG, Mohs RC, Davis KL: "A New Rating Scale for Alzheimer's Disease." *American Journal of Psychiatry* 14:1356–1364, 1984.

Brief Psychiatric Rating Scale (BPRS)

	Not Present	Mild	Moderate	Severe	Not Ratable
1. SOMATIC CONCERN: Degree of concern over present bodily health. Rate the degree to which physical health is perceived as a problem by the patient, whether complaints have a realistic basis or not.	1	OCCAS. 2 3	EXAG. 4 5	PREOCC. 6 7	0
2. ANXIETY-ANXIETY STATEMENTS: Worry, fear, or overconcern for present or future. Rate solely on the basis of verbal report of patient's own subjective experiences. Do not infer anxiety from neurotic defense mechanisms.	1	WORRIED 2 3	FEARFUL 4 5	PANICKED 6 7	0
3. EMOTIONAL WITHDRAWAL: Deficiency in relating to others; seclusiveness. Rate only the degree to which the patient gives the impression of failing to be in emotional contact with other people.	1	DOESN'T INITIATE 2 3	WITHDRAWS FROM 4 5	REPELS CONTACT 6 7	0
4. CONCEPTUAL DISORGANIZATION/DISORGANIZATION IN SPEECH: Degree to which the thought processes are confused, disconnected, or disorganized. Rate on the basis of integration of the verbal products of the patient; do not rate on the basis of the patient's subjective impression of his own level of functioning.	1	VAGUE 2 3	UNCLEAR 4 5	INCOHERENT TALK 6 7	0

	Not Present	Mild	Moderate	Severe	Not Ratable
5. GUILT FEELING/GUILT STATEMENTS: Overconcern or remorse for past behavior. Rate on the basis of the patient's subjective experiences of guilt as evidenced by verbal report with appropriate affect; do not infer guilt feelings from depression, anxiety, or neurotic defenses.	1	OVER-CONCERN 2 3	PRE-OCCUPIED 4 5	DELUSIONS OF GUILT 6 7	0
6. TENSION/TENSION BEHAVIOR: Physical and motor manifestations of tension, "nervousness," and heightened activation level. Tension should be rated solely on the basis of physical signs and motor behavior and not on the basis of subjective experiences of tension reported by the patient.	1	SEEMS TENSE 2 3	RESTLESS 4 5	AGITATED 6 7	0
7. MANNERISMS AND POSTURING: Unusual and unnatural motor behavior which causes certain mental patients to stand out in a crowd of normal people. Rate only abnormality of movements; do not rate simple heightened motor activity.	1	OCCAS. 2 3	FREQUENT 4 5	PERVASIVE 6 7	0
8. GRANDIOSITY/GRANDOISE STATEMENTS: Exaggerated self-opinion, conviction of unusual ability or powers. Rate only on the basis of patient's statements about himself or self in relation to others, not on the basis of his demeanor.	1	EXPANSIVE 2 3	SPECIAL ABILITIES 4 5	DELUSIONAL STATE 6 7	0
9. DEPRESSIVE MOOD: Despondency in mood, sadness. Rate only degree of despondency; do not rate on the basis of inferences concerning depression based upon general retardation and somatic complaints.	1	SAD 2 3	DESPON-DENT 4 5	DESPAIRING 6 7	0

	Not Present	Mild	Moderate	Severe	Not Ratable
10. HOSTILITY—STATEMENTS AND BEHAVIOR: Animosity, contempt, threats, belligerence, disdain for other people. Rate solely on the basis of reported feelings and of actions of the patient toward others; do not infer hostility from neurotic defenses, anxiety, or somatic complaints.	1	ANNOYED 2 3	HOSTILE 4 5	RAGING 6 7	0
11. SUSPICIOUSNESS: Belief (delusional or otherwise) that others have now, or have had in the past, malicious or discriminatory intent toward the patient. On the basis of verbal report and behavior, rate only those suspicions currently held, whether they concern past or present circumstances.	1	SEEMS GUARDED 2 3	SAYS DOESN'T TRUST 4 5	PARANOID DELUSIONS 6 7	0
12. HALLUCINATORY BEHAVIOR/ HALLUCINATION STATEMENTS: Perceptions without normal external stimulus correspondence. Rate only those experiences which are reported to have occurred during the rating period and which are described as distinctly different from the thought and imagery process of normal people.	1	OCCAS. WITH INSIGHT 2 3	OFTEN AND NO INSIGHT 4 5	PERVASIVE 6 7	0
13. MOTOR RETARDATION/ BEHAVIOR: Reduction in energ level, evidenced in slowed movements and speech, reduced body tone, decreased number of movements. Rate on the basis of observed behavior of the patient only; do not rate on the basis of patient's subjective impression of own energy level.	1	SLOWED 2 3	RETARDED 4 5	CATATONIC 6 7	0

	Not Present	Mild	Moderate	Severe	Not Ratable
14. UNCOOPERATIVENESS: Evidences of resistance, unfriend- liness, resentment, and lack of readiness to cooperate with ward procedures and with others.	1	RESENTS 2 3	RESISTS 4 5	REFUSES 6 7	0
15. UNUSUAL THOUGHT CONTENT: Unusual, odd, strange, or bizarre thought content. Rate here the degree of unusualness, not the degree of disorganization of thought processes.	1	ODD 2 3	BIZARRE 4 5	IMPOSSIBLE 6 7	0
16. BLUNTED AFFECT: Reduced emotional tone, apparent lack of normal feeling or involvement.	1	LOWERED FEELING 2 3	FLAT 4 5	MECHANICAL 6 7	0
17. EXCITEMENT: Heightened emotional tone, increased reactivity, agitation, impulsivity.	1	INCREASED EMOTION 2 3	INTENSE 4 5	OFF THE WALL 6 7	0
18. DISORIENTATION: Confusion or lack of proper association for person, place, or time.	1	MUDDLED 2 3	CONFUSED 4 5	DISORIENTED 6 7	0
19. LOSS OF FUNCTIONING:* Rate general level of functioning.	1	MILD LOSS 2 3	MODERATE LOSS 4 5	SEVERE LOSS 6 7	0

*Item 19 is a global scale that is not added in with the other items. Items 1 to 18 are added together to give the total score.
Source.   Reprinted with permission from Overall JE, Gorham DR: "The Brief Psychiatric Rating Scale." *Psychological Reports* 10:799–812, 1962.

CERAD Behavior Rating Scale for Dementia (BRSD)

Circle one response for each item, using following rating scale:

0 = Has not occurred since illness began;

1 = 1–2 days in past month (up to twice per week)

2 = 3–8 days in past month

3 = 9–15 days in past month (up to half the days in the past month, but not in past month)

4 = 16 days or more in past month)

8 = Occurred since illness began

9 = Unable to rate

[S] = Subject

Enter all descriptive information on the last page, with the correct question number for each response.

RATING SCALE

1. Has [S] **said** that [S] feels anxious, worried, tense or fearful? (For example, has [S] expressed worry or fear about being left alone? Has [S] said [S] is anxious or afraid of certain situations?) *If so, describe.*　0　8　1　2　9　3　4

2. Has [S] shown **physical signs** of anxiety, worry, tension or fear? (For example, is [S] easily startled? Does [S] appear nervous? Does [S] have a tense or worried facial expression?) *If so, describe.*　0　8　1　2　9　3　4

3. Has [S] appeared sad or blue or depressed?　0　8　1　2　9　3　4

Source. Reprinted with permission from Consortium to Establish a Registry for Alzheimer's Disease.

4. Has [S] expressed feelings of hopelessness
   or pessimism?   0   8   1   2
                                                         9   3   4

5. Has [S] cried within the past month?   0   8   1   2
                                                         9   3   4

6. Has [S] said that [S] feels guilty? (For
   example, has [S] blamed [S]'s self for
   things [S] did in the past?) *If yes,*
   describe nature and extent of guilt.   0   8   1   2
                                                         9   3   4

7. Has [S] expressed feelings of poor
   self-esteem? For example, has [S] said
   that [S] feels like a failure or that [S] feels
   worthless? *This item is intended to reflect*
   global loss of self-esteem rather than simply
   a concern over loss of, for example, a particular
   ability.   0   8   1   2
                                                         9   3   4

8. Has [S] said [S] feels life is not worth living?
   Or has [S] expressed a wish to die or talked
   about committing suicide? *If yes, specify*
   what subject said.   0   8   1   2
                                                         9   3   4

9. Has [S] made any suicide attempts?
   Include any suicidal gestures in rating this item. 0 8   1   2
                                                         9   3   4

10. Have there been times when [S] doesn't
    enjoy the things [S] does as much as [S]
    used to? *This item refers to any specific loss*
    of enjoyment so long as [S] actually engages
    in the activity in question. [S] need not be an
    active participant in this activity; [S] need
    only be present.   0 = No   8
                                                    1 = Yes   9

11. Do you find [S] sometimes can't seem to
    get started on things [S] used to do, even
    though [S] is capable of doing them? (For

example, do you find [S] won't start a task
or pastime on [S]'s own, but with a little
encouragement [S] goes ahead and carries
it out?) *This item refers to any failure to
initiate activities, so long as the activities
are those which S is still capable of carrying
out when given the opportunity.*

0 = No	8
1 = Yes	9

12. Has [S] seemed tired or lacking in energy?

0	8	1	2
	9	3	4

13. Has [S] had physical complaints that
seemed out of proportion to [S]'s actual
physical problems?

0	8	1	2
	9	3	4

14. Was [S]'s sleeping pattern in the past month
different from the way it was before [S]'s
dementia began? (For example, does [S]
sleep more or less than [S] used to? Does [S]
sleep at a different time of day than [S] used
to?) If yes, describe change.

0 = No	8
1 = Yes	9

15. Has [S] had difficulty falling asleep or
remaining asleep? *If yes, describe.*

0	8	1	2
	9	3	4

16. Has [S]'s appetite during the past month
changed from the way it was before [S]'s
dementia began? (For example, at meal times
does [S]'s desire to eat seem different?)
*"Appetite" refers to [S]'s response to food when
it is presented in the usual manner.*

0 = No	8
1 = Yes	9

*If yes, circle either increased or decreased
appetite according to informant's judgment.*

1 Increased
2 Decreased

17. In the past month, has [S] gained or lost
weight without intending to?

0 = No	8
1 = Yes	9

If yes, circle amount gained or lost.   Gained: 1   Up to 5 lbs
                                                     2   More than 5 lbs
                                            Lost: 1   Up to 5 lbs
                                                     2   More than 5 lbs

18. In the past month, has [S]'s sexual interest
    been different from the way it was before
    [S]'s dementia began? *If yes, describe.*   0 = No   8
                                                     1 = Yes   9

19. Has [S] shown sudden changes in [S]'s
    emotions? (For example, does [S] go from
    laughter to tears quickly?)   0   8   1   2
                                                           9   3   4

20. Have there been times when [S] was
    agitated or upset? *This item refers to observable
    signs of emotional distress, such as verbal
    comments, facial expressions, or gestures. It is
    the* **emotional component** *that distinguishes
    this item from item 21.*   0   8   1   2
                                                           9   3   4

21. Has [S] seemed restless or overactive? (For
    example, does [S] fidget or pace? Does [S]
    finger things or seem unable to sit still?)
    *When the overactive behavior is associated with
    emotional agitation that is rated in item 20, it
    should not be rated here also.*   0   8   1   2
                                                           9   3   4

22. Has [S] done things that seem to have no
    clear purpose or a confused purpose? (For
    example, does [S] open and close drawers?
    Does [S] put things in inappropriate places?
    Does [S] hoard things or rummage through
    things?) *If S's behavior shows a high level of
    motor activity rather than confusion or lack of
    purpose, it should be rated under item 21.*   0   8   1   2
                                                           9   3   4

23. Does [S] tend to say the same things
    repeatedly? *This item refers to repetitive
    statements, including questions, phrases,
    demands, etc.*   0   8   1   2
                                                           9   3   4

24. Has there been a particular time of day
    during which [S] seemed more confused
    than at other times?   0 = No   8
                                                 1 = Yes   9

If yes, circle time of day.   1   Daytime
                                  2   Evening—6:00 P.M. to bedtime
                                  3   Night

25. Has [S] done socially inappropriate things?
    (For example, does [S] make vulgar remarks?
    Does [S] talk excessively to strangers? Has
    [S] sexually exposed [S]'s self or done other
    things such as making gestures or touching
    people inappropriately?) *This item is intended
    to reflect a loss of propriety, not simply confusion.
    If inappropriate behavior can be rated under a
    more specific item, such as abusive behavior
    (item 30) or aggressive behavior (item 31),
    it should not be rated here.*   0   8   1   2
                                                           9   3   4

26. Has [S] wandered or tried to wander for
    no apparent reason? *"Wandering" includes
    wandering away from one's residence or care-
    giver, as well as within the residence. If yes,
    describe incidents.*   0   8   1   2
                                                           9   3   4

27. Has [S] tried to leave home or get away from
    whoever was taking care of [S] *with* an
    apparent purpose or destination in mind?
    If yes, describe incidents.   0   8   1   2
                                                           9   3   4

28. Have there been times when [S] was easily
    irritated or annoyed?   0   8   1   2
                                                           9   3   4

29. Has [S] been uncooperative? (For example,
does [S] refuse to accept appropriate help?
Does [S] insist on doing things [S]'s
own way?)   0   8   1   2
                                                         9   3   4

30. Has [S] been threatening or verbally
abusive toward others?   0   8   1   2
                                                         9   3   4

31. Has [S] been physically aggressive toward
people or things? (For example, has [S]
shoved or physically attacked people or
thrown or broken objects?)   0   8   1   2
                                                         9   3   4

32. Has [S] harmed [S]'s self in a way that was
not an accident or a suicide attempt? (For
example, does [S] bang [S]'s head or scratch
[S]'s self badly? *If yes, describe. This item is
intended to rate self-abusive behavior.*   0   8   1   2
                                                         9   3   4

33. Does [S] withdraw from social situations?
(For example, does [S] avoid groups of
people or prefer to be alone? Does [S]
avoid participating in activities with
others?)   0   8   1   2
                                                         9   3   4

34. Does [S] seek out more visual or physical
contact with [S]'s caregivers than before [S]'s
dementia began? (For example, has [S] seemed
"clingy"? Does [S] follow you about or seem
to want to be in the same room with you?)   0 = No   8
                                             1 = Yes   9

35. Has [S] done or said anything that suggests [S] believes people are harming, threatening, or taking advantage of [S] in some way? (For example, with no good reason has [S] thought things have been given away or stolen; has [S] thought [S] was mischarged or overcharged for purchases; has [S] seemed suspicious or wary?)

	0	8	1	2
		9	3	4

If yes, ask: If you try to correct [S], will [S] accept the truth?

0 No
1 Yes
9 N/A

36. Has [S] done or said anything that suggests [S] thinks [S's spouse] is unfaithful?

	0	8	1	2
		9	3	4

If yes, ask: If you try to correct [S], will [S] accept the truth?

0 No
1 Yes
9 N/A

37. Has [S] done or said anything that suggests [S] thinks [S's spouse or caregiver] is plotting to abandon [S]?

	0	8	1	2
		9	3	4

If yes, ask: If you try to correct [S], will [S] accept the truth?

0 No
1 Yes
9 N/A

38. Has [S] done or said anything that suggests [S] thinks [S's spouse or caregiver] is an impostor?

	0	8	1	2
		9	3	4

If yes, ask: If you try to correct [S], will [S] accept the truth?

0 No
1 Yes
9 N/A

39. Has [S] done or said anything that suggests
    [S] thinks that characters on television
    are real? (For example, has [S] talked to them,
    acted as if they could hear or see [S], or
    said that they were friends or neighbors?)   0   8   1   2
                                                        9   3   4

If yes, ask: If you try to correct [S], will [S]
    accept the truth?   0   No
                                                 1   Yes
                                                 9   N/A

40. Has [S] done or said anything that suggests
    [S] believes that there are people in or
    around the house beyond those who are
    actually there?   0   8   1   2
                                                        9   3   4

If yes, ask: If you try to correct [S], will [S]
    accept the truth?   0 No
                                                 1 Yes
                                                 9 N/A

41. Has [S] done or said anything that suggests
    that [S] believes that a dead person is still
    alive even though [S] used to know they
    were dead? *Do not rate memory problems.*
    If [S] simply cannot remember whether a
    particular person has died, it should not be
    rated as a mistaken belief.   0   8   1   2
                                                        9   3   4

If yes, ask: If you try to correct [S], will [S]
    accept the truth?   0 No
                                                 1 Yes
                                                 9 N/A

42. Has [S] done or said anything that
    suggests [S] thinks where [S] lives is not
    really [S]'s home, even though [S] used
    to consider it home?   0   8   1   2
                                                        9   3   4

If yes, ask: If you try to correct [S], will [S]
accept the truth?

0 No
1 Yes
9 N/A

43. Has [S] misidentified people? (For example,
has [S] confused one familiar person with
another, or has [S] thought that a familiar
person was a stranger?) *"Misidentification"*
means an actual belief that one person was
another, not simply a misnaming or failure
to remember who someone is, and it refers
to someone actually seen by S.

0	8	1	2
	9	3	4

44. Has [S] looked at [S]'s self in a mirror and
not recognized [S]'s self?

0	8	1	2
	9	3	4

45. Has [S] misidentified things? Has [S]
thought common things were something
else? (For example, has [S] looked at a pillow
and thought it was a person or said that a
lightbulb was a fire?) *If yes, describe.*

0	8	1	2
	9	3	4

46. Has [S] heard voices or sounds when there
was no sound? *If yes, describe.*

0	8	1	2
	9	3	4

If yes, rate for clarity. Vague 0   Clear 1

47. Has [S] seen things or people that were
not there? *If yes, describe.*

0	8	1	2
	9	3	4

If yes, rate for clarity. Vague 0   Clear 1

48. Before we stop, I want to be sure we've
     covered all of [S]'s problems, except, of
     course, for [S]'s memory problems. Has
     [S] done anything else in the past month
     that has seemed strange or been a problem?
     Has [S] said anything that suggests [S]
     has some unusual ideas or beliefs that I
     haven't asked you about? *If response*
     concerns purely cognitive symptoms, do
     not rate. If response concerns behaviors that
     can be rated under other items, do so. Any
     behavior that is rated here should be described.
     Indicate the most frequently occurring
     problem and rate it.   0   8   1   2
                                                    9   3   4

QUALITY OF INTERVIEW (RATER'S JUDGMENT)

Interview appeared valid.   0

Some questions about validity of interview,
but it is probably acceptable.   1

Information from interview is of doubtful validity.   2

Rater should record the basis for judging the interview of questionable or doubt-
ful validity.

Comments:

RESPONSE CARD

How often has it happened?

Only 1 or 2 days in past month
3 to 8 days in past month (up to twice per week)
9 to 15 days in past month (up to half the days in the month)
More than 15 days in past month (more than half the days in the month)

Cohen-Mansfield Agitation Inventory (CMAI)

Say to the Informant: *"I would like to ask you about certain specific behaviors sometimes seen in older persons. Some are verbal. Some are physical. Some are quiet behaviors and others are disruptive. I do not expect that all of these behaviors will apply to your relative (patient). I will read you a description of the 36 behaviors on this list. I will want to know how often the behavior occurred in the past two weeks. I have given you a card with a list of the behaviors I will be asking you about. I would like you to indicate the frequency of each behavior on the card."* (see behavior list)

"The frequencies listed on the card are:"

- Never
- Less than once a week but still occurring
- Once or twice a week
- Several times a week (3 or more)
- Once or twice a day
- Several times a day (3 or more)
- Several times an hour (2 or more)
- Not applicable

1. During the past two weeks, how often did [S] repeat sentences or questions? (was repetitive, whether or not addressed to any particular person)

☐ Never ☐ Less than once a week ☐ Once or twice a week ☐ Several times a week ☐ Once or twice a day ☐ Several times a day ☐ Several times an hour ☐ Not applicable

2. During the past two weeks, how often did [S] verbally interrupt or cut short others' interactions or conversations by saying something that was *relevant* to the conversation or ongoing activity?

☐ Never ☐ Less than once a week ☐ Once or twice a week ☐ Several times a week ☐ Once or twice a day ☐ Several times a day ☐ Several times an hour ☐ Not applicable

3. During the past two weeks, how often did [S] verbally interrupt or cut short others' interactions or conversations by saying something that was *not relevant* to the conversation or ongoing activity?

☐ Never ☐ Less ☐ Once or ☐ Several ☐ Once or ☐ Several ☐ Several ☐ Not
than once twice times twice times times appli-
a week a week a week a day a day an hour cable

4. During the past two weeks, how often did [S] make strange noises, including strange laughter, moaning, or crying?

☐ Never ☐ Less ☐ Once or ☐ Several ☐ Once or ☐ Several ☐ Several ☐ Not
than once twice times twice times times appli-
a week a week a week a day a day an hour cable

5. During the past two weeks, how often did [S] scream, shout, or howl?

☐ Never ☐ Less ☐ Once or ☐ Several ☐ Once or ☐ Several ☐ Several ☐ Not
than once twice times twice times times appli-
a week a week a week a day a day an hour cable

6. During the past two weeks, how often did [S] complain or whine?

☐ Never ☐ Less ☐ Once or ☐ Several ☐ Once or ☐ Several ☐ Several ☐ Not
than once twice times twice times times appli-
a week a week a week a day a day an hour cable

7. During the past two weeks, how often did [S] make unwarranted requests for attention or help? (includes nagging, pleading, calling out)

☐ Never ☐ Less ☐ Once or ☐ Several ☐ Once or ☐ Several ☐ Several ☐ Not
than once twice times twice times times appli-
a week a week a week a day a day an hour cable

8. During the past two weeks, how often was [S] negative, uncoop-erative or unwilling to participate in activities? (bad attitude, doesn't like anything, nothing is right; includes social activities, eat-ing, bathing)

☐ Never ☐ Less ☐ Once or ☐ Several ☐ Once or ☐ Several ☐ Several ☐ Not
than once twice times twice times times appli-
a week a week a week a day a day an hour cable

9. During the past two weeks, how often did [S] curse or was [S] verbally threatening or insulting? (verbal aggression; score only if intelligible words were used; otherwise score under item 5)

☐ Never ☐ Less ☐ Once or ☐ Several ☐ Once or ☐ Several ☐ Several ☐ Not
          than once   twice   times   twice   times   times   appli-
          a week   a week   a week   a day   a day   an hour   cable

10. During the past two weeks, how often did [S] spit (including during meals)? (does not include involuntary salivation or drooling)

☐ Never ☐ Less ☐ Once or ☐ Several ☐ Once or ☐ Several ☐ Several ☐ Not
          than once   twice   times   twice   times   times   appli-
          a week   a week   a week   a day   a day   an hour   cable

11. During the past two weeks, how often was [S] verbally bossy or pushy?

☐ Never ☐ Less ☐ Once or ☐ Several ☐ Once or ☐ Several ☐ Several ☐ Not
          than once   twice   times   twice   times   times   appli-
          a week   a week   a week   a day   a day   an hour   cable

12. During the past two weeks, how often did [S] make verbal sexual advances? (includes direct sexual propositioning or obvious sexual hints)

☐ Never ☐ Less ☐ Once or ☐ Several ☐ Once or ☐ Several ☐ Several ☐ Not
          than once   twice   times   twice   times   times   appli-
          a week   a week   a week   a day   a day   an hour   cable

13. During the past two weeks, how often did [S] make physical sexual advances or expose his/her sexual parts? (includes inappropriate sexual touching of self or others)

☐ Never ☐ Less ☐ Once or ☐ Several ☐ Once or ☐ Several ☐ Several ☐ Not
          than once   twice   times   twice   times   times   appli-
          a week   a week   a week   a day   a day   an hour   cable

14. During the past two weeks, how often was [S] restless or fidgety, tending to move around when in a seat, or repeatedly getting up and sitting down? (couldn't sit still)

☐ Never ☐ Less ☐ Once or ☐ Several ☐ Once or ☐ Several ☐ Several ☐ Not
          than once   twice   times   twice   times   times   appli-
          a week   a week   a week   a day   a day   an hour   cable

15. During the past two weeks, how often did [S] pace, walk repeatedly back and forth, or wander aimlessly? (includes wandering when done in a wheelchair)

☐ Never ☐ Less ☐ Once or ☐ Several ☐ Once or ☐ Several ☐ Several ☐ Not
than once twice times twice times times appli-
a week a week a week a day a day an hour cable

16. During the past two weeks, how often did [S] try to get out of doors inappropriately, sneak out, or inappropriately enter other places?

☐ Never ☐ Less ☐ Once or ☐ Several ☐ Once or ☐ Several ☐ Several ☐ Not
than once twice times twice times times appli-
a week a week a week a day a day an hour cable

17. During the past two weeks, how often did [S] dress or undress inappropriately? (such as undressing in public or repeatedly dressing and undressing; does *not* refer to inability to get dressed. If only sexual parts are exposed, rate on item 13)

☐ Never ☐ Less ☐ Once or ☐ Several ☐ Once or ☐ Several ☐ Several ☐ Not
than once twice times twice times times appli-
a week a week a week a day a day an hour cable

18. During the past two weeks, how often did [S] perform repetitious mannerisms? (includes rocking, rubbing, tapping, picking at skin)

☐ Never ☐ Less ☐ Once or ☐ Several ☐ Once or ☐ Several ☐ Several ☐ Not
than once twice times twice times times appli-
a week a week a week a day a day an hour cable

19. During the past two weeks, how often did [S] handle things inappropriately? (rummaging through drawers, picking up others' possessions or things that should not be touched)

☐ Never ☐ Less ☐ Once or ☐ Several ☐ Once or ☐ Several ☐ Several ☐ Not
than once twice times twice times times appli-
a week a week a week a day a day an hour cable

20. During the past two weeks, how often did [S] grab or snatch things from others? (including food from others' plates)

☐ Never ☐ Less ☐ Once or ☐ Several ☐ Once or ☐ Several ☐ Several ☐ Not
than once twice times twice times times appli-
a week a week a week a day a day an hour cable

21. During the past two weeks, how often did [S] hoard or collect objects?

☐ Never ☐ Less than once a week ☐ Once or twice a week ☐ Several times a week ☐ Once or twice a day ☐ Several times a day ☐ Several times an hour ☐ Not applicable

22. During the past two weeks, how often did [S] hide objects?

☐ Never ☐ Less than once a week ☐ Once or twice a week ☐ Several times a week ☐ Once or twice a day ☐ Several times a day ☐ Several times an hour ☐ Not applicable

23 During the past two weeks, how often did [S] exhibit strange movements, such as making faces (frowning or grimacing) inappropriately, or moving arms and legs aimlessly?

☐ Never ☐ Less than once a week ☐ Once or twice a week ☐ Several times a week ☐ Once or twice a day ☐ Several times a day ☐ Several times an hour ☐ Not applicable

24. During the past two weeks, how often did [S] have a temper outburst, including verbal or nonverbal expressions of anger?

☐ Never ☐ Less than once a week ☐ Once or twice a week ☐ Several times a week ☐ Once or twice a day ☐ Several times a day ☐ Several times an hour ☐ Not applicable

25. During the past two weeks, how often did [S] hit people, self or objects?

☐ Never ☐ Less than once a week ☐ Once or twice a week ☐ Several times a week ☐ Once or twice a day ☐ Several times a day ☐ Several times an hour ☐ Not applicable

26. During the past two weeks, how often did [S] kick people or objects?

☐ Never ☐ Less than once a week ☐ Once or twice a week ☐ Several times a week ☐ Once or twice a day ☐ Several times a day ☐ Several times an hour ☐ Not applicable

27. During the past two weeks, how often did [S] throw things (such as food) or knock objects off surfaces?

☐ Never ☐ Less than once a week ☐ Once or twice a week ☐ Several times a week ☐ Once or twice a day ☐ Several times a day ☐ Several times an hour ☐ Not applicable

28. During the past two weeks, how often did [S] tear or destroy objects or property?

☐ Never ☐ Less than once a week ☐ Once or twice a week ☐ Several times a week ☐ Once or twice a day ☐ Several times a day ☐ Several times an hour ☐ Not applicable

29. During the past two weeks, how often did [S] grab on to or cling to people physically?

☐ Never ☐ Less than once a week ☐ Once or twice a week ☐ Several times a week ☐ Once or twice a day ☐ Several times a day ☐ Several times an hour ☐ Not applicable

30. During the past two weeks, how often did [S] push other people?

☐ Never ☐ Less than once a week ☐ Once or twice a week ☐ Several times a week ☐ Once or twice a day ☐ Several times a day ☐ Several times an hour ☐ Not applicable

31. During the past two weeks, how often did [S] bite people or things?

☐ Never ☐ Less than once a week ☐ Once or twice a week ☐ Several times a week ☐ Once or twice a day ☐ Several times a day ☐ Several times an hour ☐ Not applicable

32. During the past two weeks, how often did [S] scratch people, self, or things?

☐ Never ☐ Less than once a week ☐ Once or twice a week ☐ Several times a week ☐ Once or twice a day ☐ Several times a day ☐ Several times an hour ☐ Not applicable

33. During the past two weeks, how often did [S] hurt him/herself by using a harmful object? (cutting, burning or by other means)

☐ Never ☐ Less than once a week ☐ Once or twice a week ☐ Several times a week ☐ Once or twice a day ☐ Several times a day ☐ Several times an hour ☐ Not applicable

34. During the past two weeks, how often did [S] hurt others by using a harmful object? (cutting, burning or by other means)

☐ Never ☐ Less than once a week ☐ Once or twice a week ☐ Several times a week ☐ Once or twice a day ☐ Several times a day ☐ Several times an hour ☐ Not applicable

35. During the past two weeks, how often did [S] appear to fall intentionally? (includes from bed or wheelchair)

☐ Never ☐ Less ☐ Once or ☐ Several ☐ Once or ☐ Several ☐ Several ☐ Not
    than once   twice   times   twice   times   times   appli-
    a week   a week   a week   a day   a day   an hour   cable

36. During the past two weeks, how often did [S] attempt to or did [S] actually eat or drink nonfood substances?

☐ Never ☐ Less ☐ Once or ☐ Several ☐ Once or ☐ Several ☐ Several ☐ Not
    than once   twice   times   twice   times   times   appli-
    a week   a week   a week   a day   a day   an hour   cable

37. During the past two weeks, did [S] engage in any other inappropriate behavior?

☐ Never ☐ Less ☐ Once or ☐ Several ☐ Once or ☐ Several ☐ Several ☐ Not
    than once   twice   times   twice   times   times   appli-
    a week   a week   a week   a day   a day   an hour   cable

If yes, please describe: _____

_____

_____

_____

_____

38. Did agitated behavior(s) occur most often:
    ☐ Morning
    ☐ Afternoon
    ☐ Evening
    ☐ No time more than others
    ☐ Different times for different behaviors

Cohen-Mansfield Agitation Inventory Behavior List

*Please indicate the
frequency of each behavior:*

- Never
- Less than once a week but still occurring
- Once or twice a week
- Several times a week (3 or more)
- Once or twice a day
- Several times a day (3 or more)
- Several times an hour (2 or more)
- Not applicable (unable to do)

1. Repeats sentences or questions (was **repetitive,** whether or not addressed to any particular person)?

2. Verbally **interrupts** or cuts short others' interactions or conversations saying something that was *relevant*?

3. Verbally interrupts or cuts short others' interactions or conversations saying something that was *not relevant*?

4. Makes **strange noises,** including strange laughter, moaning, or crying?

5. **Screams,** shouts, or howls?

6. **Complains** or whines?

7. Makes unwarranted **requests for attention** or help?

8. **Negative,** uncooperative, or unwilling to participate in activities?

9. **Cursing, verbally threatening,** or **insulting?**

10. **Spits** (including during meals)?

11. **Verbally bossy** or **pushy?**

12. Makes **verbal sexual advances?**

13. Makes **physical sexual advances?**

14. **Restless** or fidgety, or tends to move around when in a seat or repeatedly gets up and sits down?

15. **Paces,** walks repeatedly back and forth, or **wanders** aimlessly?

16. Tries to **get out** of doors inappropriately, sneaks out or **inappropriately enters other places?**

17. **Dresses** or **undresses** inappropriately?

18. Performs **repetitive mannerisms?**

19. **Handles things** inappropriately?

20. **Grabs** or **snatches things** from others?

21. **Hoards** or collects objects?

22. **Hides** objects?

23. Exhibits **strange movements?**

24. Has **temper outbursts?**

25. **Hits** people, self, or objects?

26. **Kicks** people or objects?

27. **Throws things** such as food or knocks objects off surfaces?

28. **Tears** or **destroys objects** or property?

29. **Grabs on to** or **clings to people** physically?

30. **Pushes** other persons?

31. **Bites** people or things?

32. **Scratches** people or things?

33. **Hurts him/herself** by using a **harmful object** (cutting, burning, or by other means)?

34. **Hurts others** by using a **harmful object** (cutting, burning, or by other means)?

35. **Falls intentionally?**

36. **Eats** or **drinks nonfood substances?**

37. Engages in **any other inappropriate behavior?**

Abnormal Involuntary Movement Scale (AIMS)

Before conducting the formal examination below, observe patients unobtrusively at rest in a hard, firm, armless chair. Then ask the following questions or make the following requests:

1. "Is there anything in your mouth such as gum or candy? If so, please remove it."

2. "How are your teeth?" "Do you wear dentures?" "Do your teeth or dentures bother you?"

3. "Do you notice any movements in your mouth, face, hands, or feet? If so, describe them." "How much do they bother you at present, and how much do they interfere with your activities?"

4. "Please sit with your hands on your knees, legs slightly apart and feet flat on the floor." (Observe for large body movements)

5. "Please let your hands to hang down between your legs" or (if wearing a dress) "Let your hands hang over your knees." (Observe hands and other body areas)

6. "Please open your mouth." (Do twice, observing tongue at rest)

7. "Please stick out your tongue." (Do twice, noting abnormalities of tongue movement)

8. "Tap your thumb with each finger of the same hand as fast as you can." (Do 15 seconds for each finger of both hands, one hand at a time. Observe face and leg movements)

9. "Please stand up." (Observe all body areas, including hips, in profile)

10. "Please stretch your arms out in front of you with your palms down." (Observe trunk, legs, and mouth)

11. "Please walk a few steps, turn, and walk back to the chair." (Do twice, observing hands and gait)

Circle the highest severity noted. 0 = none; 1 = minimal; 2 = mild; 3 = moderate; 4 = severe.

1.	Muscles of facial expression (frowning, blinking, grimacing)	0	1	2	3	4
2.	Lips and perioral area (puckering, pouting, smacking)	0	1	2	3	4
3.	Jaw (chewing, clenching, mouth opening, lateral motion)	0	1	2	3	4
4.	Tongue	0	1	2	3	4
5.	Upper extremities (choreic [rapid, purposeless, spontaneous, irregular] and athetoid [slow, irregular, complex, serpentine] movements only)	0	1	2	3	4
6.	Lower extremities	0	1	2	3	4
7.	Trunk (squirming, rocking, twisting)	0	1	2	3	4
8.	Global severity of abnormal movements	0	1	2	3	4
9.	Incapacity from abnormal movements	0	1	2	3	4
10.	Patient's awareness of abnormal movements	0	1	2	3	4

10. 0 = none; 1 = aware, no distress; 2 = aware, mild distress; 3 = aware, moderate distress; 4 = aware, severe distress

11. Current problem with teeth or dentures?   No 0 Yes 1

Source.   Adapted from Guy 1976.

Resources

NATIONAL AGENCIES

Alzheimer's Disease Education and Referral (ADEAR)
1-800-438-4380

This agency is contracted through the National Institute on Aging. ADEAR maintains an online database and functions as a clearinghouse for publications and information on Alzheimer's disease. It has publications from the federally funded Alzheimer's Disease Centers and other sources.

Elderlink
217-785-3356 or 1-800-252-8966 (Illinois only)

A national telephone information and referral program for elderly people sponsored by the National Association of State Units on Aging. Primary objective is to assist long-distance caregivers in locating services for a relative or friend.

Alzheimer's Association (National Office)
70 East Lake Street
Chicago IL 60601-5997
1-800-621-0379 or 1-800-272-3900
(Illinois only, 1-800-572-6037)

A privately funded national voluntary organization with chapters nationwide. The national office can be contacted for information on many issues regarding Alzheimer's disease, as well as referral to the nearest local chapter.

National Association of Private Geriatric Care Managers
602-881-8008 (call for care managers in your area)

Private Case Managers are certified to provide an array of assessment and social services ranging from obtaining in-home health help to linking with financial, legal, and other long-term care services.

National Council on the Aging, Inc.
202-479-1200

Provides various brochures on care and resources for older adults. Publishes the *Directory of Adult Day Care in America*, which includes a listing of state adult day-care associations.

National Health Information Center
P.O. Box 133
Washington, DC 20013-1133
1-800-336-4797

Healthfinder series provides a starting point for consumers and health professionals looking for information on home health care. Currently available books and additional organizations that can provide further information are cited. Financial issues and how to find home health care providers are discussed.

National Stroke Association (NSA)
8480 East Orchard Road
Suite 1000
Englewood, CO 80111-5015
303-771-1700 or 1-800-787-6537

A nonprofit organization whose mission is to reduce the incidence and impact of stroke on individuals and on society. It supports stroke research in all areas, develops and distributes educational materials, and is an information and referral clearinghouse.

Huntington's Disease Society of America (HDSA)
140 W. 22nd Street
New York, NY 10011
1-800-345-4372 or 212-242-1968

A national voluntary organization providing support and services to patients and families. HDSA also supports research and education and disseminates information. There is also a network of local chapters across the United States.

National Head Injury Foundation (NHIF)
333 Turnpike Road
Southborough, MA 01772
1-800-444-6443

An advocacy organization whose mission is to improve the quality of life for persons with head injuries and their families, and to develop programs to prevent head injuries. To fulfill its mission, the NHIF focuses its efforts on education, support and information, public awareness, prevention, research, and training.

National Organization of Rare Disorders (NORD)
100 Route 37
P.O. Box 8923
New Fairfield, CT 06812-8923
203-746-6927

A federation of voluntary health organizations dedicated to helping people with rare "orphan" diseases. NORD is a clearinghouse for information and is committed to the identification, treatment, and cure of rare disorders through programs of education, advocacy, research, and service.

National Parkinson Foundation (NPF)
1501 NW 9th Avenue
Miami, FL 33136
1-800-327-4545 (in Florida, 1-800-433-7022)

Provides educational services and information in the form of support groups, publications, and workshops. NPF also supports Parkinson's disease research.

United Parkinson Foundation (UPF)
833 W. Washington Boulevard
Chicago, IL 60607
312-733-1893

UPF supports research and provides educational services and information.

The American Parkinson Disease Association, Inc.
60 Bay Street Suite 401
Staten Island, NY 10301
1-800-223-2732

APDA supports research and produces educational materials including a newsletter and various pamphlets covering issues such as nutrition in Parkinson's disease and mobility aids.

United Seniors Health Cooperative
202-393-6222

A private nonprofit organization furnishing members with information and assistance in obtaining services and negotiates for discounts and special services. Computerized "Benefits Outreach and Screening Service," which identifies a person's potential eligibility for more than 50 federal, state, and local funding programs. Annual Fee.

STATE AGENCIES

State Department on Aging

(See state governmental listings in local telephone directories.)

These agencies in each state funnel federal dollars to local area agencies on aging for disbursement to community agency services and programs for elders. Some programs may be dementia specific. This agency is a good entry point for information and referral for aging services.

State Department of Human Services

Provides linkage to state-administered and subsidized programs including community care and adult day care, elder abuse and neglect programs, nursing home, and other residential care programs under Title XX.

State Alzheimer's Programs

Several states have Alzheimer's programs that provide a variety of services including information and referral. These states include California, Connecticut, Delaware, Florida, Kansas, Massachusetts, Missouri, New Hampshire, New Jersey, New York, North Carolina, Pennsylvania, Texas, and Wisconsin.

Nursing Home Ombudsman Programs

Information available regarding quality of care in nursing homes, lists of nursing homes, checklists, etc. Contact the nearest Area Agency on Aging for information on the ombudsman program in your area.

References

Abernethy DR: Psychotropic drugs and the aging process: pharmacokinetics and pharmacodynamics, in Clinical Geriatric Psychopharmacology, 2nd Edition. Edited by Salzman C. Baltimore, MD, Williams & Wilkins, 1992, pp 61–76

Adams RD, Victor M: Principles of Neurology, 4th Edition. New York, McGraw-Hill, 1989

Adams RD, Victor M, Mancall EL: Central pontine myelinolysis. Archives of Neurology and Psychiatry 81:154–172, 1959

Adams RD, Fisher CM, Hakim S, et al: Symptomatic occult hydrocephalus with "normal" cerebrospinal fluid pressure: a treatable syndrome. N Engl J Med 273:117–126, 1965

Adem A: Putative mechanisms of action of tacrine in Alzheimer's disease. Acta Neurol Scand 139:69–74, 1992

Agency for Health Care Policy and Research: Urinary Incontinence in Adults: Clinical Practice Guidelines. Rockville, MD, U.S. Department of Health and Human Services, 1992

Aisen PS, Davis KL: Inflammatory mechanisms in Alzheimer's disease: implications for therapy. Am J Psychiatry 151:1105–1113, 1994

Ajmani A, Habte-Gabr E, Zarr M, et al: Cerebral blood flow SPECT with Tc-99m exametazine correlates in AIDS dementia complex stages: a preliminary report. Clin Nucl Med 16:656–659, 1991

Akiyama H, Harrop R, McGeer PL, et al: Crossed cerebellar and uncrossed basal ganglia and thalamic diaschisis in Alzheimer's disease. Neurology 39:541–548, 1989

Alarcon R, Franceschini J: Hyperparathyroidism and paranoid psychoses. Br J Psychiatry 145:477–486, 1984

Albert ML, Feldman RG, Willis AL: The "subcortical dementia" of progressive supranuclear palsy. J Neurol Neurosurg Psychiatry 37:121–130, 1974

Albert MS: Cognitive function, in Geriatric Neuropsychology. Edited by Albert MS, Moss MB. New York, Guilford, 1988, pp 33–53

Albert MS, Heaton RK: Intelligence testing, in Geriatric Neuropsychology. Edited by Albert MS, Moss MB. New York, Guilford, 1988, pp 13–32

Albert MS, Moss MB: Geriatric Neuropsychology. Edited by Albert MS, Moss MB. New York, Guilford, 1988

Alexopoulos GS, Meyers BS, Young RC: The course of geriatric depression with "reversible dementia": a controlled study. Am J Psychiatry 150:1693–1699, 1993

Altshuler L: Bipolar disorder: are repeated episodes associated with neuroanatomic and cognitive changes? Biol Psychiatry 33:563–565, 1993

Altshuler L, Conrad A, Kovelman JA, et al: Hippocampal pyramidal cell orientation in schizophrenia. Arch Gen Psychiatry 44:1094–1098, 1987

Alvarez WC: Little Strokes. New York, Lippincott, 1966

Alvir JMJ, Lieberman JA, Safferman AZ, et al: Clozapine-induced agranulocytosis: incidence and risk factors in the United States. N Engl J Med 329:162–167, 1993

Alzheimer A: Uber eine eigenartige Erkrankung der Hirnrinde. Allgemeine Zeitschrift fur Psychiatr 64:146–148, 1907

Amaducci L, the SMID group: Phosphatidylserine in the treatment of Alzheimer's disease: results of a multicenter study. Psychopharmacol Bull 24:130–134, 1988

Amano T, Meyer JS: Prostaglandin utilization and cerebrovascular control in patients with headache. Headache 22:52–59, 1978

American Academy of Neurology AIDS Task Force: Nomenclature and case definitions for neurologic manifestations of human immunodeficiency virus-type 1 (HIV-1) infection. Neurology 41:778–785, 1991

American Bar Association Commission on the Mentally Disabled: Exercising Judgment for the Disabled: Report of an Inquiry Into Limited Guardianship. Washington, DC, American Bar Association, 1979

American Psychiatric Association: Diagnostic and Statistical Manual: Mental Disorders. Washington, DC, American Psychiatric Association, 1952

American Psychiatric Association: Diagnostic and Statistical Manual of Mental Disorders, 3rd Edition, Revised. Washington, DC, American Psychiatric Association, 1987

American Psychiatric Association: Tardive Dyskinesia: A Task Force Report. Washington, DC, American Psychiatric Association, 1992

American Psychiatric Association: Diagnostic and Statistical Manual of Mental Disorders, 4th Edition. Washington, DC, American Psychiatric Association, 1994

American Psychiatric Association Task Force on Quantitative Electrophysiologic Assessment: Quantitative electroencephalography: a report on the present state of computerized EEG techniques. Am J Psychiatry 148:961–964, 1991

Ancoli-Israel S, Parker L, Sinaee R, et al: Sleep fragmentation in patients from a nursing home. J Gerontol 44:M18–21, 1989

Andreasen NC: Nuclear magnetic resonance imaging, in Brain Imaging: Applications in Psychiatry. Edited by Andreasen NC. Washington, DC, American Psychiatric Press, 1989, pp 6–122

Annas GJ: Privacy rules for DNA databanks. JAMA 270:2346–2350, 1993

Annell AL: Lithium in the treatment of children and adolescents. Acta Psychiatr Scand 207:19–33, 1969

Appel SH: A unifying hypothesis for the cause of amyotropic lateral sclerosis, parkinsonism, and Alzheimer disease. Ann Neurol 10:499–505, 1981

Applebaum PS, Roth LH: Competency to consent to research. Arch Gen Psychiatry 39:951–958, 1982

Araujo DM, Lapchak PA, Robitaille Y, et al: Differential alteration of various cholinergic markers in cortical and subcortical regions of human brain in Alzheimer's disease. J Neurochem 50:1914–1923, 1988

Aretaeus: The Extant Works of Aretaeus, the Cappadocian (circa A.D. 200). Edited by London AF. Sydenham Society, 1861

Arispe N, Pollard HB, Rojas E: Giant multilevel cation channels formed by Alzheimer disease amyloid β-protein [AβP-(1-40)] in bilayer membranes. Proc Natl Acad Sci U S A 90:10573–10577, 1993

Aronson M: Understanding Alzheimer's Disease: What Is It, How to Cope With It, Future Directions. New York, Scribner's, 1988

Aspirin Myocardial Infarction Study Research Group: A randomized controlled trial of aspirin in persons recovering from myocardial infarction. JAMA 243:661–669, 1980

Astrom S, Nilsson M, Norber A, et al: Staff burnout in dementia care: relations to empathy and attitudes. Int J Nurs Stud 8:65–75, 1991

Au R, Albert ML, Obler LK: The relationship of aphasia to dementia. Aphasiology 2:161–173, 1988

Austrom MG, Thompson RF Jr, Hendrie HC: Foci of increased T2 signal intensity in MR images of healthy elderly subjects: a follow-up study. J Am Geriatr Soc 38:1133–1138, 1990

Ayd FJ Jr: Prescribing anxiolytics and hypnotics for the elderly. Psychiatric Annals 24:91–97, 1994

Aylward EH, Henderer JD, McArthur JC, et al: Reduced basal ganglia volume in HIV-1–associated dementia: results from quantitative neuroimaging. Neurology 43:2099–2104, 1993

Bachman DL, Wolf PA, Linn R, et al: Prevalence of dementia and probable senile dementia of the Alzheimer type in the Framingham study. Neurology 42:115–119, 1992

Baddeley AD, Della Sala S, Spinnler H: The two-component hypothesis of memory deficit in Alzheimer's disease. J Clin Exp Neuropsychol 3:372–380, 1991

Bahro M, Silber E, Sunderland T: How do patients with Alzheimer's disease cope with their illness? A clinical experience report. J Am Geriatr Soc 43:41–46, 1995

Baily J, Gilbert E, Herweyer S: To find a soul. Nursing 22:63–64, 1992

Baker AC, Ko L-W, Blass JP: Systemic manifestations of Alzheimer's disease. Age 11:60–65, 1988

Baldessarini RJ: Chemotherapy in Psychiatry. Cambridge, MA, Harvard University Press, 1977

Ball MJ: Pathological similarities between Alzheimer's disease and Down's syndrome: is there a genetic link? Integrative Psychiatry 5:159–170, 1987

Balldin J, Gottfries CG, Karlsson I, et al: Dexamethasone suppression test and serum prolactin in dementia disorders. Br J Psychiatry 143:277–281, 1983

Ballenger JC, Post RM: Carbamazepine in manic-depressive illness: a new treatment. Am J Psychiatry 137:782–790, 1975

Baltes MM, Zerbe MB: Independence training in nursing home residents. Gerontologist 16:416–432, 1976

Barnes R, Raskind M: Strategies for diagnosing and treating agitation in the aging. Geriatrics 35:111–119, 1980

Barry PB, Moskowitz MA: The diagnosis of reversible dementia in the elderly. Arch Intern Med 148:1914–1918, 1988

Bartol MA: Nonverbal communication in patients with Alzheimer's disease. Journal of Gerontologic Nursing 5:23–31, 1979

Bartus RT: Physostigmine and recent memory: effects on young and aged non-human primates. Science 206:1087–1089, 1979

Bartus RT: Effects of cholinergic agents on learning and memory in animal models of aging, in Alzheimer's Disease: A Report of Progress in Research. Edited by Corkin S, Davis KL, Growdon JH. New York, Raven, 1982, pp 271–280

Bartus RT, Dean RL: The cholinergic hypothesis of geriatric memory dysfunction. Science 217:408–412, 1982

Bartus RT, Dean RL, Pontecorvo MJ, et al: The cholinergic hypothesis: a historical overview, current perspective and future directions. Ann N Y Acad Sci 44:332–358, 1985

Bauer J, Ganter U, Strauss S, et al: The participation of interleukin-6 in the pathogenesis of Alzheimer's disease. Res Immunol 143:650–657, 1992

Baum C, Edwards DF, Morrow-Howell M: Identification and measurement of productive behaviors in senile dementia of the Alzheimer type. Gerontologist 33:403–408, 1993

Beauchamp TL, Childress JF: Principles of Bioethics, 3rd Edition. New York, Oxford University Press, 1989

Beck AT, Ward CH, Mendelson M, et al: An inventory for measuring depression. Arch Gen Psychiatry 4:561–571, 1961

Becker JT: Working memory and secondary memory deficits in Alzheimer's disease. J Clin Exp Neuropsychol 10:739–753, 1988

Becker R, Giacobini E, Elble R, et al: Potential pharmacotherapy of Alzheimer's disease: a comparison of various routes of administration. Acta Neurol Scand 116:19–32, 1988

Behl C, Davis J, Cole GM, et al: Vitamin E protects nerve cells from amyloid β protein toxicity. Biochem Biophys Res Commun 186:944–950, 1992

Behl C, Davis JB, Lesley R, et al: Hydrogen peroxide mediates amyloid beta protein toxicity. Cell 77:817–827, 1994

Beller SA, Overall JE, Rhoades HM, et al: Long-term outpatient treatment of senile dementia with oral physostigmine. J Clin Psychiatry 49:400–404, 1988

Belmont Report: Ethical Principles and Guidelines for the Protection of Human Subjects of Research. Washington, DC, U.S. Government Printing Office, 1978

Bender AD, Post A, Meier JP, et al: Plasma protein binding of drugs as a function of age in adult human subjects. J Pharm Sci 64:1711–1713, 1975

Benson D: Aphasia, in Clinical Neuropsychology. Edited by Heilman KM, Valenstein E. New York, Oxford University Press, 1985, pp 17–48

Benson DF, Kuhl DE, Hawkins RA, et al: The fluorodexyglucose F-18 scan in Alzheimer's and multi-infarct dementia. Arch Neurol 40:711–714, 1983

Beresford TP, Low D, Hall RCW: Alcohol withdrawal, in Manual of Psychiatric Consultation and Emergency Care. Edited by Guggenheim, FG, Weiner MF. New York, Jason Aronson, 1984, pp 202–210

Berger JR, Levy RM: The neurologic complications of human immunodeficiency virus infection. Med Clin North Am 77:1–23, 1993

Bergman M, Blumenfield VG, Cascardo D, et al: Age-related decrement in hearing for speech: sampling and logitudinal studies. J Gerontol 31:533–538, 1976

Bernstein BE, Weiner MF: The many faces of competence. Tex Med 76:54–57, 1980

Bierer LM, Aisen PS, Davidson M, et al: A pilot study of oral physostigmine plus yohimbine in patients with Alzheimer's disease. Alzheimer Dis Assoc Disord 7:98–104, 1993

Bigler ED: Diagnostic Clinical Neuropsychology. Austin, TX, University of Texas Press, 1984

Binetti G, Magni E, Cappa SF: Semantic memory in Alzheimer's disease: an analysis of category fluency. J Clin Exp Neuropsychol 17:82–89, 1995

Blackford RC, LaRue A: Criteria for diagnosing age associated memory impairment: proposed improvements from the field. Developmental Neuropsychology 5:298–300, 1989

Blansjaar BA, Takens H, Zwinderman AH: The course of alcohol amnestic disorder: a three-year follow-up study of clinical signs and social disabilites. Acta Psychiatr Scand 86:240–246, 1992

Blass JP, Hanin I, Barclay L, et al: Red blood cell abnormalities in Alzheimer disease. J Am Geriatr Soc 33:401–405, 1985

Blessed G, Tomlinson BE, Roth M: The association between quantitative measures of dementia and of senile change in the cerebral gray matter of elderly subjects. Br J Psychiatry 114:797–811, 1968

Bleuler E: Textbook of Psychiatry. New York, Macmillan, 1924

Bliwise DL, Tinklenberg J, Yesavage JA, et al: REM latency in Alzheimer's disease. Biol Psychiatry 25:320–328, 1989

Board of Directors of the American Association for Geriatric Psychiatry, Clinical Practice Committee of the American Geriatrics Society, Committee on Long-Term Care and Treatment for the Elderly, American Psychiatric Association: Psychotherapeutic medications in the nursing home. J Am Geriatr Soc 40:946–949, 1992

Boast CA, Leventer S, Sabb A, et al: Biochemical and behavioral characterization of a novel cholinergic agonist, SR 95639. Pharmacol Biochem Behav 39:287–92, 1991

Bolla KI, Lindgren KN, Bonaccorsy C, et al: Memory complaints in older adults. Arch Neurol 48:61–64, 1991

Bolla-Wilson K, Robinson RG, Starkstein SE, et al: Lateralization of dementia of depression in stroke patients. Am J Psychiatry 146:627–634, 1989

Boller F, Lopez OC, Moossy J: Diagnosis of dementia: clinicopathologic correlation. Neurology 39:76–79, 1989

Bondareff W, Mountjoy CQ, Roth M: Loss of neurons of origin of the adrenergic projection to the cerebral cortex (nucleus locus ceruleus) in senile dementia. Neurology 32:164–168, 1982

Bonder BR: Psychotherapy for individuals with Alzheimer disease. Alz Dis Assoc Disord 8 (suppl 3):75–81, 1994

Bonte FJ, Stokely EM: Single-photon tomographic study of regional cerebral blood flow after stroke: concise communication. J Nucl Med 22:1049–1053, 1981

Bonte FJ, Ross ED, Chehabi HH, et al: SPECT study of regional cerebral blood flow in Alzheimer disease. J Comput Assist Tomogr 10:579–583, 1986a

Bonte FJ, Devous MD, Stokely EM, et al: Testing vasoreactivity with SPECT study of regional cerebral blood flow in patients with Alzheimer or cerebrovascular disease. J Comput Assist Tomogr 10:579–583, 1986b

Bonte FJ, Devous MD, Reisch JS, et al: The effect of acetazolamide on regional cerebral blood flow in patients with Alzheimer's disease or stroke as measured by single-photon emission computed tomography. Invest Radiol 24:99–103, 1989

Bonte FJ, Tintner R, Weiner MF, et al: Brain blood flow in the dementias: SPECT with histopathologic correlation. Radiology 186:361–365, 1993

Bornstein RA: Methodological and conceptual issues in the study of cognitive change in HIV infection, in Neuropsychology of HIV Infection. Edited by Grant I, Martin A. New York, Oxford, 1994, pp 146–160

Bornstein RA, Nasrallah MD, Para MF, et al: Rate of CD4 decline and neuropsychological performance in HIV infection. Arch Neurol 48:704–707, 1991

Bosch EP, Hart MN: Late adult onset metachromatic leukodystrophy. Arch Neurol 35:475–477, 1978

Bottomley PA: Human in vivo NMR spectroscopy in diagnostic medicine: clinical tool or research probe? Radiology 170:1–15, 1989

Bowen DM, Neary D: Cerebral biopsy in the study of Alzheimer's disease. Bulletin of Clinical Neuroscience 50:44–48, 1985

Bowen DM, Smith CB, White P, et al: Neurotransmitter related enzymes and indices of hypoxia in senile dementia and other abiotrophies. Brain 99:459–496, 1976

Bowen DM, Allen SJ, Benton JS, et al: Biochemical assessment of serotonergic and cholinergic dysfunction and cerebral atrophy in Alzheimer's disease. J Neurochem 41:266–272, 1983

Braak H, Braak E: Neuropathological staging of Alzheimer's disease. Acta Neuropathol (Berl) 82:239–259, 1991

Braga MF, Harvey AL, Rowan EG: Effects of tacrine, velnacrine (HP029), suronacrine (HP128), and 3,4 diaminopyridine on skeletal neuromuscular transmission in vitro. Br J Pharmacol 102:909–915, 1991

Branchey L, Branchey M, Zucker D, et al: Association between low plasma tryptophan and blackouts in male alcoholic patients. Alcoholism 9:393–395, 1985

Branconnier RJ: The efficacy of the cerebral metabolic enhancers in the treatment of senile dementia. Psychopharmacol Bull 19:212–219, 1983

Branconnier RJ, Cole JO, Dessain EC, et al: The therapeutic efficacy of piracetam in Alzheimer's disease: preliminary observations. Psychopharmacol Bull 19:726–730, 1983b

Brandt JA, Bylsma FW: The dementia of Huntington's disease, in Neuropsychology of Alzheimer's Disease and Other Dementias. Edited by Parks RW, Zec RF, Wilson RS. New York, Oxford, 1993, pp 265–282

Brawley B: Alzheimer's disease: designing the physical environment. American Journal of Alzheimer's Care and Related Disease and Research 7:3–8, 1992

Breitner JCS, Folstein MF: Familial Alzheimer dementia: a prevalent disorder with specific clinical features. Psychol Med 14:63–80, 1984

Breitner JCS, Magruder-Habib K, Murphy EA: Risk factor intervention in Alzheimer's disease: delay of onset by five years will halve morbidity (abstract). Biol Psychiatry 25:66A, 1989

Breitner JCS, Gau BA, Welsh KA, et al: Inverse relationship of anti-inflammatory treatments and Alzheimer's disease: initial results of a co-twin control study. Neurology 44:227–232, 1994

Brenner RP, Reynold CF, Ulrich RF: Diagnostic efficiency of computerized spectral versus visual EEG analysis in elderly normal, demented and depressed subjects. Electroencephalogr Clin Neurophysiol 69:110–117, 1988

Breslau J, Starr A, Sicotte N, et al: Topographic EEG changes with normal aging and SDAT. Electroencephalogr Clin Neurophysiol 72:281–289, 1989

Brew BJ, Bhalla RB, Paul M, et al: Cerebrospinal fluid beta 2-microglobulin in patients with AIDS dementia complex: an expanded series including response to zidovudine treatment. AIDS 6:461–465, 1992

Brewster ME: Noninvasive drug delivery to the brain. Neurobiol Aging 10:638–639, 1989

Brierley JB, Corsellis JAN, Hierons R, et al: Subacute encephalitis of later adult life mainly affecting the limbic areas. Brain 83:357–370, 1960

Brink CA: Absorbent pads, garments, and management strategies. J Am Geriatr Soc 38:368–373, 1990

Broderick DF, Wippold FJ, Clifford DB, et al: White matter lesions and cerebral atrophy on MR images in patients with and without AIDS dementia complex. American Journal of Roentgenology 161:177–181, 1993

Brody B: The family at risk, in Alzheimer's Disease Treatment and Family Stress: Directions for Research. Edited by Light E, Lebowitz B. Rockville, MD, U.S. Department of Health and Human Services, 1989, pp 2–49

Brown GL, Ballenger C, Minichiello MD, et al: Human aggression and its relation to cerebrospimal fluid 5-hydroxyindol acetic acid, 3-methoxy-4-hydroxyphenylglycol, and homovaillic acid, in Psychopharmacology of Aggression. Edited by Sandler M. New York, Raven, 1979, pp 131–148

Brown TH, Chapman PF, Kairiss EW, et al: Long-term synaptic potentiation. Science 242:724–728, 1988

Bruce G, Heinrich G: Production and characterization of biologically active recombinant human nerve growth factor. Neurobiol Aging 10:89–94, 1989

Brufani M, Marta M, Pomponi M: Anticholinesterase activity of a new carbamate, heptylphysostigmine, in view of its use in patients with Alzheimer-type dementia. Eur J Biochem 157:115–120, 1986

Brugge K, Katzman R, Hill LR, et al: Serological α1-antichymotrypsin in Down's syndrome and Alzheimer's disease. Ann Neurol 32:193–197, 1992

Brun A: Frontal lobe degeneration of non-Alzheimer type; I: neuropathology. Archives of Gerontology and Geriatrics 6:193–208, 1987

Brunetti A, Berg G, DiChiro G, et al: Reversal of brain metabolic abnormalities following treatment of AIDS dementia complex w3'-azido-2',3'-dideoxythymidine (AZT, zidovudine): a PET-FDG study. J Nucl Med 30:581–590, 1989

Bruno G, Mohr E, Gillespie M, et al: RS-86 therapy of Alzheimer's disease. Arch Neurol 43:659–661, 1985

Buccafusco JJ, Jackson WJ, Terry AV Jr: Effects of concomitant cholinergic and adrenergic stimulation on learning and memory performance by primates. Life Sci 51:7–12, 1992

Buchsbaum MS, Wu J, DeLisi E, et al: Frontal cortex and basal ganglia metabolic rates assessed by positron emission tomography with [^{18}F]-2-deoxyglucose in affective illness. J Affect Disord 10:137–152, 1986

Buckley NJ, Bonner TI, Buckley A, et al: Antagonist binding properties of five cloned muscarinic receptors expressed in CHO-K1 cells. Mol Pharmacol 35:469–476, 1989

Bulbena A, Berrios GE: Pseudodementia: facts and figures. Br J Psychiatry 148:87–94, 1986

Burger LJ, Rowan J, Goldensohn ES: Creutzfeldt-Jakob disease: an electroencephalographic study. Arch Neurol 26:428–433, 1972

Burke WJ, Folks DG, Roccaforte WH, et al: Serotonin reuptake inhibitors for the treatment of coexisting depression and psychosis in dementia of the Alzheimer type. Am J Geriatr Psychiatry 2:352–354, 1994

Burns A, Philpot M: Capgras' syndrome in a patient with dementia. Br J Psychiatry 150:876–877, 1987

Burns A, Luthert P, Levy R, et al: Accuracy of clinical diagnosis of Alzheimer's disease (abstract). BMJ 301:1026, 1990a

Burns A, Jacoby R, Levy R: Psychiatric phenomena in Alzheimer's disease. Br J Psychiatry 157:72–94, 1990b

Burnside I: Working With the Elderly: Group Process and Techniques, 2nd Edition. Belmont, CA, Wadsworth, 1984

Burnside I: Nursing care, in Treatment for the Alzheimer Patient: The Long Haul. Edited by Jarvik LF, Winograd CH. New York, Springer, 1988, pp 39–58

Buschke H, Fuld P: Evaluating storage, retention and retrieval in disordered memory and learning. Neurology 11:1019–1025, 1974

Butters N, Granholm E, Salmon D, et al: Episodic and semantic memory: a comparison of amnestic and dementia patients. J Clin Exp Neuropsychol 9:479–497, 1987

Buxbaum JD, Oishi M, Chen HI, et al: Effect of CDP-choline on cognition and immune function in Alzheimer's disease and multi infarct dementia. Ann N Y Acad Sci 695:321–323, 1992

Cacabelos R, Alvarez XA, Franco MA, et al: Effect of CDP-choline on cognition and immune function in Alzheimer's disease and multi-infarct dementia. Ann N Y Acad Sci 695:321–323, 1993

Calkins MP: Design for Dementia: Planning Environments for the Elderly and the Confused. Owings Mills, MD, National Health Publishing, 1988

Calkins MP: Blueprint for a specialized Alzheimer's disease nursing home. Workshop hosted by the Massachusetts Alzheimer's Disease Research Center, Boston, MA, May 11–13, 1989a

Calkins MP: Designing cues for wanderers. Provider 15:7–10, 1989b

Calkins MP: Proper environment may be therapeutic to influence dementia patients' behavior. Group Practice Journal 40:58–67, 1991

Calkins MP: Toward a new conceptualization of factors influencing supportive residential facilities for the elderly, Area of Concentration Exam. Milwaukee, WI, University of Wisconsin-Milwaukee, 1993

Calkins MP, Namazi KH, Rosner TT, et al: Home Modifications: Responding to Dementia. Milwaukee, WI, The Research Center of the Corinne Dolan Alzheimer Center at Heather Hill, 1990

Cantor NL: Legal Frontiers of Death and Dying. Bloomington, IN, Indiana University Press, 1987

Caplan LR, Schoene WC: Clinical findings of subcortical arteriosclerotic encephalopathy (Binswanger disase). Neurology 28:1206–1215, 1978

Capruso DX, Levin HS: Cognitive impairment following closed head injury. Neurol Clin North Am 10:879–893, 1992

Caroff SN: The neuroleptic malignant syndrome. J Clin Psychiatry 41:79–83, 1980

Carr D, Jackson TW, Madden DJ, et al: The effect of age on driving skills. J Am Geriatr Soc 40:567–573, 1992

Carroll BJ, Feinberg M, Greden JF, et al: A specific laboratory test for the diagnosis of melancholia: standardization, validation, and clinical utility. Arch Gen Psychiatry 38:15–22, 1981

Carta A, Calvani A: Acetyl l-carnitine: a drug able to slow the progress Alzheimer disease. Ann N Y Acad Sci 640:228–232, 1991

Caserta M, Lund D, Wright S, et al: Caregivers to dementia patients: the utilization of community services. Gerontologist 29:209–214, 1987

Cassem N: Cardiovascular effects of antidepressants. J Clin Psychiatry 43:22–28, 1982

Cauley J, Eichner J, Kamboh I, et al: Apo E allele frequencies in younger (42–50) vs older (age 65–90) women. Genet Epidemiol 10:27–34, 1993

Cautela J: Behavior therapy in geriatrics. J Genet Psychol 108:9–17, 1966

Cella SG, Imbimbo BP, Pieretti F, et al: Eptastigmine augments basas and GHRH stimulated growth hormone release in young and old dogs. Life Sci 53:389–395, 1993

Celsus AC: De Medicina (circa A.D. 100). Translated by Greive J. London, UK, Wilson & Durham, 1756

Centers for Disease Control: Sexually transmitted diseases treatment guidelines. MMWR 38 (suppl 5–8):5–15, 1989

Chafetz PK, West HL: Longitudinal control group evaluation of a special care unit for dementia patients: initial findings. Paper presented at the annual meeting of the Gerontological Society of America, Washington, DC, November 18–22, 1987

Chang TMS, Barre P: Effect of desferrioxamine on removal of aluminum and iron by coated charcoal haemoperfusion and haemodialysis. Lancet 1:1051–1053, 1983

Chapron DJ, Cameron IR, White LB, et al: Observations on lithium distribution in the elderly. J Am Geriatr Soc 30:651–655, 1982

Chatellier G, Lacomblez L: Tacrine (tetrahydroaminoacridin; THA) and lecithin in senile dementia of the Alzheimer's type: a multi-center trial. BMJ 300:495–499, 1990

Chen JY, Stern Y, Sano M, et al: Cumulative risks of developing extrapyramidal signs, psychosis, or myoclonus in the course of Alzheimer's disease. Arch Neurol 48:1141–1143, 1991

Chenoweth B, Spencer B: Dementia: the experience of family caregivers. Gerontologist 26:267–272, 1986

Chesrow EJ, Kaplitz SE, Vetra H, et al: Double-blind study of oxazepam in the management of geriatric patients with behavioral problems. Clinical Medicine 72:1001–1005, 1965

Chiarello RJ, Cole JO: The use of psychostimulants in general psychiatry. Arch Gen Psychiatry 44:286–295, 1987

Chouinard G, de Montigny C, Annable L: Tardive dyskinesia and antiparkinson medication. Am J Psychiatry 136:228–229, 1979

Christensen H, Hadzi-Pavlovic D, Jacomb P: The psychometric differentiation of dementia from normal aging: a meta-analysis. J Consult Clin Psychol 3:147–155, 1991

Christie JE, Blackburn IM, Glen AIM, et al: Effects of choline and lecithin on CSF choline levels and cognitive functions in patients with pre-senile dementia of the Alzheimer type, in Nutrition and the Brain, Vol 5. Edited by Barbeau A, Growdon JH, Wurtman RJ. New York, Raven, 1979, pp 377–387

Christie JE, Shering A, Ferguson J, et al: Physostigmine and arecholine: effects of intravenous infusions in Alzheimer's disease. Br J Psychiatry 138:46–50, 1981

Chui HC: Dementia: a review emphasizing clinicopathologic correlation and brain-behavior relationships. Arch Neurol 46:806–814, 1989

Citron M, Vigo-Pelfrey C, Teplow DB, et al: Excessive production of amyloid protein by peripheral cells of symptomatic and presymptomatic patients carrying the Swedish familial Alzheimer disease mutation. Proc Natl Acad Sci 91:11993–11997, 1994

Civil RH, Whitehouse PJ, Lanska DJ, et al: Degenerative dementias, in Dementia. Edited by Whitehouse P. Philadelphia, PA, FA Davis, 1993, pp 167–214

Clairfield AM: The reversible dementias: do they reverse? Ann Intern Med 109:476–486, 1988

Clark RF, Goate AM: Molecular genetics of Alzheimer's disease. Arch Neurol 50:1164–1172, 1993

Claus JJ, Ludwig C, Mohr E, et al: Nootropic drugs in Alzheimer's disease: symptomatic treatment with pramiracetam. Neurology 41:570–574, 1991

Clayton RM, Sedowofia SKA, Rankin JM, et al: A long term effect of aluminum in the fetal mouse brain. Life Sci 51:1921–1928, 1992

Cohen U, Day K: Contemporary Environments for People with Dementia. Baltimore, MD, Johns Hopkins Press, 1993

Cohen D, Eisdorfer C: The Loss of Self: A Family Resource for the Care of Alzheimer's Disease and Related Disorders. New York, WW Norton, 1986

Cohen EL, Wurtman RJ: Brain acetylcholine: control by dietary choline. Science 191:561–562, 1976

Cohen MB, Metter EJ, Graham LS, et al: Differential diagnosis of dementia with "pure" I-123 iodoamphetamine and a clinical camera. J Nucl Med 24:106, 1983

Cohen ML, Golde TE, Usiak MF, et al: In situ hybridization of nucleus basalis neurons shows increased β-amyloid mRNA in Alzheimer disease. Proc Natl Acad Sci U S A 85:1227–1231, 1988

Cohen RM, Weingartner H, Smallberg SA, et al: Effort and cognition in depression. Arch Gen Psychiatry 39:593–597, 1982

Cohen U, Weisman J: Holding on to Home. Baltimore, MD, Johns Hopkins University Press, 1991

Cohen-Mansfield J: Agitated behaviors in the elderly; II: preliminary results in the cognitively deteriorated. J Am Geriatr Soc 34:711–721, 1986

Cohen-Mansfield J, Billig N: Agitated behaviors in the elderly; I: a conceptual review. J Am Geriatr Soc 34:711–721, 1986

Cohen-Mansfield J, Marx MS: Do past experiences predict agitation in nursing home residents? Int J Aging Hum Dev 28:285–293, 1989

Colenda CC: Buspirone in treatment of agitated dementia patient (letter). Lancet 1:1169, 1988

Collerton D: Cholinergic function and intellectual decline in Alzheimer's disease. Neuroscience 19:1–28, 1986

In re Colyer, 660 P2d 738, 748, 1983

In re Conroy, 486 A2d 1209 (NJ 1985)

Cook L: Biochemical, neurophysiological and cognitive effects of an enhancer of stimulus-induced release of acetylcholine: DuP 996 (3,3-Bis(4-pyridinyl-methyl)-1-phenylindolin-2-one). Paper presented at the annual meeting of the American College of Neuropharmacology, Puerto Rico, December 1988

Cook L, Nickolson VJ, Steinfels GF, et al: Cognition enhancement by the acetylcholine releaser DuP 996. Drug Development Research 19:301–304, 1990

Cook P, James I: Cerebral vasodilators. N Engl J Med 305:1508–1513, 1981

Coons D: A residential unit for persons with dementia. Contract report prepared for the Office of Technology Assessment. Washington, DC, U.S. Government Printing Office, 1986

Coons D: Specialized Dementia Care Units. Baltimore, MD, Johns Hopkins University Press, 1991

Cooper AJ: Medroxprogesterone acetate as a treatment for sexual acting out in organic brain syndrome (letter). Am J Psychiatry 145:1179, 1988

Cooper AJL, Plum F: Biochemistry and physiology of brain ammonia. Physiol Rev 67:440–519, 1987

Cooper BA, Gowland C, McIntosh J: The use of color in the environment of the elderly to enhance function. Clin Geriatr Med 2:151–163, 1986

Cooper JK, Mungas D, Weiler PG: Relation of cognitive status and abnormal behaviors in Alzheimer's disease. J Am Geriatr Soc 38:867–870, 1990

Coppell DB, Burton D, Becker J, et al: Relationship of cognitions associated with coping reactions to depression in spousal caregivers of Alzheimer's disease patients. Cognitive Therapy Research 9:253–266, 1985

Corder EH, Saunders AM, Strittmatter WJ: Gene dose of apoliprotein E type 4 allele and the risk of Alzheimer's disease in late onset families. Science 261:921–923, 1993

Corder EH, Saunders AM, Risch NJ, et al: Protective effect of apolipoprotein E type 2 allele for late onset Alzheimer disease. Nature Genetics 7:180–184, 1994

Cornfeldt M, Wirtz-Burgger, Szewczak M, et al: HP 749: a pharmacologic profile of the therapeutic agent for Alzheimer's disease (abstract). Society for Neuroscience Abstracts 16:612, 1990

Corsellis JAN: Mental Illness and the Aging Brain. London, UK, Oxford University Press, 1962

Crapper DR, Krishnan SS, Dalton AJ: Brain aluminum distribution in Alzheimer's disease and experimental neurofibrillary degeneration. Science 180:511–513, 1973

Crapper DR, Dalton AJ, Skopitz M: Alzheimer degeneration in Down's syndrome. Arch Neurol 33:618–623, 1975

Crapper McLachlan DR, Dalton AJ, Kruck TP, et al: Intramuscular desferriox-amine in patients with Alzheimer's disease. Lancet 337:1304–1308, 1991

Creditor MC: Hazards of hospitalization of the elderly. Ann Intern Med 118:219–223, 1993

Crellin R, Bottiglieri T, Reynolds EH: Folates and psychiatric disorders: clinical potential. Drugs 45:623–636, 1993

Croisile B, Trillet M, Fondarai J, et al: Long-term and high-dose piracetam treatment of Alzheimer's disease. Neurology 43:301–305, 1993

Cronin-Colomb A, Corkin S, Rizzo JF, et al: Visual dysfunction in Alzheimer's disease: relation to normal aging. Ann Neurol 29:41–52, 1991

Crook T: Central nervous system stimulants: appraisal of use in geropsychiatric patients. J Am Geriatr Soc 27:476–477, 1979

Crook T, Bartus RT, Ferris SH, et al: Age-associated memory impairment. Proposed diagnostic criteria and measures of clinical change: report of a National Institute of Mental Health Work Group. Developmental Neuropsychology 2:261–276, 1986

Crook T, Wilner E, Rothwell A, et al: Noradrenergic intervention in Alzheimer's disease. Psychopharmacol Bull 28:67–70, 1992

Crum RM, Anthony JC, Bassett SS, et al: Population-based norms for the Mini-Mental State Examination by age and educational level. JAMA 269:2386–2391, 1993

Cross AJ, Crow TJ, Ferrier IN, et al: The selectivity of the reduction of serotonin S2 receptors in Alzheimer-type dementia. Neurobiol Aging 7:3–7 1986

Cruzan v Director, Missouri Dept of Health, et al, 110 SCt 2841, 1990

Crystal HA, Ortof E, Frishman WH, et al: Serum vitamin B_{12} levels and incidence of dementia in a healthy elderly population: a report from the Bronx Longitudinal Aging Study. J Am Geriatr Soc 42:933–936, 1994

Cummings BJ, Su JH, Geddes J, et al: Aggregation of the amyloid precursor protein within degenerating neurons and dystrophic neurites in Alzheimer's disease. Neuroscience 48:763–777, 1992Cummings JL: Clinical Neuropsychiatry. New York, Grune & Stratton, 1985

Cummings JL: Multi-infarct dementia: diagnosis and management. Psychosomatics 28:117–125, 1987

Cummings JL: Introduction, in Subcortical Dementia. Edited By Cummings JL. New York, Oxford University Press, 1990, pp 4–16

Cummings JL: Depression and Parkinson's disease: a review. Am J Psychiatry 149:443–454, 1992

Cummings JL, Mahler ME: Cerebrovascular dementia, in Neurobehavioral Aspects of Cerebrovascular Disease. Edited by Bornstein RA, Brown GM. New York, Oxford University Press, 1991, pp 131–149

Cummings JL, Benson F, LoVerme S Jr: Reversible dementia: illustrative cases, definition, and review. JAMA 243:2434–2439, 1980

Cummings JL, Ross W, Absher J, et al: Depressive symptoms in Alzheimer's disease: assessment and determinants. Alz Dis Assoc Disord 9:87–93 1995

Curl A: Agitation and the older adult. J Psychosoc Nurs Ment Health Serv 27:12–14, 1989

Cutler NR, Haxby J, Narang PK, et al: Evaluation of an analogue of somatostatin (L363,586) in Alzheimer's disease (leter). N Engl J Med 312:75, 1985

Cutler NR, Murphy MF, Nash RJ, et al: Clinical safety, tolerance and plasma levels of the oral anticholinesterase 1,2,3,4-tetrahydro-9-aminoacrdin-1-olmaleate (HP 029) in Alzheimer's disease: preliminary findings. J Clin Pharmacol 30:556–561 1990a

Cutler NR, Sedman AJ, Prior P, et al: Steady state pharmacokinetics of tacrine in patients with Alzheimer's disease. Psychopharmacol Bull 26:231–234, 1990b

Cutler NR, Sramek JJ, Murphy MF: Implications of the study population in the early evaluation of anticholinesterase inhibitors for Alzheimer's disease. Ann Pharmacother 26:1118–1122, 1992a

Cutler NR, Sramek JJ, Murphy MF, et al: Alzheimer's patients should be included in phase I clinical trials to evaluate compounds for Alzheimer's disease. J Geriatr Psychiatry Neurol 5:192–194, 1992b

Dal-Bianco P, Maly J, Wober Ch, et al: Galanthamine treatment in Alzheimer's disease. J Neural Transm Suppl 33:59–63, 1991

Davidson M, Mohs RC, Hollander E, et al: Lecithin and piracetam in patients with Alzheimer's disease. Biol Psychiatry 22:112–114, 1987

Davidson M, Zamislany Z, Mohs RC, et al: 4-Aminopyridine in the treatment of Alzheimer's disease. Biol Psychiatry 23:485–490, 1988

Davidson M, Bierer LM, Kaminsky R, et al: Combined administration of physostigmine and clonidine to patients with dementia of the Alzheimer type: a pilot safety study. Alzheimer Dis Assoc Disord 1:1–4, 1989

Davies CA, Mann DM, Sumpter PQ, et al: A quantitative morphometric analysis of the neuronal and synaptic content of the frontal and temporal cortex in patients with Alzheimer's disease. J Neurol Sci 78:151–164, 1987

Davies DF, Shock N: Age changes in glomerular filtration rate, effective renal plasma flow, and the tubular excretory capacity in adult males. J Clin Invest 29:496–506, 1950

Davies P, Maloney AJF: Selective loss of central cholinergic neurons in Alzheimer's disease (letter). Lancet 2:1403, 1976

Davis RJ, Cummings JL: Clinical variants of tardive dyskinesia. Neuropsychiatry, Neuropsychology and Behavioral Neurology 1:31–38, 1988

Davis KL, Powchik P: Tacrine. Lancet 345:625–630, 1995

Davis KL, Mohs RC, Tinklenberg JR, et al: Physostigmine: improvement of long-term memory processes in normal humans. Science 201:272–274, 1978

Davis KL, Hollander E, Davidson M, et al: Induction of depression with oxotremorine in Alzheimer's disease. Am J Psychiatry 144:468–471, 1987

Davis KL, Thal L, Gamzu ER, et al: A double-blind placebo-controlled multicenter study of tacrine for Alzheimer's disease. N Engl J Med 327:1253–1259, 1992

Davis R, Raby C, Callahan MJ, et al: Subtype selective muscarinic agonists; potential therapeutic agents for Alzheimer's disease. Prog Brain Res 98:439–445, 1993a

Davis RE, Emmerling MR, Jaen JC, et al: Therapeutic intervention in dementia. Crit Rev Neurobiol 7:41–83, 1993b

Davis RJ, Cummings JL: Clinical variants of tardive dyskinesia. Neuropsychiatry, Neuropsychology, and Behavioral Neurology 1:31–38, 1988

DeKosky ST, Scheff SW: Synapse loss in frontal cortex biopsies in Alzheimer's disease: correlation with cognitive severity. Ann Neurol 27:457–464, 1990

DeKosky ST, Harbaugh RE, Schmitt FA, et al: Cortical biopsy in Alzheimer's disease: diagnostic accuracy and neurochemical, neuropathological and cognitive correlations. Ann Neurol 32:625–632, 1992

de la Morena E: Efficacy of CDP-choline in the treatment of senile alterations in memory. Ann N Y Acad Sci 640:233–236, 1993

Delabar J-M, Goldgaber D, Lamour Y, et al: β-Amyloid gene duplication in Alzheimer's disease and karyotypically normal Down syndrome. Science 235:1390–1392, 1987

DeLamos GP, Clements WR, Nickels E: Effect of diazepam suspension in geriatric patients hospitalized for psychiatric illness. J Am Geriatr Soc 13:355–359, 1967

Delis DC, Kramer JH, Kaplan E, et al: California Verbal Learning Test: Manual. San Antonio, TX, The Psychological Corporation, 1987

DeLong AJ: The micro-spatial structure of the older person: some implications of planning the social and spatial environment, in Spatial Behavior of Older People. Edited by Pastalan LA, Carson DH. Ann Arbor, MI, University of Michigan, Institute of Gerontology, 1970, pp 68–87

Dening TR: The neuropsychiatry of Wilson's disease: a review. Int J Psychiatry Med 21:135–148, 1991

Dening TR, Berrios GE: Wilson's disease: psychiatric symptoms in 195 cases. Arch Gen Psychiatry 46:1126–1134, 1989

Denny-Brown D, Meyer JS, Horenstein S: Amorphosynthesis from left parietal lesion. Arch Neurol 71:302–313, 1954

Derouesne C, Rancurel G, LePoncin-Lafitte M, et al: Variability of cerebral blood flow defects in Alzheimer's disease on 123-iodo-isopropyl-amphetamine and single-photon emission tomography (letter). Lancet 1:1282, 1985

DeSarno P, Pomponi M, Giacobini E, et al: The effect of heptylphysostigmine, a new cholinesterase inhibitor, on the central cholinergic system of the rat. Neurochem Res 14:971–977, 1989

De Smet Y, Ruberg M, Serdaru M, et al: Confusion, dementia and anticholinergics in Parkinson's disease. J Neurol Neurosurg Psychiatry 45:1161–1164, 1982

Deutsch LH, Byslma FW, Rovner BW: Psychosis and physical aggression in probable Alzheimer's disease. Am J Psychiatry 148:1159–1163, 1991

Devous MD Sr: Single-photon emission computer tomography, in Brain Imaging: Applications in Psychiatry. Edited by Andreasen NC. Washington, DC, American Psychiatric Press, 1989, pp 147–234

Devous MD, Bonte FJ: Initial evaluation of cerebral blood flow imaging with a high-resolution, high-sensitivity three-headed SPECT system (PRISM) (letter). J Nucl Med 29:912, 1988

Devous MD, Stokely EM, Chehabi HH, et al: Normal distribution of regional cerebral blood flow measured by dynamic single-photon emission tomography. J Cereb Blood Flow Metab 6:95–104, 1986

De Wied D: The importance of vasopressin in memory. Trends Neurosci 7:62–63, 1984

Dhingra U, Rabins PV: Mania in the elderly: a 5–7 year follow-up. J Am Geriatr Soc 39:581–583, 1991

Dietch JT, Hewett LJ, Jones S: Adverse effects of reality orientation. J Am Geriatr Soc 37:974–976, 1989

In re Dinnerstein, 380 NE2nd 134 (Mass App Ct 1978)

Dobbs MN, Shroyer JL, Anderson GM: Aging and perception of light and color in the institutional environment. Housing and Society 15:262–265, 1988

Dolezal V, Tucek S: Positive and negative effects of tacrine (tetrahydroaminoacridine) and methoxytacrine on the metabolism of acetylcholine in brain cortical prisms incubated under "resting" conditions. J Neurochem 56:1207–15, 1991

Doods HN, Quirion R, Mihm R, et al: Therapeutic potential of CNS-active M2 antagonists: novel structures and pharmacology. Life Sci 52:497–503, 1993

Doughty DB: Urinary and Fecal Incontinence: Nursing Management. Philadelphia, PA, Mosby, 1992

Drachman DA, Leavitt J: Memory impairment in the aged: storage versus retrieval deficit. Journal of Experimental Psychology 93:302–308, 1972

Drachman DA, Leavitt J: Human memory and the cholinergic system. Arch Neurol 30:113–121, 1974

Dreisbach RH: Handbook of Poisoning: Prevention, Diagnosis and Treatment, 12th Edition. Los Altos, CA, Lange, 1987

Drickamer MA, Lach MS: Should patients with Alzheimer's disease be told their diagnosis? N Engl J Med 326:947–951, 1992

Drinka JK, Smith JC, Drinka PJ: Correlates of depression and burden for informal caregivers of patients in a geriatrics referral clinic. J Am Geriatr Soc 35:522–525, 1987

Drukarch B, Kits S, Van der Meer EG, et al: 9-Amino-1,2,3,4-tetrahydroacridine (THA), an alleged drug for the treatment of Alzheimer's disease, inhibits acetylcholinesterase activity and slow outward K+ current. Eur J Pharmacol 141:153–157, 1987

Drukarch B, Leysen JE, Stoof JC: Further analysis of the neuropharmacological profile of 9-amino-1,2,3,4-tetrahydroacridine (THA), an alleged drug for the treatment of Alzheimer's disease. Life Sci 42:1011–1117, 1988

Duara R, Grady C, Haxby J, et al: Positron emission tomography in Alzheimer's disease. Neurology 36:879–887, 1986

Dube A, Mitchell E: Accidental strangulation from vest restraints. Journal of Gerontological Nursing 4:15–17, 1986

Duffy FH, Burchfiel JL, Lombroso CT: Brain electrical activity mapping (BEAM): a method for extending the clinical utility of EEG and evoked potential data. Ann Neurol 5:309–332, 1979

Dunne JW, Leedman PJ, Edis RH: Inobvious stroke: a cause of delirium and dementia. Aust N Z Med 16:771–778, 1986

Durnbaugh T, Haley B, Roberts S: Feeding behaviors in mid-stage Alzheimer's disease: a review. American Journal of Alzheimer's Care and Related Disease and Research 8:22–27, 1993

Dysken MW, Mendels J, LeWitt P, et al: Milacemide: a placebo-controlled study in senile dementia of the Alzheimer type. J Am Geriatr Soc 40:503–506, 1992

Eagger SA, Levy R, Sahakian BJ: Tacrine in Alzheimer's disease. Lancet 337:989–992, 1991

Engel GE: Psychological Development in Health and Disease. Philadelphia, PA, WB Saunders, 1962

Engel GE, Romano J: Delirium, a syndrome of cerebral insufficiency. J Chron Dis 9:260–277, 1959

Engel GE, Schmale AH: Conservation withdrawal: a primary regulatory process of organismic homeostasis, in Physiology, Emotion and Psychosomatic Illness: CIBA Foundation Symposium No 8. Amsterdam, Elsevier-Excerpta Medica, 1972

Ensinger HA, Doods HN, Immel Sehr AR, et al: WAL 2014—a muscarinic agonist with preferential neuron-stimulating properties. Life Sci 52:473–480,1993

Enz A, Boddeke H, Gray J, et al: Pharmacologic and clinicopharmacologic properties of SDZ ENA 713, a centrally selective acetycholinesterase inhibitor. Ann N Y Acad Sci 640:272–275, 1991

Enz A, Shapiro G, Supavilai P, et al: SDZ ENS 163 is a selective M$_1$ agonist and induces release of acetylcholine. Naunyn Schmiedebergs Arch Pharmacol 345:282–287, 1992

Enz A, Boddeke H, Sauter A, et al: SDZ ENS 163 a novel pilocarpine-like drug: pharmacological in vitro and in vivo profile. Life Sci 52:513–520, 1993

Erkinjuntti T, Fuqiang G, Lee DH, et al: Lack of difference in brain hyperintensities between patients with early Alzheimer's disease and control subjects. Arch Neurol 51:260–268, 1994

Ertel W, Morrison MH, Ayala A, et al: Chloroquine attenuates hemorrhagic shock induced suppression of Kupffer cell antigen presentation and major histocompatibility complex class II antigen expression through blockade of tumor necrosis factor and prostaglandin release. Blood 78:1781–1788, 1991

Esquirol JED: Mental Maladies: A Treatise on Insanity (1845). Translated by Hunt EK. New York, Hafner Publishing Company, 1965

Estus S, Golde TE, Younkin SG: Normal processing of the Alzheimer's disease amyloid beta protein precursor generates potentially amyloidogenic carboxyl terminal derivatives. Ann N Y Acad Sci 674:138–148, 1992

Etcheberrigaray R, Ito E, Oka K, et al: Potassium channel dysfunction in fibroblasts identifies patients with Alzheimer disease. Proc Natl Acad Sci U S A 90:8209–8213, 1993

Etienne PE: Treatment of Alzheimer's disease with lecithin, in Alzheimer's Disease. Edited by Reisberg B. New York, Free Press, 1983, pp 353–354

Etienne PE, Dastoor D, Goldapple E, et al: Adverse effects of medical and psychiatric workup in six demented geriatric patients. Am J Psychiatry 138:520–521, 1981

Evans DA, Funkenstein HH, Albert MS, et al: Prevalence of Alzheimer's disease in a community population of older persons: higher than previously reported. JAMA 262:2551–2556, 1989

Farlow M, Gracon SI, Hershey LA, et al: A controlled trial of tacrine in Alzheimer's disease. JAMA 268:2523–2529, 1992

Faulstich ME: Psychiatric aspects of AIDS. Am J Psychiatry 144:551–556, 1987

Feil N: Validation therapy. Geriatr Nurs 13:129–133, 1992

Feltner DE, Hertzman M: Progress in the treatment of tardive dyskinesia: theory and practice. Hosp Community Psychiatry 33:25–34, 1993

Fernandez F, Levy JK, Galizzi H: Response of HIV-related depression to psychostimulants: case reports. Hosp Community Psychiatry 39:628–631, 1988a

Fernandez F, Adams F, Levy JK: Cognitive impairment of AIDS-related complex and its response to psychostimulants. Psychosomatics 28:38–46, 1988b

Fielding S, Cornfeldt ML, Szewczak MR, et al: HP-029, a new drug for the treatment of Alzheimer's disease: its pharmacological profile. Paper presented at IV World Congress on Clinical Pharmacology and Therapeutics, West Berlin, July, 1989

Fields WS, Lemak NA, Frankowski RF, et al: Controlled trial of aspirin in cerebral ischemia II. Surgical group. Stroke 18:325–334, 1987

Filip V, Vachek J, Albrecht V, et al: Pharmacokinetics and tolerance of 7-methoxytacrine following the single dose administration in healthy volunteers. Int J Clin Pharmacol Ther Toxicol 29:431–436, 1991

Filley CM, Heaton RK, Rosenberg NL: White matter dementia in chronic toluene abuse. Neurology 40:532–534, 1990

Fillit HM, Kemeny E, Luine V, et al: Antivascular antibodies in the sera of patients with senile dementia of the Alzheimer's type. J Gerontol 42:180–184, 1987

Fillit H, Ding W, Buee L, et al: Elevated circulating tumor necrosis factor levels in Alzheimer's disease. Neurosci Lett 129:318–320, 1991

Finch CE: Catecholamine metabolism in the brains of aging mice. Brain Res 52:261–276, 1973

Fine A, Dunnett SB, Bjorkland A, et al: Cholinergic ventral forebrain grafts into the neocortex improve passive avoidance memory in a rat model of Alzheimer's disease. Proc Natl Acad Sci U S A 82:5227–5229, 1985

Finkel MJ, Halperin JJ: Nervous system Lyme borreliosis revisited. Arch Neurol 49:102–107, 1992

Fischhof PK, Saletu B, Ruether E, et al: Therapeutic efficacy of pyritinol in patients with SDAT and MID. Neuropsychobiology 26:65–70, 1992

Fishbain DA, Rotundo D: Frequency of hypoglycemic delirium in a psychiatry emergency service. Psychosomatics 29:346–348, 1988

Fisher JW: Legal aspects of the psychosocial management of the demented patient. Psychiatric Annals 24:197–201, 1994

Fisher LJ, Raymon HK, Gage FH: Cells engineered to produce acetylcholine: therapeutic potential for Alzheimer's disease. Ann N Y Acad Sci 695:278–84, 1993a

Fisher LJ, Heldman E, Gurwitz D, et al: Selecting signaling via unique M1 muscarinic agonists. Ann N Y Acad Sci 695:300–303, 1993b

Fitzgerald GA: Dipyridamole. N Engl J Med 316:1247–1257, 1987

Flynn DD, Weinstein DA, Mash DC: Loss of high-affinity agonist binding to M1 muscarinic receptors in Alzheimer's disease: implications for the failure of cholinergic replacement therapies. Ann Neurol 29:256–262, 1991

Folsom CF: Mental diseases, in A System of Practical Medicine. Edited by Pepper W, Starr L. Philadelphia, PA, Lea Bros, 1886, pp 99–104

Folstein MF, McHugh PR: Dementia syndrome of depression, in Alzheimer's Disease: Senile Dementia and Related Disorders. Edited by Terry RD, Bick KL. New York, Raven, 1978, pp 87–93

Folstein MF, Folstein SE, McHugh PR: Mini-mental State: a practical method for grading the cognitive state of patients for the clinician. J Psychiatr Res 12:189–198, 1975

Folstein MF, Bassett SS, Anthony JC, et al: Dementia: case ascertainment in a community survey. J Gerontol 46:M132–M138, 1991

Foote SL, Bloom FE, Aston-Jones G: Nucleus locus ceruleus: new evidence of anatomic and physiologic specificity. Physiol Rev 63:844–914, 1983

Forette F, Henry JF, Orgogozo JM, et al: Reliability of clinical criteria for the diagnosis of dementia: a longitudinal multicenter study. Arch Neurol 46:646–648, 1989

Fornazzari L, Wilkinsin DA, Kapur BM, et al: Cerebellar, cortical and functional impairment in toluene abusers. Acta Neurol Scand 67:319–329, 1983

F"rstl H, Burns A, Luthert P, et al: The Lewy-body variant of Alzheimer's disease: clinical and pathological findings. Br J Psychiatry 162:385–392, 1993

Foster JR: Use of lithium in elderly psychiatric patients: a review of the literature. Lithium 3:77–93, 1992

Foster NL, Chase TN, Fedio P, et al: Alzheimer's disease: focal cortical changes shown by positron emission tomography. Neurology 33:961–965, 1983

Fovall P, Dysken MW, Davis JM: Treatment of Alzheimer's disease with choline salts, in Alzheimer's Disease. Edited by Reisberg B. New York, Free Press, 1983, pp 346–352

Francis PT, Cross AJ, Bowen DM: Neurotranmitters and neuropeptides, in Alzheimer Disease. Edited by Terry RD, Katzman R, Bick KL. New York, Raven, 1994, pp 247–261

Fraser CL, Arieff AI: Metabolic encephalopathy as a complication of renal failure: mechanisms and mediators. New Horizons 2:518–526, 1994

Fraser P, Nguyen JT, Inouye H, et al: Alpha 1-antichymotrypsin binding to Alzheimer's A beta peptides is sequence specific and induces fibril disaggregation in vitro. J Neurochem 61:298–305, 1993

Freeman SE, Dawson RM: Tacrine: a pharmacological review. Prog Neurobiol 36:257–277, 1991

Freud A: The Ego and the Mechanisms of Defense. New York, International Universities Press, 1946

Frieden PM, Walus LR, Watson P, et al: Blood-brain barrier penetration and in vivo activity of an NGF conjugate. Science 259:373–377, 1993

Friedland RP: Alzheimer's disease, clinical and biological heterogeneity. Ann Intern Med 109:298–311, 1988

Friedland RP: "Normal"-pressure hydrocephalus and the saga of treatable dementias. JAMA 262:2577–2581, 1989

Friedland RP: Epidemiology, education, and the ecology of Alzheimer's disease. Neurology 43:246–249, 1993

Friedland RP, Brun A, Budinger TF: Pathological and positron emission tomographic correlations in Alzheimer's disease (letter). Lancet 1:228, 1985

Friedman E, Sherman KA, Ferris SH, et al: Clinical response to choline plus piracetam in senile dementia: relation to red-cell choline levels. N Engl J Med 304:1490–1491, 1981

Friedman JH, Lannon MC: Clozapine in the treatment of psychosis in Parkinson's disease. Neurology 39:1219–1221, 1989

Frisoni GB, Govoni S, Geroldi C, et al: Gene dose of the E4 allele of alipoprotein E and disease progression in sporadic late-onset Alzheimer's disease. Ann Neurol 35:596–604, 1995

Fryer JH: Studies of body composition in men aged 60 and over, in Biological Aspects of Aging. Edited by Shock NW. New York, Columbia University Press, 1962

Gabuzda DH, Levy SR, Chiappa KH: Electroencephalography in AIDS and AIDS-related complex. Clin Electroencephalogr 19:1–6, 1988

Gajdusek DC, Gibbs CJ Jr, Alpers M: Experimental transmission of a kuru-like syndrome to chimpanzees. Nature 209:794–796, 1966

Games D, Adams D, Alessandrini R, et al: Alzheimer-type neuropathology in transgenic mice overexpressing V717F β-amyloid precursor protein. Nature 373:523–527, 1995

Gandy S, Czernik AJ, Greengard P: Phosphorylation of Alzheimer disease amyloid precursor protein peptide by protein kinase C and Ca2+ +/calmodulin-dependent protein kinase II. Proc Natl Acad Sci U S A 85:6218–6221, 1988

Garcia CA, Reding MJ, Blass JP: Overdiagnosis of dementia. J Am Geriatr Soc 29:407–410, 1981

Gardos G, Cole JO, Salomon M, et al: Clinical forms of severe tardive dyskinesia. Am J Psychiatry 144:895–902, 1986

Gatti G, Barzaghi N, Acuto G, et al. A comparative study of free plasma choline levels following intramuscular administration of L alpha glycerylphosphorylcholine and citicoline in normal volunteers. Int J Clin Pharmacol Ther Toxicol 30:331–5, 1992

Gauthier S, Leblanc R, Quirion R, et al: Transmitter-replacement therapy in Alzheimer's disease using intracerebroventricular infusions of receptor agonists. Can J Neurol Sci 13:394–402, 1986

Gauthier S, Bouchard R, Lamontagne A, et al: Tetrahydroaminoacridine-lecithin combination treatment in patients with intermediate-stage Alzheimer's disease. N Engl J Med 323:1272–1276, 1990

Gearing M, Mirra SS, Hedreen JC, et al: The Consortium to Establish a Registry for Alzheimer's Disease (CERAD); part X: neuropathology confirmation of the clinical diagnosis of Alzheimer's disease. Neurology 45:461–466, 1994

Gelenberg AJ, Van Putten T, Lavori PW, et al: Anticholinergic effects on memory: benztropine versus amantadine. J Clin Psychopharmacol 9:180–185, 1989

Gemmell HG, Sharp EF, Evans NTS et al: Single photon emission tomography with I-123 isopropylamphetamine in Alzheimer's disease and multi-infarct dementia (letter). Lancet 2:1348, 1984

Gent M, Blakely JA, Easton JD: The Canadian American Ticlopidine Study (CATS) in thromboembolic stroke. Lancet 1:1215–1220, 1989

Gentleman SM, Graham DI, Roberts GW: Molecular pathology of head trauma: altered β APP metabolism and the aetiology of Alzheimer's disease, in Progress in Brain Research. Edited by Kogure K, Hossmann K-A, Siesjo BK. New York, Elsevier, 1993, pp 237–246

George LK: The Dynamics of Caregiver Burden. Final report submitted to the AARP Andrus Foundation, December 1984

George LK, Gwyther LP: Caregiver well-being: a multidimensional examination of family caregivers of demented adults. Gerontologist 26:253–259, 1986

Georgotas A, McCue RE, Cooper T, et al: Clinical predictors of response to antidepressants in elderly patients. Biol Psychiatry 22:733–740, 1987a

Georgotas A, McCue RE, Friedman E, et al: Response of depressive symptoms to nortriptyline, phenelzine and placebo. Br J Psychiatry 151:102–106, 1987b

Gerdner LA: The effects of individualized music on elderly patients who are confused and agitated. Unpublished master's thesis, University of Iowa, Iowa City, IA, 1992

German DC, White CL III, Sparkman DR: Alzheimer's disease: neurofibrillary tangles in nuclei that project to the cerebral cortex. Neuroscience 21:305–312, 1987

Gerner RH: Geriatric depression and treatment with trazodone. Psychopathology 20:82–91, 1987

Gershon S: The use of lithium salts in psychiatric disorders. Diseases of the Nervous System 29:51–62, 1968

Gerson SC, Plotkin DA, Jarvik LF: Antidepressant drug studies, 1964 to 1985: empirical evidence for aging patients. J Clin Psychopharmacol 8:311–322, 1988

Gerson SL: Clozapine-deciphering the risks. N Engl J Med 329:204–205, 1993

Geula C, Mesulam M-M: Cholinergic systems and related neuropathological predilection patterns in Alzheimer's disease, in Alzheimer's Disease. Edited by Terry RD, Katzman R, Bick KL. New York, Raven, 1994, pp 263–291

Gibbs CJ Jr, Gajdusek GC, Asher DM, et al: Creutzfeldt-Jakob disease (spongiform encephalopathy): transmission to the chimpanzee. Science 161:388–389, 1968

Gibbs CV, Joy A, Heffner R, et al: Clinical and pathological features and laboratory confirmation of Creutzfeldt-Jakob disease in a recipient of pituitary derived growth hormone. N Engl J Med 313:734–738, 1985

Gillen RW, Golden CG, Eyde, DR: Use of Luria-Nebraska Neuropsychological Battery with elderly populations. Clinical Gerontologist 1:3–21, 1983

Gilley DW: Behavioral and affective disturbances in Alzheimer's disease, in Neuropsychology of Alzheimer's Disease and Other Dementias. Edited by Parks RW, Zec RF, Wilson RS. New York, Oxford University Press, 1993, pp 112–137

Giurgea CE: Vers une pharmacologie de l'activite integrative du cerveaux. Tentative du concept nootrope en psychopharmacologie. Acta Pharmacologica (Paris) 25:115–157, 1972

Glass D, Singer J: Urban Stress: Experiments in Noise and Social Stressors. New York, Academic Press, 1972

Glass JD, Wesselingh SL, Selnes OA, et al: Clinical-neuropathologic correlation in HIV-associated dementia. Neurology 43:2230–2237, 1993

Glenner GG, Wong CW: Alzheimer's disease: initial report or the purification and characterization of a novel cerebrovascular amyloid protein. Biochem Biophys Res Commun 120:885–890, 1984

Gnaedinger N: Housing Alzheimer's Disease at Home. Toronto, Canada, Canada Housing and Mortgage Corporation, 1989

Goedert M: Tau protein and the neurofibrillar pathology of Alzheimer's disease. Trends Neurosci 16:460, 1993

Gold K, Rabins PV: Isolated visual hallucinations and the Charles Bonnet syndrome: a review of the literature and presentation of six cases. Compr Psychiatry 30:90–98, 1989

Golden CJ: The value of neuropsychological testing to the physician. S D J Med 29:9–11, 1976

Golden CJ, Purisch AD, Hammeke TA: Luria-Nebraska Psychological Battery: Forms I and II (Manual). Los Angeles, CA, Western Psychological Services, 1985

Golden CJ, Strider MA, Ariel R, et al: Neuropsychology and medical disorders, in Handbook of Clinical Neuropsychology, Vol 2. Edited by Filskove SB, Boll TJ. New York, Wiley, 1986, pp 257–278

Goldgaber D, Lerman MI, McBride OW, et al: Characterization and chromosomal localization of a cDNA encoding brain amyloid of Alzheimer's disease. Science 235:877–880, 1987

Goldgaber D, Goldfarb L, Brown P, et al: Mutations in familial Creutzfeldt-Jakob disease and Gerstmann-Straussler-Scheinker syndrome. Exp Neurol 106:204–206, 1989

Goldin S, MacDonald JE: The Ganser state. J Ment Sci 101:267–280, 1955

Goldmeier D, Hay P: A review and update on adult syphilis, with particular reference to treatment. Int J STD AIDS 4:70–82, 1993

Goldstein K: After Effects of Brain Injuries in War. New York, Grune & Stratton, 1942

Golombok S, Moodley P, Lader M: Cognitive impairment in long-term benzodiazepine users. Psychol Med 18:365–374, 1988

Goodglass H, Kaplan E: The Assessment of Aphasia and Related Disorders. Philadelphia, PA, Lea & Febiger, 1972

Gottfries CG, Roos BE, Winblad B: Monoamine and monoamine metabolites in the human brain post mortem in senile dementia. Aktuelle Gerontologie 6:429–435, 1976

Gottfries CG, Adolfsson R, Aquilonius SM, et al: Biochemical changes in dementia disorders of the Alzheimer type (AD/SDAT). Neurobiol Aging 4:261–271, 1983

Gouvier WD, Maxfield MW, Schweitzer JR: Psychometric prediction of driving performance among the disabled. Arch Phys Med Rehabil 70:745–750, 1989

Granacher RP, Baldessarini RJ: The usefulness of physostigmine in neurology and psychiatry, in Clinical Neuropharmacology, Vol 1. Edited by Klawans HL. New York, Raven, 1976

Granato JE, Stern BJ, Ringel A, et al: Neuroleptic malignant syndrome: successful treatment with dantrolene and bromocriptine. Ann Neurol 14:89–90, 1983

Granholm E, Jeste DV: Cognitive impairment in schizophrenia. Psychiatric Annals 24:484–490, 1994

Gray F, Gherardi R, Marshall A, et al: Adult polyglucosan body disease (APBD). Neuropathology and Experimental Neurology 47:459–474, 1988

Green RC, Goldstein FC, Auchus AP, et al: Treatment trial of oxiracetam in Alzheimer's disease. Arch Neurol 49:1135–1136, 1992

Greenamyre JT, Young AB: Review: excitatory amino acids and Alzheimer's disease. Neurobiol Aging 10:593–602, 1989

Greenberg AS, Coleman M: Depressed 5-hydroxyindole associated with hyperactive and aggressive behavior. Arch Gen Psychiatry 33:331–336, 1976

Greendyke RM, Kanter DR: Therapeutic effects of pindolol on behavioural disturbances associated with organic brain disease: a double-blind study. J Clin Psychiatry 47:423–426, 1986

Greendyke RM, Schuster DB, Wooten JA: Propranolol in the treatment of assaultive patients with organic brain disease. J Clin Psychopharmacol 4:282–285, 1984

Greenwald BS, Mathe AA, Mohs RC, et al: Cortisol and Alzheimer's disease; II: dexamethasone suppression, dementia severity, and affective symptoms. Am J Psychiatry 143:442–446, 1986

Greenwald BS, Kramer-Ginsberg E, Marin DB, et al: Dementia with coexistent major depression. Am J Psychiatry 146:1472–1478, 1989

Griffin WS, Stanley LC, Ling C, et al: Brain interleukin 1 and S-100 immunoreactivity are elevated in Down syndrome and Alzheimer disease. Proc Natl Acad Sci U S A 86:7611–7615, 1989

Gronwall DM: A paced auditory serial addition task: a measure of recovery from concussion. Percept Mot Skills 44:367–373, 1977

Gross JS, Weintraub NT, Neufeld RR, et al: Pernicious anemia in the demented patient without anemia or macrocytosis: a case for early recognition. J Am Geriatr Soc 34:612–614, 1986

Growdon JH, Corkin S, Huff FJ, et al: Piracetam combined with lecithin in the treatment of Alzheimer's disease. Neurobiol Aging 7:269–276, 1986

Gueldner SH, Spradley J: Outdoor walking lowers fatigue. Journal of Gerontologic Nursing 14:6–12, 1988

Guilleminault C, Eldridge FL, Dement WC: Insomnia with sleep apnea: a new syndrome. Science 181:856–858, 1973

Gurian B, Rosowsky E: Methylphenidate treatment of minor depression in very old patients. Am J Geriatr Psychiatry 1:171–174, 1993

Gusella JF, Wexler NS, Conneally PM, et al: A polymorphic DNA marker genetically linked to Huntington's disease. Nature 306:234–238, 1983

Gusella JF, MacDonald ME, Ambrose CM, et al: Molecular genetics of Huntington's disease. Arch Neurol 50:1157–1163, 1993

Gustafson Y, Berggren D, Brannstrom B, et al: Acute confusional states in elderly patients treated for femoral neck fracture. J Am Geriatr Soc 36:525–530, 1988

Gutteridge JMC, Westermarck T, Halliwell B: Oxygen radical damage in biological systems, in Free Radicals, Aging and Degenerative Diseases, Modern Aging Research, Vol 8. Edited by Johnson JE, Walford R, Harman D, et al. New York, Alan R Liss, 1986, pp 99–139

Guy W: ECDEU Assessment Manual for Psychopharmacology (DHEW Publ No ADM-76-388). Washington, DC, U.S. Department of Health, Education and Welfare, 1976

Haass C, Selkoe DJ: Cellular processing of β-amyloid precursor protein and the genesis of amyloid β-peptide. Cell 75:1039–1042, 1993

Haass C, Schlossmacher MG, Hung AY, et al: Amyloid beta peptide is produced by cultured cells during normal metabolism. Nature 359:322–325, 1992

Hachinski VC, Lassen NA, Marshall J: Multi-infarct dementia, a cause of mental deterioration in the elderly. Lancet 2:207–210, 1978

Hachinski VC, Potter P, Merskey H: Leuko-araiosis. Arch Neurol 44:21–23, 1987

Hales RE, Silver JM, Yudofsky SC: Beta-blocking agents and the treatment of aggresssion, in Alzheimer's Disease: Treatment and Long-Term Management. Edited by Cummings JL, Miller BL. New York, Marcel Dekker, 1990, pp 109–123

Haley WE, Brown SL, Levine EG: Family caregiver appraisals of patient behavioral disturbance in senile dementia. Aging and Human Development 25:25–33, 1987

Hall G: Challenges in feeding patients with chronic dementia. Clinical Applied Nutrition 1:1795–1802, 1991

Hall GH: Caring for people with Alzheimer's disease using the conceptual model of progressively lowered stress threshold in the clinical setting. Nurs Clin North Am 29:129–141, 1994

Hall GR, Buckwalter KC: Progresively lowered stress threshold: a model for care of adults with Alzheimer's disease. Arch Psychiatr Nurs 1:399–406, 1987

Hall G, Kirschling M, Todd S: Sheltered Freedom: a special care unit in an ICF. Geriatric Nursing 7:132–136, 1986

Hallak M, Giacobini E: A comparison of the effects of two inhibitors on brain cholinesterase. Neuropharmacology 26:521–530, 1987

Hammerstrom DC, Zimmer B: The role of lumbar puncture in the evaluation of dementia: the University of Pittsburgh study. J Am Geriatr Soc 33:397–400, 1985

Hamos JE, DeGennaro LJ, Drachman DA: Synaptic loss in Alzheimer's disease and other dementias. Neurology 39:355–361, 1989

Hansen L, Salmon D, Galasko D, et al: The Lewy body variant of Alzheimer's disease: a clinical and pathologic entity. Neurology 40:1–8, 1990

Harbaugh RE: Intracerebroventricular bethanecol administration in Alzheimer's disease: preliminary results of a double-blind study. Journal of Neurotransmission 24:271–277, 1987

Hardy JA, Higgins GA: Alzheimer's disease: the amyloid cascade hypothesis. Science 256:184–185, 1992

Haroutunian V, Kanof PD, Davis KL: Pharmacologic alleviation of cholinergic lesion induced memory deficits in rats. Life Sci 37:945–952, 1985

Haroutunian V, Kanof PD, Tsuboyama G, et al: Restoration of cholinomimetic activity by clonidine in cholinergic plus adrenergic lesioned rats. Brain Res 507:251–256, 1990

Harrison PJ, Barton AJL, Proctor AW, et al: The effects of Alzheimer's disease, other dementias, and premortem course on beta-amyloid precursor protein messenger RNA in frontal cortex. J Neurochem 62:635–644, 1994

Harrow M, Amdur MJ: Guilt and depressive disorders. Arch Gen Psychiatry 25:240–246, 1971

Hartvig P, Askmark H, Aquilonius SM, et al: Clinical pharmacokinetics of intravenous and oral 9 amino 1,2,3,4 tetrahydroacridine, tacrine. Eur J Clin Pharmacol 38:259–263, 1990

Harwart D: The treatment of chronic cerebrovascular insufficiency: a double-blind study with pentoxyphylline ("Trental" 400). Curr Med Res Opin 6:73–84, 1979

Hass WK, Easton JD, Adams HP Jr: A randomized trial comparing ticlopidine hydrochloride with aspirin for the prevention of strokes in high-risk patients. N Engl J Med 321:501–507, 1989

Hathaway SR, McKinley JC: Manual for Administration and Scoring the Minnesota Multiphasic Personality Inventory—2. Minneapolis, MN, The University of Minnesota Press, 1989

Haupt M, Kurz A: Reversibility of dementia in hypothyroidism. J Neurol 240:333–335, 1993

Haxby JV, Grady CL, Koss E, et al: Heterogeneous anterior posterior metabolic patterns in dementia of the Alzheimer type. Neurology 38:1853–1863, 1988

Hayden MR, Martin WRW, Stoessl AJ, et al: Positron emission tomography in the early diagnosis of Huntington's disease. Neurology 36:888–894, 1986

Hayes PE, Kristoff CA: Adverse reactions to five new antidepressants. Clin Pharm 5:471–480, 1986

Hayman MA, Adams R: Capgras' syndrome and cerebral dysfunction. Br J Psychiatry 130:68–71, 1977

Health Care Financing Administration: Medicare and Medicaid: requirements for long term care facilities. Federal Register 56:48865–48921, September 26, 1991

Health Care Financing Administration: State Operations Manual. Baltimore, MD, United States Department of Health and Human Services, 1992

Heaton RK: Wisconsin Card Sorting Test Manual. Odessa, FL, Psychological Assessment Resources, 1981

Heaton RK, Grant I, Matthews CG: Differences in neuropsychological test performance associated with age, education, and sex, in Neuropsychological Assessment of Neuropsychiatric Disorders. Edited by Grant I, Adams KM. New York, Oxford University Press, 1986, pp 13–32

Heaton RK, Grant K, Matthews CG: Comprehensive Norms for an Expanded Halstead-Reitan Battery: Demographic Corr Sections, Research Findings, and Clinical Applications. Odessa, FL, Psychological Assessment Resources, 1991

Heaton RK, Grant I, Butters N, et al: The HNRC 500 neuropsychology of HIV infection at different disease stages. J Int Neuropsych Soc 1:231–251, 1995

Hector M, Burton JR: What are the psychiatric manifestations of vitamin B_{12} deficiency? J Am Geriatr Soc 36:1105–1112, 1988

Hefti F: Nerve growth factor promotes survival of septal cholinergic neurons after fimbrial transsections. J Neurosci 6:2155–2162, 1986

Heilman KM, Valenstein E (eds): Clinical Neuropsychology. New York, Oxford University Press, 1985

Heinonen O, Soininen H, Syrjanen S, et al: β-Amyloid protein immunoreactivity in skin is not a reliable marker of Alzheimer's disease. Arch Neurol 51:799–804, 1994

Heiss WD, Kessler J, Slansky I, et al: Activiation PET as an instrument to determine therapeutic efficacy in Alzheimer's disease. Ann N Y Acad Sci 695:327–331, 1993

Hellen C: Eating: an Alzheimer's activity. American Journal of Alzheimer's Care and Related Disorders and Research 5:5–9, 1990

Hellman RS, Tikofsky RS, Collier BD, et al. Alzheimer disease: quantitative analysis of I-123-iodoamphetamine SPECT brain imaging. Radiology 172:183–188, 1989

Henderson VW, Paganini-Hill A, Emanuel CK, et al: Estrogen replacement therapy in older women: comparison between Alzheimer's disease cases and nondemented control subjects. Arch Neurol 51:896–900, 1993

Hernandez M, Miller J: How to reduce falls. Geriatric Nursing 7:97–102, 1986

Herr SS, Hopkins BL: Health care decision making for persons with disabilities: an alternative to guardianship. JAMA 271:1017–1022, 1994

Herrmann N, Eryavec G: Buspirone in the management of agitation and aggression associated with dementia. Am J Geriatr Psychiatry 1:249–253, 1993

Herting RL: Milacemide and other drugs active at glutamate NMDA receptors as potential treatment for dementia. Ann N Y Acad Sci 640:237–240, 1991

Hestad K, McArthur JH, Dal Pan GJ, et al: Regional brain atrophy in HIV-1 infection: association with specific neuropsychological test performance. Acta Neurol Scand 88:112–118, 1993

Heston L, White JA, Mastri R: Pick's disease: clinical genetics and natural history. Arch Gen Psychiatry 44:409–411, 1987

Hewick DS, Newbury PA: Age: its influence on lithium dosage and plasma levels (letter). Br J Clin Pharmacol 3:354, 1976

Heyman A, Wilkinson WE, Heyden S, et al: Risk of stroke in asymptomatic persons with cervical arterial bruits. N Engl J Med 302:838–841, 1980

Heyman A, Wilkinson WE, Hurwitz BJ, et al: Early onset Alzheimer's disease: clinical predictors of institutionalization and death. Neurology 37:980–984, 1987

Hiatt LG: Environmental design and memory impaired older people, in A Guidebook for Long Term Care Providers. Edited by Altman HJ. Phoenix, AZ, Alzheimer's Disease and Related Disorders Association, Phoenix Chapter, 1987a

Hiatt LG: Environmental design and mentally impaired older people, in Alzheimer's Disease: Problems, Prospects and Perspectives. New York, Plenum, 1987b

Higgins LS, Rodems JM, Catalano R: Early Alzheimer disease-like histopathology increases in frequency with aqe in mice transgenic for β-APP751. Proc Natl Acad Sci USA 92:4402–4406, 1995

Hinds TR, Kukull WA, Vanbelle G, et al: Relationship between serum alpha 1-antichymotrypsin and Alzheimer's disease. Neurobiol Aging 15:21–27, 1994

Hof P, Morrison JH: The cellular basis of cortical disconnection in Alzheimer disease and related dementing conditions, in Alzheimer Disease. Edited by Terry RD, Katzman R, Bick KL. New York, Raven, 1994, pp 197–229

Hof PR, Bouras C, Perl DP: Age-related distribution of neuropathologic changes in the cerebral cortex of patients with Down's syndrome. Arch Neurol 52:379–391, 1995

Hofman A, Schulte W, Tanja TA, et al: History of dementia and Parkinson's disease in 1st-degree relatives of patients with Alzheimer's disease. Neurology 39:1589–1592, 1989

Holden U: Neuropsychology and Aging. New York, University Press, 1988

Hollander E, Davidson M, Mohs RC, et al: RS 86 in the treatment of Alzheimer's disease: cognitive and biological effects. Biol Psychiatry 22:1067–1079, 1987

Holman B: Perfusion and receptor SPECT in the dementias. J Nucl Med 27:855–860, 1986

Holton A, George K: The use of lithium in severely demented patients with behavioral disturbance. Br J Psychiatry 146:99–100, 1985

Hom J: General and specific cognitive dysfunctions in patients with Alzheimer's disease. Arch Clin Neuropsychol 7:121–133, 1992

Hom J: Brain tumors and dementia, in Neuropsychology of Alzheimer's Disease and Other Dementias. Edited by Parks RW, Zec RF, Wilson RS. New York, Oxford University Press, 1993, pp 210–234

Honer WG, Prohovnik I, Smith G, et al: Scopolamine reduces frontal cortex perfusion. J Cereb Blood Flow Metab 8:635–641, 1989

Honer WG, Dickson DW, Gleeson J, et al: Regional synaptic pathology in Alzheimer's disease. Neurobiol Aging 13:375–382, 1992

Houlihan DJ, Mulsant BH, Sweet RA, et al: A naturalistic study of trazodone in the treatment of behavioral complications of dementia. Am J Geriatric psychiatry 2:78–85, 1994

Hsiao KK, Scott M, Foster D, et al: Spontaneous neurodegeneration in transgenic mice with mutant prion protein. Science 250:1587–1596, 1990

Hsu RS, Di Leo EM, Chesson SM: Determination of HP 749, a potential therapeutic agent for Alzheimer's disease, in plasma by high-performance liquid chromatography. J Chromatography 572:352–359, 1991

Huber SJ, Shuttleworth EC: Neuropsychological assessment of subcortical dementia, in Subcortical Dementia. Edited by Cummings J. New York, Oxford University Press, 1990, pp. 71–86

Huff FJ, Antuono P, Murphy M, et al: Potential clinical use of an adrenergic/cholinergic agent (HP 128) in the treatment of Alzheimer's disease. Ann N Y Acad Sci 640:263–267, 1991

Hughes CP, Berg L, Danziger WL: A new clinical scale for the staging of dementia. Br J Psychiatry 140:566–572, 1982

Hughes JR, Williams JG, Currier RD: An ergot alkaloid preparation (Hydergine) in the treatment of dementia: critical review of the clinical literature. J Am Geriatr Soc 24:490–497, 1976

Hunt E: Experimental perspectives: theoretical memory models, in Handbook for Clinical Memory Assessment of Older Adults. Edited by Poon LW. Washington, DC, American Psychological Association, 1986, pp 43–54

Hunt L, Morris JC, Edwards D, Wilson BS: Driving performance in persons with mild senile dementia of the Alzheimer type. J Am Geriatr Soc 41:747–753, 1993

Husain MM, Nemeroff CB: Neuropeptides and Alzheimer's disease. J Am Geriatr Soc 38:918–925, 1990

Hussian R, Brown D: Use of two-dimensional grid patterns to limit hazardous ambulation in demented patients. J Gerontol 42:558–560, 1987

Hussian RA, Davis RL: Responsive Care: Behavioral Interventions with Elderly Persons. Champaign, IL, Research Press, 1985

Hwang AS, Magraw RM: Syndrome of inappropriate secretion of antidiuretic hormone due to fluoxetine (letter). Am J Psychiatry 146:399, 1989

Hyde TM, Nawroz S, Goldberg TE, et al: Is there cognitive decline in schizophrenia? A cross-sectional study. Br J Psychiatry 164:494–500, 1994

Hyman BT, West HL, Harr SD, et al: Quantitative neuropathology in Alzheimer disease: neuronal loss in high order association cortex parallels dementia. Neurobiol Aging 15:S141, 1994

Hyman BT, West HL, Rebeck W, et al: Neuropathological changes in Down's syndrome hippocampal formation. Arch Neurol 52:373–378, 1995

Ikeda T, Yamammoto K, Takahashi K, et al: Treatment of Alzheimer-type dementia with intravenous mecobalamin. Clin Ther 14:426–437, 1992

Incalzi RA, Gemma A, Marra C, et al: Chronic obstructive pulmonary disease. An original model of cognitive decline. Am Rev Resp Dis 148:418–424, 1993

Ingvar DH, Risberg J: Increase of regional cerebral blood flow during mental effort in normals and in patients with focal brain disorders. Exp Brain Res 3:195–211, 1967

Iversen LL: Approaches to the cholinergic therapy in Alzheimer's disease. Prog Brain Res 98:423–426, 1993

Jagust WJ, Budinger TF, Reed BR: The diagnosis of dementia with single photon emission computed tomography. Arch Neurol 44:258–262, 1987

Jefferson JW, Greist JH, Ackerman DL: Lithium Encyclopedia for Clinical Practice, 2nd Edition. Washington, DC, American Psychiatric Press, 1986

Jenike MA: Treatment of rage and violence in elderly patients with propranolol. Geriatrics 38:29–34, 1983

Jenike MA: Handbook of Geriatric Psychopharmacology. Littleton, MA, PSG Publishing Company, 1985

Jenike MA, Albert MS: The dexamethasone suppression test in patients with presenile and senile dementia of the Alzheimer's type. J Am Geriatr Soc 32:441–444, 1984

Jenike MA, Albert MS, Baer L: Oral physostigmine as a treatment for Alzheimer disease: a long-term outpatient trial. Alzheimer Dis Assoc Disord 4:226–231, 1990

Jeste DV, Lohr JB: Hippocampal pathologic findings in schizophrenia: a morphometric study. Arch Gen Psychiatry 46:1019–1024, 1989

Joachim CL, Morris JH, Selkoe DJ: Clinically diagnosed Alzheimer disease: autopsy results in 150 cases. Ann Neurol 25:50–56, 1988

Joachim CL, Morris JH, Selkoe DJ: Amyloid β-protein deposition in tissues other than brain in Alzheimer's disease. Nature 341:226–230, 1989a

Joachim CL, Morris JH, Selkoe DJ: Diffuse senile plaques occur commonly in the cerebellum in Alheimer's disease. Am J Pathol 135:309–319, 1989b

Jobst KA, Hindley NJ, King E, et al: The diagnosis of Alzheimer's disease: a question of image? J Clin Psychiatry 55 (suppl 11):22–31, 1994

Johnson KA, Mueller ST, Walshe TM, et al: Cerebral perfusion imaging in Alzheimer's disease: use of single photon emission computed tomography and iofetamine hydrochloride I-23. Arch Neurol 44:165–168, 1987

Johnson S, McNeill T, Cordell B, et al: Relation of neuronal APP-751/APP-695 mRNA ratio and neuritic plaque density in Alzheimer's disease. Science 248:854–857, 1990

Jolles J: Neuropeptides and the treatment of cognitive deficits in aging and dementia. Prog Brain Res 70:429–441, 1986

Jones RW, Wesnes KA, Kirby J: Effects of NMDA modulation in scopolamine dementia. Ann N Y Acad Sci 640:241–244, 1991

Jose CJ, Barton JR, Perez-Cruet J: Hyponatremic seizures in psychiatric patients. Biol Psychiatry 14:839–843, 1979

Joyce EM, Levy R: Treatment of mood disorder associated with Binswanger's disease. Br J Psychiatry 154:259–261, 1989

Kahn D, Stevenson E, Douglas CJ: Effect of sodium valproate in three patients with organic brain syndromes. Am J Psychiatry 145:1010–1011, 1988

Kahana B, Kahana J: Stress reactions, in Clinical Geropsychology: New Directions in Assessment and Treatment. Edited by Lewinsohn PW, Teri L. New York, Pergamon, 1983

Kaplitz SE: Withdrawn, apathetic geriatric patients responsive to methylphenidate. J Am Geriatr Soc 23:271–276, 1975

Karlinsky H, Schulman K: The clinical use of ECT in old age. J Am Geriatr Soc 32:183–186, 1984

Kaszniak AW, Poon LW, Riege W: Assessing memory deficits: an information-processing approach, in Handbook for Clinical Memory Assessment of Older Adults. Edited by Poon LW. Washington, DC, American Psychological Association, 1986, pp 168–188

Katz IR, Simpson GM, Jethanandani V, et al: Steady state pharmacokinetics of nortriptyline in the frail elderly. Neuropsychopharmacology 2:229–236, 1989

Katzman R: Diagnosis and management of dementia, in Principles of Geriatric Neurology. Edited by Katzman R, Rowe JW. Philadelphia, Davis FA, 1992, pp 167–206

Keck PE Jr, Pope HG Jr, McElroy SL: Frequency and presentation of neuroleptic malignant syndrome: a prospective study. Am J Psychiatry 144:1344–1346, 1987

Keller H: Malnutrition in institutionalized elderly: how and why? J Am Geriatr Soc 41:1212–1218, 1993

Kety SS, Schmidt CF: The nitrous oxide method for quantitative determination of cerebral blood flow in man: theory, procedure and normal values. J Clin Invest 27:476–483, 1948

Khachaturian Z: Diagnosis of Alzheimer's disease. Arch Neurol 42:1097–1105, 1985

Kidd M: Paired helical filaments in electron microscopy of Alzheimer's disease. Nature 197:192–193, 1963

Kiloh LG: Pseudo-dementia. Acta Psychiatr Scand 37:336–351, 1961

King DA, Caine DA: Depression, in Subcortical Dementia. Edited by Cummings JL. New York, Oxford University Press, 1990, pp 218–230

Kirk A, Kertesz A: On drawing impairment in Alzheimer's disease. Arch Neurology 48:73–77, 1991

Kisilevsky R, Lemieux LJ, Fraser PE, et al: Arresting amyloidosis in vivo using small-molecule anionic sulphonates or sulphates; implications for Alzheimer's disease. Nature Medicine 1:143–148, 1995

Klein M: Envy and Gratitude. London, Tavistock, 1957

Klotz U, Avant GR, Hoyumpa A, et al: The effects of age and liver disease on disposition and elimination of diazepam in adult man. J Clin Invest 55:347–359, 1975

Knapp MJ, Knopman DS, Solomon PR, et al: A 30-week randomized controlled trial of high-dose tacrine in patients with Alzheimer's disease. JAMA 271:985–991, 1994

Knoll J: The pharmacological profile of (-)Deprenyl (Selegiline) and its relevance for humans: a personal review. Pharmacol Toxicol 70:317–324, 1992

Kochansky GE: Psychiatric rating scales for assessing psychopathology in the elderly: a critical review, in Psychiatric Symptoms and Cognitive Loss in the Elderly. Edited by Raskin A, Jarvik LF. New York, Wiley, 1979, pp 125–156

Koelle GB, Koelle WA, Smyrl EG, et al: Histochemical and pharmacological evidence of the function of butyrylcholin- esterase, in Cholinergic Mechanisms and Psychopharmacology. Edited by Jenden DJ. New York, Plenum, 1977, pp 125–137

Koelle GB, Massoulie J, Eugene D, et al: Distribution of the molecular forms of acetylcholinesterase and butyryl-cholinesterase in nervous tissue of the cat. Proc Natl Acad Sci U S A 84:7749–7752, 1987

Koff TH: New Approaches to Health Care for an Aging Population. San Francisco, CA, Jossey-Bass, 1988

Koivisto K, Reinikainen KJ, Hanninen T, et al: Prevalence of ageassociated memory impairment in a randomly selected population from eastern Finland. Neurology 45:741–747, 1995

Kolb B, Whishaw IQ: Fundamentals of Human Neuropsychology. San Francisco, CA, WH Freeman, 1980

Koss E: Neuropsychology of aging and dementia, in Neuropsychology, Vol 15 (Handbook of Perception). Edited by Zaidel D. New York, Academic Press, 1994, pp 247–270

Koss E, Weiffenbach JM, Haxby JV, et al: Olfactory detection and identification performance are dissociated in early Alzheimer's disease. Neurology 38:1228–1232, 1988

Koss E, Haxby JV, DeCarli C, et al: Patterns of performance preservation and loss in healthy aging. Developmental Neuropsychology 7:99–113, 1991

Koss E, Patterson MB, Ownby R, et al: Memory evaluation in Alzheimer's disease: caregivers' appraisals and objective testing. Arch Neurol 50:92–97, 1993

Kovacs JA, Kovacs AA, Polis M, et al: Cryptococcosis in the acquired immunodeficiency syndrome. Ann Intern Med 103:533–538, 1985

Kraepelin E: Lectures on Clinical Psychiatry, 2nd Edition. Translated by Johnstone T. New York, William Wood, 1913

Kragh-Sorensen P, Lolk A: Neuropeptides and dementia. Prog Brain Res 72:269–277, 1987

Kral VA: Types of memory function in senescence. Psychiatr Res Rep 11:30–40, 1959

Kral VA: Benign senile forgetfulness in Alzheimer's disease, in Senile Dementia and Related Disorders. Edited by Katzman R, Terry RD, Bick KL. New York, Raven, 1978, pp 47–51

Krop HD, Block AJ, Cohen E: Neuropsychological effects of continuous oxygen therapy in chronic obstructive pulmonary disease. Chest 64:317–322, 1973

Kumar V, Smith RC, Reed K, et al: Plasma levels and effects of nortriptyline in geriatric depressed patients. Acta Psychiatr Scand 75:20–28, 1987

Kumar A, Schapiro MB, Grady CL, et al: Anatomic, metabolic, neuropsychological and molecular genetic studies of three pairs of identical twins discordant for dementia of the Alzheimer type. Arch Neurol 48:160–168, 1991

Kumar A, Gottlieb G: Frontotemporal dementias: a new clinical syndrome? Am J Geriatr Psychiatry 1:95–108, 1993

LaBarge E, Smith DS, Dick L, et al: Agraphia in dementia of the Alzheimer's type. Arch Neurol 49:1151–1156, 1992

Lachner G, Satzger W, Engel RR: Verbal memory tests in the differential diagnosis of depression and dementia: discriminative power of seven test variations. Arch Clin Neuropsychol 9:1–13, 1994

LaFerla FM, Tinkle BT, Bieberich CJ, et al: The Alzheimer's A peptide induces neurodegeneration and apoptotic cell death in transqenic mice. Nature Genetics 9:21–29, 1995

Lamberty GJ, Bieliauskas LA: Distinguishing between depression and dementia in the elderly: a review of neuropsychological findings. Arch Clin Neuropsychol 8:149–170, 1993

Larson EB, Reifler BV, Featherstone HJ, et al: Dementia in elderly outpatients: a prospective study. Ann Intern Med 100:417–423, 1984

Larson E, Kukull WA, Buchner D, et al: Adverse drug reactions associated with global cognitive impairment in elderly persons. Ann Intern Med 107:169–173, 1987

LaRue A: Research issues and neuropsychology, in Treatments for the Alzheimer Patient. Edited by Jarvik LF, Winograd CH. New York, Springer, 1988, pp 173–185

LaRue A, Spar J, Hill CD: Cognitive impairment in late-life depression: clinical correlates and treatment implications. J Affect Disord 11:179–184, 1986

Lawton MP: Ecology and Aging, in Spatial Behavior of Older People, Edited by Pastalan LA and Carson DH. Ann Arbor, MI, University of Michigan-Wayne State University Institute of Gerontology, 1970, pp 40–67

Lawton MP: Environment and Aging. Monterey, CA, Brooks Cole, 1980

Lawton MP: Sensory deprivation and the effect of the environment on management of the patient with senile dementia, in Clinical Aspects of Alzheimer's Disease and Senile Dementia, Edited by Miller N, Cohen G. New York, Raven, 1981, pp 227–250

Lawton MP: Competence, environmental press and the adaptation of older people, in Aging and the Environment: Theoretical Approaches. Edited by Lawton MP, Windley PG, Byerts TO. New York, Springer, 1982

Lawton MP: Environmental approaches to research and treatment of Alzheimer's disease, in Alzheimer's Disease, Treatment and Family Stress: Directions for Research. Edited by Light E, Lebowitz B. Washington, DC, National Institute of Mental Health, 1989, pp 340–362

Lawton MP, Nahemow L: Ecology and the aging process, in Psychology of Adult Development and Aging. Edited by Eisdorfer C, Lawton MP. Washington, DC, American Psychological Association, 1973

Lazarus R: Psychological Stress and the Coping Process. New York, McGraw-Hill, 1966

Learoyd BM: Psychotropic drugs and the elderly patient. Med J Aust 1:1131–1133, 1972

Lehrich JP: Unnamed agents of Creutzfeldt-Jakob disease and Kuru, in Principles and Practice of Infectious Disease. Edited by Mandell GC, Douglas RG, Bennett JE. New York, Wiley, 1985, pp 1041–1043

Leuchter A, Holschneider D: Quantitative electroencephalography: neurophysiological alterations in normal aging and geriatric neuropsychiatric disorders, in The American Psychiatric Press Textbook of Geriatric Neuropsychiatry. Edited by Coffey CE, Cummings JL. Washington, DC, American Psychiatric Press, 1994, pp 215–240

Levin HS, Benton AL, Grossman RG: Neurobehavioral Consequences of Closed Head Injury. New York, Oxford University Press, 1982

Levy R, Little A, Chuaqui-Kidd P, et al: Early results from double blind placebo controlled trial of high-dose phosphatidylcholine in Alzheimer's disease. Lancet 1:987–988, 1983

Levy RM, Bredesen DE, Rosenblum ML: Neurological manifestations of the acquired immune deficiency syndrome (AIDS): experience at USCF and review of the literature. J Neurosurg 62:475–495, 1985

Lewin K: Field Theory in Social Science. New York, Harper, 1951

Lewinsohn PM, Dancher BG, Kikel S: Visual imagery as a mnemonic aid for brain-injured persons. J Consult Clin Psychol 45:717–723, 1977

Lezak MD: Neuropsychological assessment, 2nd Edition. New York, Oxford University Press, 1983

Libbon DJ, Glosser G, Malamut L, et al: Age, executive functions, and visuospatial functioning in health older adults. Neuropsychology 8:38–43, 1994

Light E, Lebowitz B: Alzheimer's Disease Treatment and Family Stress: Directions for Research. Washington, DC, U.S. Department of Health and Human Services, 1989

Linden M: Group psychotherapy with institutionalized senile women. Int J Group Psychother 3:150–170, 1953

Lindvall O, Rehncrona S, Brundin P, et al: Human fetal dopamine neurons grafted into the striatum in two patients with severe Parkinson's disease. Arch Neurol 46:615–631, 1989

Lines CR, Dawson C, Preston GC, et al: Memory and attention in patients with senile dementia of the Alzheimer type and in normal elderly subjects. J Clin Exp Neuropsychol 13:691–702, 1991

Lipinski JF, Zubenko GS, Cohen BM, et al: Propranolol and the treatment of neuroleptic-induced akathisia. Am J Psychiatry 141:412–415, 1984

Lipowski ZJ: Organic mental disorders: introduction and review of syndromes, in Comprehensive Textbook of Psychiatry/III, Vol 2. Edited by Kaplan HI, Freedman AM, Sadock BJ. Baltimore, MD, Williams & Wilkins, 1980, pp 1359–1391

Lipowski ZJ: Delirium (acute confusional states). JAMA 258:1789–1792, 1987

Lipton SA, Gendelman HE: Dementia associated with the acquired immunodeficiency syndrome. N Engl J Med 332:934–939, 1995

Little A, Levy R, Chuaqui-Kidd P, et al: A double-blind, placebo-controlled trial of high-dose lecithin in Alzheimer's disease. J Neurol Neurosurg Psychiatry 48:736–742, 1985

Loew DM, Weil C: Hydergine in senile mental impairment. Gerontology 28:54–74, 1982

Luby J: Infections of the central nervous system. Am J Med Sci 304:379–391, 1992

Lucas-Blaustein MJ, Filipp L, Dungan C, et al: Driving in patients with dementia. J Am Geriatr Soc 36:1087–1091, 1988

Luft BJ, Remington JS: Toxoplasmic encephalitis in AIDS. Clin Inf Dis 15:211–222, 1992

Lund C, Sheafor ML: Is your patient about to fall? Journal of Gerontologic Nursing 11:37–41, 1985

Lynn J (ed): By No Extraordinary Means. Bloomington, IN, Indiana University Press, 1986

Lynn J, Childress JF: Must patients always be given food and water? in By No Extraordinary Means. Edited by Lynn J. Bloomington, IN, Indiana University Press, 1986, pp 47–60

Mace N, Rabins P: The 36-Hour Day: A Family Guide to Coping for Persons with Alzheimer's Disease, Related Dementing Illnesses, and Memory Loss in Later Life. Baltimore, MD, Johns Hopkins University Press, 1981 (revised edition, 1991)

MacInnes WD, Robbins DE: Brief neuropsychological assessment of memory, in Essentials of Neuropsychological Assessment. Edited by Hartlage LC, Asken MJ, Hornsby JL. New York, Springer, 1987, pp 175–196

MacInnes WD, Gillen RW, Golden CG, et al: Aging and performance on the Luria-Nebraska Neuropsychological Battery. Int J Neurosci 9:179–190, 1983

MacKeith IG, Perry RH, Fairbairn AF, et al: Operational criteria for senile dementia of Lewy body type (SDLT). Psychol Med 22:911–922, 1992

Madrazzo I, Drucker-Colin R, Diaz V, et al: Open microsurgical autograft of adrenal medulla to the right caudate nucleus in two patients with intractable Parkinson's disease. N Engl J Med 316:831–834, 1987

Mahurin RK, Feher EP, Nance ML, et al: Cognition in Parkinson's disease and related disorders, in Neuropsychology of Alzheimer's Disease and Other Dementias. Edited by Parks RW, Zec RF, Wilson RS. New York, Oxford University Press, 1993, pp 308–349

Maini CL, Pigorini F, Pau FM, et al: Cortical cerebral blood flow in HIV-1-related dementia complex. Nucl Med Commun 11:639–648, 1990

Maj M, Satz P, Janssen R, et al: WHO Neuropsychiatric aids study, cross-sectional phase; II: neuropsychological and neurological findings. Arch Gen Psychiatry 51:51–61, 1994

Maletta GJ, Winegarden T: Reversal of anorexia by methylphenidate in apathetic, severely demented nursing home patients. Am J Geriatr Psychiatry 1:234–243, 1993

Maltby N, Broe AG, Creasey H, et al: Efficacy of tacrine and lecithin in mild to moderate Alzheimer's disease: double blind trial. BMJ 308:879–883, 1994

Manaster A: Therapy with the senile geriatric patient. Int J Group Psychother 22:250–257, 1972

Maneulidis EE, DeFigueireda JM, Kim JH, et al: Transmission studies from blood of Alzheimer's disease patients and healthy relatives. Proc Natl Acad Sci U S A 85:4898–4901, 1988

Mann AH, Graham N, Ashby D: Psychiatric illness in residential homes for the elderly: a survey of one London borough. Age Ageing 13:257–265, 1984

Mann DM: The pathological association between Down syndrome and Alzheimer disease. Mech Ageing Dev 31:213–255, 1988

Mann DM, Esiri MM: The site of the earliest lesions of Alzheimer's disease (letter). N Engl J Med 318:789–790, 1988

Mann DM, Esiri MM: The pattern of acquisition of plaques and tangles in the brains of patients under 50 years of age with Down's syndrome. J Neurol Sci 89:169–179, 1989

Mann DM, Lincoln J, Yates PO, et al: Changes in the monoamine containing neurons of the human CNS in senile dementia. Br J Psychiatry 136:533–541, 1980

Mann DM, Marcyniuk B, Yates PO, et al: The progression of the pathological changes of Alzheimer's disease in frontal and temporal neocortex examined both at biopsy and at autopsy. Neuropathol Appl Neurobiol 14:177–195, 1988

Mansheim P: Treatment with propranolol of the behavioral sequelae of brain damage (letter). J Clin Psychiatry 42:132, 1981

Marcyniuk B, Mann DM, Yates PO: The topography of cell loss from locus coeruleus in Alzheimer's disease. J Neurol Sci 76:335–345, 1986

Marder SR, Meibach RC: Risperidone in the treatment of schizophrenia. Am J Psychiatry 151:825–835, 1994

Marsden CD, Harrison MJG: Outcome of investigation of patients with presenile dementia. BMJ 2:229–252, 1972

Marsden CD, Tarsey D, Baldessarini RJ: Spontaneous and drug-induced movement disorders in psychotic patients, in Psychiatric Aspects of Neurologic Disease. Edited by Benson DF, Blumer D. New York, Grune & Stratton, 1975, pp 219–265

Martignoni M, Bono G, Blandini E, et al: Monoamines and related metabolites levels in the cerebrospinal fluid of patients with dementia of Alzheimer type. Influence of treatment with l-deprenyl. J Neural Transm 3:15–25, 1991

Martin EM, Wilson RS, Penn RD, et al: Cortical biopsy results in Alzheimer's disease: correlation with cognitive deficits. Neurology 37:1201–1204, 1987

Martin PR, Adinoff B, Eckardt MJ, et al: Effective pharmacotherapy of alcoholic amnestic disorder with fluvoxamine. Arch Gen Psychiatry 46:617–621, 1989

Martyn CN, Barker DJP, Osmond C, et al: Geographical relation between Alzheimer's disease and drinking water. Lancet 1:59–62, 1989

Mash DC, Flynn DD, Potter LT: Loss of M2 muscarinic receptors in the cerebral cortex in Alzheimer's disease and experimental cholinergic denervation. Science 228:1115–1117, 1985

Masliah E, Terry RD, Mallory M, et al: Diffuse plaques do not accentuate synapse loss in Alzheimer's disease. Am J Pathol 137:1293–1297, 1990

Masliah E, Terry RD, Alford M, et al: Cortical and subcortical patterns of synaptophysin-like immunoreactivity in Alzheimer's disease. Am J Pathol 138:235–246, 1991

Massachusetts General Hospital: Case records of the Massachusetts General Hospital (Case 30-1985). N Engl J Med 313:249–257, 1985

Massey EW: Neuropsychiatric manifestations of porphyria. J Clin Psychiatry 41:208–213, 1980

Mattes JA: Metoprolol for intermittent explosive disorder. Am J Psychiatry 142:1108–1109, 1985

Mattis S: Dementia Rating Scale. Odessa, FL, Psychological Assessment Resources, 1988

Mayeux R, Stern Y, Rosen J, et al: Depression, intellectual impairment and Parkinson's disease. Neurology 31:645–650, 1981

Mayeux R, Ottman R, Maestre G, et al: Synergistic effects of traumatic head injury and apolipoprotein-E4 in patients with Alzheimer's disease. Neurology 45:555–557, 1995

Mazure CM, Druss BG, Cellar JS: Valproate treatment of older psychotic patients with organic mental syndromes and behavioral dyscontrol. J Am Geriatr Soc 40:914–916, 1992

McArthur JC, Hoover DR, Bacellar H, et al: Dementia in AIDS patients: incidence and risk factors: Multicenter AIDS Cohort Study. Neurology 43:2245–2252, 1993

McClannahan L, Risley T: Design of living environment for nursing home residents: recruiting attendance at activities. Gerontologist 14:236–240, 1974

McClosky JC, Bulechek GM (eds): Nursing Interventions Classifications (NIC). St. Louis, MO, Mosby, 1992

McCormick KA, Burgio KL: Incontinence: an update on nursing care measures. Journal of Gerontological Nursing 10:16–23, 1984

McCormick KA, Scheve AAS, Leahy E: Nursing management of urinary incontinence in geriatric inpatients. Nurs Clin North Am 23:231–264, 1988

McDonald EM, Mann AH, Thomas HC: Interferons as mediators of psychiatric morbidity. Lancet 2:1175–1177, 1987

McDonald RJ: Hydergine: a review of 26 clinical studies. Pharmacopsychiatry 12:407–422, 1979

McEntee WJ, Crook TH: Age-associated memory impairment: a role for catecholamines. Neurology 40:526–530, 1990

McEvoy JP, McCue M, Spring B, et al: Effect of amantadine and trihexyphenidyl on memory in elderly normal volunteers. Am J Psychiatry 144:573–577, 1987

McGeer PL, McGeer EG: Complement proteins and complement inhibitors in Alzheimer's disease. Res Immunol 143:621–624, 1992

McGeer PL, Kamo H, Harrop R, et al: Comparison of PET, MRI and CT with pathology in a proven case of Alzheimer's disease. Neurology 36:1569–1574, 1986

McGeer PL, Akiyama H, Itagaki S, et al: Immune system response in Alzheimer's disease. Can J Neurol Sci 16:516–527, 1989

McGeer PL, McGeer E, Rogers J, et al: Anti-inflammatory drugs and Alzheimer's disease (letter). Lancet 335:1037, 1990

McGeer PL, Rogers J, McGeer EG: Neuroimmune mechanisms in Alzheimer disease pathogenesis. Alz Dis Assoc Disord 8:149–158, 1994

McGovern RJ, Koss E: The use of behavior modification with Alzheimer patients: values and limitations. Alz Dis Assoc Disord 8(suppl 3):82–91, 1995

McKeith IG, Fairbairn AF, Bothwell RA, et al: An evaluation of the predictive validity and inter-rater reliability of clinical diagnostic criteria for senile dementia of Lewy body type. Neurology 44:872–877, 1994

McKhann G, Drachman D, Folstein M, et al: Clinical diagnosis of Alzheimer's disease: report of the NINCDS-ADRDA work group under the auspices of the Department of Health and Human Services Task Force on Alzheimer's disease. Neurology 34:939–944, 1984

McLean S, Maher G: Medicine, Morals and the Law. Aldershot, Hampshire, UK, Gower Publishing Co, 1983

Meda L, Cassatella MA, Szendrei GI, et al: Activation of microglial cells by amyloid protein and interferon-Y. Nature 374:647–650, 1995

Mehler MF, Horoupian DS, Davies P, et al: Reduced somatostatin-like immunoreactivity in cerebral cortex in nonfamilial dysphasic dementia. Neurology 37:1448–1453, 1987

Mellow AM, Solano-Lopez C, Davis S: Sodium valproate in the treatment of behavioral disturbance in dementia. J Geriatr Psychiatry Neurol 6:205–209, 1993

Melnick VL, Dubler NN: Alzheimer's Dementia: Dimensions in Human Research. Clifton, NJ, Humana Press, 1985

Mena EE, Desai MC: High affinity [3H]THA (tetrahydroaminoacridine) binding sites in rat brain. Pharmacol Res 8:200–203, 1991

Mendez MF, Ashla-Mendez M: Differences between multi-infarct dementia and Alzheimer's disease on unstructured neuropsychological tasks. J Clin Exp Neuropsychol 13:923–932, 1991

Mendez MF, Mendez MA, Martin R, et al: Complex visual disturbances in Alzheimer's disease. Neurology 40:439–443, 1990

Meneilly GS, Greenspan JL, Rowe J, et al: Endocrine systems, in Geriatric Medicine, 2nd Edition. Edited by Rowe J, Besdine RW. Boston, MA, Little Brown, 1988, pp 402–430

Menza M, Blake J, Goldberg L: Affective symptoms and adrenoleukodystrophy: a report of two cases. Psychosomatics 29:442–445, 1988

Merriam AE, Aronson MK, Gaston P, et al: The psychiatric symptoms of Alzheimer's disease. J Am Geriatr Soc 36:7–12, 1988

Mesulam M-M: Slowly progressive aphasia without generalized dementia. Ann Neurol 11:592–598, 1982

Metter EJ, Wilson RS: Vascular dementias, in Neuropsychology of Alzheimer's Disease and Other Dementias. Edited by Parks RW, Zec RF, Wilson RS. New York, Oxford University Press, 1993, pp 416–437

Metter EJ, Riege WH, Kameyama M, et al: Cerebral metabolic relationships for selected brain regions in Alzheimer's, Huntington's, and Parkinson's diseases. J Cereb Blood Flow Metab 4:500–506, 1981

Meyer JS, Rogers RL, McClintic K, et al: Randomized clinical trial of daily aspirin therapy in multi-infarct dementia: a pilot study. J Am Geriatr Soc 37:549–555, 1989

Miguel EC, Pereira RM, Pereira CA, et al: Psychiatric manifestations of systemic lupus erythematosus: clinical features, symptoms, and signs of central nervous system activity in 43 patients. Medicine 73:224–232, 1994

Mihara M, Ohnishi A, Tomono Y, et al: Pharmacokinetics of E2020, a new compound for Alzheimer's disease, in healthy male volunteers. Int J Clin Pharmacol Ther Toxicol 31:223–229, 1993

Milberg WP, Hebben N, Kaplan E: The Boston process approach to neuropsychological assessment, in Neuropsychological Assessment of Neuropsychiatric Disorders. Edited by Grant I, Adams KM. New York, Oxford University Press, 1986, pp 65–86

Miller BL, Cummings JL, Villanueva-Meyer J, et al: Frontal lobe degeneration: clinical, neuropsychological, and SPECT characteristics. Neurology 41:1374–1382, 1991

Miller RJ, Snowdon J, Vaughan R: The use of the Cohen-Mansfield agitation inventory in the assessment of behavioral disorders in nursing homes. J Am Geriatr Soc 43:546–549, 1995

Miller TP, Fong K, Tinklenberg JR: An ACTH 4-9 analog (Org 2766) and cognitive performance: high dose efficacy and safety in dementia of the Alzheimer's type. Biol Psychiatry 33:307–309, 1993

Mirra SS, Heyman A, McKeel D, et al: The consortium to establish a registry for Alzheimer's disease (CERAD); Part II: standardization of the neuropathologic assessment of Alzheimer's disease. Neurology 41:479–486, 1991

Mizuki Y, Yamada M, Kato I, et al: Effects of aniracetam, a nootropic drug, in senile dementia—a preliminary report. Kurume Med J 31:135–143, 1984

Mohr E, Schlegel J, Fabbrini G, et al: Clonidine treatment of Alzheimer's disease. Arch Neurol 46:376–378, 1989

Mohr E, Knott V, Herting RL, et al: Cycloserine treatment in Alzheimer's disease. Abstr Neuropsychopharm 9:96s–97s, 1993

Mohr E, Feldman H, Gauthier S: Canadian guidelines for the development of antidementia therapies: a conceptual summary. Can J Neurol Sci 22:62–71, 1995

Mohs RC, Davis KL: The experimental pharmacology of Alzheimer's disease and related dementias, in Psychopharmacology: Third Generation of Progress. Edited by Meltzer HY. New York, Raven, 1987, pp 921–928

Mohs RC, Rosen WG, Greenwald BS, et al: Neuropathologically validated scales for Alzheimer's disease, in Assessment in Geriatric Psychopharmacology. Edited by Crook T, Ferris S, Bartus R. New Canaan, CT, Mark Powley Associates, 1983, pp 37–46

Mohs RC, Breitner JCS, Silverman JM, et al: Alzheimer's disease: morbid risk among first-degree relatives approximates 50% by 90 years of age. Arch Gen Psychiatry 44:405–408, 1987

Monsch AU, Bondi MW, Butters N, et al: Comparisons of verbal fluency tasks in the detection of dementia of the Alzheimer type. Arch Neurol 49:1253–1258, 1992

Monsch AU, Bondi MW, Butters N, et al: A comparison of category and letter fluency in Alzheimer's disease and Huntington's disease. Neuropsychology 8:25–30, 1994

Moran PM, Higgins LS, Cordell B, et al: Age-related learning deficits in transgenic mice expressing the 751-amino acid isoform of human β-amyloid precursor protein. Proc Natl Acad Sci USA 92:5341–5345, 1995

Morris RG: Working memory in Alzheimer-type dementia. Neuropsychology 8:544–554, 1994

Morris JC, Rubin EH, Morris EJ, et al: Senile dementia of the Alzheimer's type: an important risk factor for serious falls. J Gerontol 42:412–417, 1987

Morris JC, Heyman A, Mohs RC, et al: The Consortium to Establish a Registry for Alzheimer's Disease (CERAD); Part I: clinical and neuropsychological assessment of Alzheimer's disease. Neurology 39:1159–1165, 1989

Morris JC, Cole M, Banker BQ, et al: Hereditary dysphasic dementia and the Pick-Alzheimer spectrum. Ann Neurol 16:455–466, 1994

Mortimer JA: Alzheimer's disease and senile dementia: prevalence and incidence, in Alzheimer's Disease. Edited by Reisberg B. New York, Free Press, 1983

Mortimer JA, von Duijn CM, Clayton D, et al: Head trauma as a risk factor for Alzheimer's disease: a collaborative re-analysis of case-control studies. Int J Epidemiol 20:528–535, 1991

Moser HW, Moser AE, Singh I, et al: Adrenoleukodystrophy: survey of 303 case: biochemistry, diagnosis and therapy. Ann Neurol 16:628–641, 1985

Moss MB, Albert MS: Alzheimer's disease and other dementing disorders, in Geriatric Neuropsychology. Edited by Moss MB, Albert MS. New York, Guilford, 1988, pp 145–178

Mouradian MM, Mohr E, Williams AJ, et al: No response to high-dose muscarinic agonist therapy in Alzheimer's disease. Neurology 38:606–608, 1988

Mouradian MM, Blin J, Giuffra M, et al: Somatostatin replacement therapy for Alzheimer dementia. Ann Neurol 30:610–613, 1991

Mullan M, Houlden H, Windelspecht M: A locus for familial early onset Alzheimer's disease on the long arm of chromosome 14 proximal to the alpha 1 antichymotrypsin gene. Nature Genet 2:340–343, 1992

Murphy DGM, Bottomley PA, Salerno JA, et al: An in-vivo study of phosphorus and glucose metabolism in Alzheimer's disease using magnetic resonance spectroscopy and PET. Arch Gen Psychiatry 50:341–349, 1993

Murphy MF, Hardiman ST, Nash RJ, et al: Evaluation of HP 029 (velnacrine maleate) in Alzheimer's disease. Ann N Y Acad Sci 640:253–262, 1991

Murray HA: Explorations in Personality. New York, Oxford University Press, 1938

Musilkova J, Tucek S: The binding of cholinesterase inhibitors tacrine (tetrahydroaminoacridine) and 7-methoxytacrine to muscarinic acetylcholine receptors in rat brain in the presence of eserine. Neurosci Lett 125:113–116, 1991

Naidich TP, Daniels DL, Haughton VM, et al: Hippocampal formation and related structures of the limbic lobe: anatomic-MR correlation. Radiology 162:747–754, 1987

Nakahara N, Iga Y, Mizobe F, et al: Amelioration of experimental amnesia (passive avoidance failure) in rodents by selective M1 agonist AF102B. Jpn J Pharmacol 48:502–505, 1988

Namazi KH, Johnson BD: Pertinent autonomy for residents with dementias: modification of the physical environment to enhance independence. American Journal of Alzheimer's Care and Related Disease and Research 7:16–21, 1992

Namazi KH, Rosner TT, Calkins MP: Visual barriers to prevent ambulatory Alzheimer's patients from exiting through an emergency door. Gerontologist 29:699–702, 1989

Namazi KH, Rosner TT, Rechlin L: Long-term memory cuing to reduce visuo-spatial disorientation in Alzheimer's disease patients in a special care unit. American Journal of Alzheimer's Care and Related Disease and Research 6:10–15, 1991

Natori K, Okazaki Y, Irie T, et al: Pharmacological and biochemical assessment of SM-10888, a novel cholinesterase inhibitor. Jpn J Pharmacol 53:145–155, 1990

Navia BA: The AIDS dementia complex, in Subcortical Dementia. Edited by Cummings J. New York, Oxford University Press, 1990, pp 181–198

Navia BA, Jordan BD, Price RN: The AIDS dementia complex; I: clinical features. Ann Neurol 19:517–524, 1986a

Navia BA, Cho ES, Petito CK, et al: The AIDS dementia complex; II: neuropathology. Annals of Neurology 19:525–535, 1986b

Neary D: Dementia of frontal lobe type. J Am Geriatr Soc 38:71–72, 1990

Neary D, Snowden JS, Mann DM, et al: Alzheimer's disease: a correlative study. J Neurol Neurosurg Psychiatry 49:229–237, 1986

Neary B, Snowden JS, Mann DMA, et al: Dementia of the frontal lobe type. J Neurol Neurosurg Psychiatry 51:353–361, 1988

Newhouse PA, Sunderland T, Tariot PN, et al: Intravenous nicotine in Alzheimer's disease: a pilot study. Psychopharmacology 95:171–175, 1988

Niendorf HP, Dinger JC, Haustein J, et al: Tolerance of Gd-DTPA: a clinical experience, in Contrast Media in MRI. Edited by Dinger JC, Bydder G, Bucheler E, et al. Berlin, Medicom, 1990, pp 31–39

Nilsson K, Palmstierna T, Wistedt B: Aggressive behavior in hospitalized psychogeriatric patients. Acta Psychiatr Scand 78:172–175, 1988

Nitsch RM, Slack BE, Wurtman RJ, et al: Release of Alzheimer amyloid precursor derivatives stimulated by activation of muscarinic acetylcholine receptors. Science 258:304–307, 1992

Nitsch RM, Rebeck GW, Deng M, et al: Cerebrospinal fluid levels of amyloid-protein in Alzheimer's disease: inverse correlation with severity of dementia and effect of apoliprotein E genotype. Ann Neurol 37:512–518, 1995

Noelker L: Incontinence in elderly cared for by family. Gerontologist 27:194–200, 1987

Noetzel MJ: Dementia in Down syndrome, in Handbook of Dementing Illnesses. Edited by Morris JC. New York, Marcel Dekker, 1994, pp 243–264

Nordberg A, Nilsson Hakansson L, et al: Multiple actions of THA on cholinergic neurotransmission in Alzheimer brains. Prog Clin Biol Res 317:1169–1178, 1989

Nordgren I, Holmstedt B: Metrifonate: a review, in Current Research in Alzheimer Therapy. Edited by Giacobini E, Becker R. New York, Taylor & Francis, 1988, pp 281–288

Nuremberg Code: Trials of war criminals before the Nuremberg Military Tribunals under Control Council Law N. 10, Vol 2. Washington, DC, U.S. Government Printing Office, 1949

Nutritional Screening Initiative: Report of Nutrition Screening; I: Toward a Common View. Washington, DC, The Nutrition Screening Initiative, 1991

Oberholzer AF, Hendriksen C, Monsch AU, et al: Safety and effectiveness of low-dose clozapine in psychchogeriatric patients: a preliminary study. Int Psychogeriatr 4:187–195, 1992

Obler LK, Albert ML: Language in the Elderly Aphasic and in the Dementing Patient. New York, Academic Press, 1981

Obrist WD, Chivian E, Cronquist S, et al: Regional cerebral blood flow in senile and presenile dementia. Neurology 20:315–322, 1970

O'Connor JF, Musher DM: Central nervous sysytem involvement in systemic lupus erythematosus: a study of 150 cases. Arch Neurol 14:157–164, 1966

Office of Technology Assessment: Losing a Million Minds: Confronting the Tragedy of Alzheimer's Disease and Other Dementias. Washington, DC, Office of Technology Assessment, 1987

Ohtsubo K, Izumiyama N, Shimada H, et al: Three-dimensional structure of Alzheimer's neurofibrillary tangles of the aged human brain revealed by the quick-freeze, deep-etch and replica method. Acta Neuropathol 79:480–485, 1990

Oka A, Belliveau MF, Rosenberg PA, et al: Vulnerability of oligodendroglia to glutamate: pharmacology, mechanisms, and prevention. J Neurosci 13:141–153, 1993

Okazaki Y, Natori K, Irie T, et al: Effect of a novel CNS-selective cholinesterase inhibitor, SM-10888, on habituation and passive avoidance responses in mice. Jpn J Pharmacol 53:211–220, 1990

Olsen RV, Ehrenkrantz E, Hutchings B: Homes That Help. Newark, NJ, New Jersey Institute of Technology, 1993

Olsen WL, Longo FM, Mills CM, et al: White matter disease in AIDS: findings at MR imaging. Radiology 169:445–448, 1988

Olsho LW, Harkins SW, Lenhardt ML: Aging and the auditory system, in Handbook of the Psychology of Aging, 2nd Edition. Edited by Birren JE, Schaie KW. New York, Van Nostrand Reinhold, 1985

Olson L, Hoffer BJ: The potential use of neurotrophic factiors in the treatment of Alzheimer's disease, in Alzheimer's Disease, New Treatment Strategies. Edited by Khachaturian ZS, Blass JP. New York, Marcel Dekker, 1993, pp 125–134

Olton DS, Wenk GL: Dementia: animal models of the cognitive impairments produced by the degeneration of the basal forebrain cholinergic system, in Psychopharmacology: The Third Generation of Progress. Edited by Meltzer HY. New York, Raven, 1987, pp 941–953

Ono S, Saito Y, Ohgane N, et al: Heterogeneity of muscarinic heteroreceptors in the rat brain: effects of a novel M1 agonist, AF102B. Eur J Pharmacol 155:77–84, 1988

Overall JE, Gorham DR: The Brief Psychiatric Rating Scale. Psychol Rep 10:799–812, 1962

Overall JE, Gorham DR: The Brief Psychiatric Rating Scale (BPRS): recent developments in ascertainment and scaling. Psychopharmacol Bull 24:97–98, 1988

Overman W Jr, Stoudemire A: Guidelines for legal and financial counseling of Alzheimer's disease patients and their families. Am J Psychiatry 145:1495–1500, 1988

Padget BL, Walker DL, ZuRhein GM, et al: Cultivation of papova-like virus from human brain with progressive multifocal leukoencephalopathy. Lancet 1:1257–1260, 1971

Paganini-Hill A, Henderson VW: Estrogen deficiency and risk of Alzheimer's disease in women. Am J Epidemiol 140:256–261, 1994

Pajeau AK, Roman GC: HIV encephalopathy and dementia. Psychiatr Clin North Am 15:455–466, 1992

Palmer AM: Excitatory amino acid neurons and receptors in Alzheimer's Disease, in Neurobiology of the NMDA receptor: From Chemistry to Clinic. Edited by Kozikowski AP, Barrionuevo G. New York, VCH Publishers, 1991, pp 203–237

Palmert MR, Polisny MB, Witker DS, et al: The β amyloid precursor of Alzheimer's disease has soluble derivatives found in human brain and cerebrospinal fluid. Proc Natl Acad Sci U S A 86:6338–6342, 1989

Panella J Jr: Day Care Programs for Alzheimer's Disease and Related Disorders. New York, Demos, 1987

Pappola MA, Omar RA, Kim KS, et al: Immunohistochemical evidence of antioxidant stress in Alzheimer's disease. Am J Pathol 140:621–628, 1992

Pardridge WM: Strategies for drug delivery through the blood-brain barrier. Neurobiol Aging 10:636–637, 1989

Parker WD, Parks JK: Cytochrome *c* oxidase in Alzheimer's disease brain: purification and characterization. Neurology 45:482–486, 1995

Parkinson IS, Ward MK, Kerr DNS: Dialysis encephalopathy, bone disease and anemia: the aluminum intoxication syndrome during regular hemodialysis. J Clin Pathol 34:1285–1294, 1981

Parks RW, Haxby JV, Grady CL: Positron emission tomography in Alzheimer's disease, in Neuropsychology of Alzheimer's Disease and Other Dementias. Edited by Parks RW, Zec RF, Wilson RS. New York, Oxford University Press, 1993, pp 459–488

Parnetti L, Abate G, Bartorelli L, et al: Multicentre study of L-α-glyceryl-phosphorylcholine vs ST200 among patients with probable senile dementia of Alzheimer's type. Drugs Ageing 3:159–164, 1993

Parsons OA, Butters N, Nathan PE (eds): Neuropsychology of Alcoholism: Implications for Diagnosis and Treatment. New York, Guilford, 1987

Pastalan LA: Privacy preferences among relocated institutionalized elderly, in Man-Environment Interaction: Evaluation and Application, Edited by Carson D. Washington, DC, Environmental Design Research Association, 1974, pp 73–82

Patten BM: The ancient art of memory—usefulness in treatment. Arch Neurol 26:25–31, 1972

Patterson JV, Michalewski HJ, Starr A: Latency variability of the components of auditory event-related potentials to infrequent stimuli in aging, Alzheimer-type dementia and depression. Electroencephalogr Clin Neurophysiol 71:450–460, 1988

Paulman RG, Kennelly KJ: Test anxiety and ineffective test taking: different names, same construct? Journal of Educational Psychology 76:279–288, 1984

Paykel ES, Brayne C, Huppert FA, et al: Incidence of dementia in a population older than 75 years in the United Kingdom. Arch Gen Psychiatry 51:325–332, 1994

Pearce BD, Potter LT: Coupling of m1 muscarinic receptors to G protein in Alzheimer's disease. Alzheimer Dis Assoc Disord 5:163–172, 1991

Pearlman CA: Neuroleptic malignant syndrome: a review of the literature. J Clin Psychopharm 6:257–273, 1986

Pearson RCA, Esiri MM, Hiorns RW, et al: Anatomical correlates of the distribution of the pathological changes in the neocortex of Alzheimer's disease. Proc Natl Acad Sci U S A 82:4531–4534, 1985

Pellegrino ED: Is truth telling to the patient a cultural artefact? JAMA 268:1734–1735, 1992

Penn RD, Goetz CG, Tanner CM, et al: The adrenal medullary transplant operation for Parkinson's disease: clinical observation in five patients. Neurosurgery 22:999–1004, 1988a

Penn RD, Martin EM, Wilson RS, et al: Intraventricular bethanecol infusion of Alzheimer's disease: results of a double blind and escalating dose trials. Neurology 38:219–222, 1988b

Pentecost AR: Designing for the aging: subtleties and guidelines. Contemporary Administration 6:43–46, 1984

Pericak-Vance MA, Bebout JL, Gaskell PC Jr, et al: Linkage studies in familial Alzheimer disease: evidence for chromosome 19 linkage. Am J Hum Genet 48:1034–1050, 1991

Perl DP, Brody AR: Alzheimer's disease: X-ray spectrometric evidence of aluminum accumulation in neurofibrillary Al++ tangle-bearing neurons. Science 208:297–299, 1980

Perlmutter LS, Scott SA, Barron E, et al: MHC Class II-positive microglia in human brain: association with Alzheimer lesions. J Neurosci Res 33:549–558, 1992

Perr IN: The many faces of competence, in Law and the Mental Health Professional. Edited by Barton WE, Sanborn CJ. New York, International Universities Press, 1978, pp 211–234

Perry EK: Nerve growth factor and the basal forebrain cholinergic system: a link in the etiopathology of neurodegenerative dementias? Alzheimer Dis Assoc Disord 4:1–13, 1990

Perry EK, Perry RH, Blessed G, et al: Necropsy evidence of central cholinergic deficits in senile dementia (letter). Lancet 1:189, 1977

Perry EK, Tomlinson BE, Blessed G: Correlation of cholinergic abnormalities with senile plaques and mental test scores in senile dementia. BMJ 2:1457–1459, 1978

Petersen RC, Smith GE, Ivnik RJ: Apoliprotein E status as a predictor of the development of Alzheimer's disease in memory-impaired individiuals. JAMA 273:1274–1278, 1995

Petrie WM, Ban TA: Propranolol in organic agitation (letter). Lancet 1:324, 1981

Peyser M, Edwards KR, Poser CM, et al: Cognitive function in patients with multiple sclerosis. Arch Neurol 37:577–579, 1980

Piaget J: The Construction of Reality in the Child. New York, Basic Books, 1954

Piccinin FL, Finali G, Piccirilli M: Neuropsychological effects of l-deprenyl in Alzheimer's type dementia. Clin Neuropharmacol 13:147–163, 1990

Pincus JH: Folic acid deficiency, a cause of subacute combined system degeneration, in Folic Acid in Neurology, Psychiatry and Internal Medicine. Edited by Botez MI, Reynolds EH. New York, Raven, 1979, pp 427–433

Pinel P: A Treatise on Insanity (1806). New York, Hafner Publishing Company, 1962

Pinkston EM, Linsk NL: Care of the Elderly: A Family Approach. New York, Pergamon, 1984

Pollack CP, Perlick D: Sleep problems and institutionalization of the elderly. J Geriatr Psychiatry Neurol 4:204–210, 1991

Poon LW: Differences in human memory with aging: nature, causes and clinical implications, in Handbook of the Psychology of Aging, 2nd Edition. Edited by Birren JE, Schaie KW. New York, Van Nostrand Reinhold, 1985, pp 427–462

Portegies P, Enting RH, de Gans J, et al: Presentation and course of AIDS dementia complex: 10 years of follow-up in Amsterdam. AIDS 7:669–675, 1993

Post SG: Alzheimer disease and physician-assisted suicide. Alz Dis Rel Disord 7:65–68, 1993

Post SG: Genetics, ethics and Alzheimer's disease. J Am Geriatr Soc 42:782–786 1994

Post SG, Foley JM: Biological markers and truth-telling. Alzheimer Dis Assoc Disord 6:201–204, 1992

Powell LS, Courtice K: Alzheimer's Disease: A Guide for Families. Reading, MA, Addison-Wesley, 1983

Pratt C, Schmall V, Wright S, et al: Burden and coping strategies of caregivers to Alzheimer's patients. Family Relations 34:27–33, 1985

Prichard JAC: A Treatise on Insanity. Philadelphia, PA, Haswell, Barrington, and Haswell, 1837

Prigatano GP, Parsons O, Levin DC, et al: Neuropsychological test performance in mildly hypoxemic patients with chronic obstructive pulmonary disease. J Consult Clin Psychol 51:108–116, 1983

Proctor AW, Palmer AM, Francis PT, et al: Evidence of glutamatergic denervation and possible abnormal metabolism in Alzheimer's disease. J Neurochem 50:790–802, 1988

Propper R, Cooper B, Rufo B, et al: Continuous administration of desferrioxamine in patients with iron overload. N Engl J Med 297:418–423, 1977

Proshansky HM, Ittleson WH, Rivlin LG: Freedom of choice and behavior in a physical setting, in Environmental Psychology. Edited by Proshansky HM, Ittleson WH, Rivlin LG. New York, Holt Reinhart Winston, 1970, pp 173–178

Prusiner SB: Novel proteinaceous infectious particles cause scrapie. Science 216:136–143, 1982

Public Law 101-508, Sections 4206 (Medicare) and 4751 (Medicaid), 104 Stat 1388, 1990

Puri K, Hsu RS, Ho I, et al: Single dose safety, tolerance, and pharmakokinetics of HP029 in healthy young men. J Clin Pharmacol 29:278–284, 1989

Pynoos J, Ohta R: Home Environment Management for Alzheimer's Caregivers: A Program of Research and Dissemination to Reduce Burden and Increase Safety and Functioning, Final Report. Los Angeles, CA, Andrus Gerontology Center, 1988

Pynoos J, Cohen E, Davis L, et al: Home modifications: improvements that extend independence, in Housing the Aged: Design Directives and Policy Implications. Edited by Regnier V, Pynoos J. New York, Elsevier, 1987, pp 277–303

Rabins PV, Mece NL, Lucas MJ: The impact of dementia on the family. JAMA 248:333–335, 1982

Raffaele KC, Berardi A, Morris P, et al: Effects of acute infusion of the muscarinic cholinergic agonist arecoline on verbal memory and visuo-spatial function in dementia of the Alzheimer type. Progress in Neuropsychobiological Psychiatry 15:643–648, 1991a

Raffaele KC, Berardi A, Asthana S, et al: Effects of long-term continuous infusion of the muscarinic cholinergic agonist arecoline on verbal memory in dementia of the Alzheimer type. Psychopharmacol Bull 27:315–319, 1991b

Rainer M, Mark TH, Haushofer A: Galanthamium hydrobromicum in treatment of senile dementia (Alzheimer's disease). Presented at IV World Congress on Clinical Pharmacology and Therapeutics, West Berlin, July 28–30, 1989

Ramasubbu R, Kennedy SH: Factors complicating the diagnosis of depression in cerebrovascular disease; part II: neurological deficits and various assessment methods. Can J Psychiatry 39:601–607, 1994

Randels PM, Marco LA, Ford DI, et al: Lithium and lecithin treatment in Alzheimer's disease: a pilot study. Hillside Journal of Clinical Psychiatry 6:139–147, 1984

Rapelji D, Papp R, Crawford L: Creating a therapeutic part for the mentally frail. Dimensions in Health Services 58:12–15, 1981

Rauch RA, Jinkins JR: Infections of the central nervous system. Curr Opin Radiol 3:16–24, 1991

Ravizza L, Ferrero P, Eva C, et al: Peripheral cholinergic changes and pharmacological aspects in Alzheimer's disease, in Current Research in Alzheimer Therapy. Edited by Giacobini E, Becker R. New York, Taylor & Francis, 1988, pp 355–363

Reding M, Haycox J, Blass J: Depression in patients referred to a dementia clinic. Arch Neurol 42:894–896, 1985

Reese HW, Rodeheaver D: Problem solving and complex decision making, in Handbook of the Psychology of Aging, 2nd Edition. Edited by Birren JE, Schaie KW. New York, Van Nostrand Reinhold, 1985, pp 474–499

Reim B, Glass D, Singer J: Behavioral consequences of exposure to uncontrollable and unpredictable noise. Journal of Applied Social Psychology 1:44–56, 1971

Reinboth J, Gyldevand T: Pilot Study of Falls in an Extended Care Setting. Iowa City, IA, University of Iowa, 1982

Reisberg B, Borenstein J, Salob S, et al: Behavioral symptoms in Alzheimer's disease: phenomenology and treatment. J Clin Psychiatry 48:9–15, 1987

Reisberg B, Franssen E, Sclan SG, et al: Stage specific incidence of potentially remediable behavioral symptoms in aging and Alzheimer's disease: a study of 120 patients using the BEHAVE-AD. Bulletin of Clinical Neuroscience 54:95–112, 1989

Reitan RM, Wolfson D: The Halstead-Reitan Neuropsychological Test Battery. Tucson, AZ, Neuropsychology Press, 1993

Reynolds CF, Perel JM, Kupfer DJ, et al: Open-trial response to anti depressant treatment in elderly patients with mixed depression and cognitive impairment. Psychiatry Res 21:111–122, 1987

Richardson JC, Steele J, Olszewski J: Supranuclear ophthalmoplegia, pseudobulbar palsy, nuchal dystonia and dementia. Transactions of the American Neurological Association 88:25–29, 1963

Riley C: Evaluation of a new nutritional supplement for patients with Alzheimer's disease. J Am Diet Assoc 90:433–5, 1990

Roberts GW, Gentleman SM, Lynch A, et al: βA4 amyloid protein deposition in brain after head trauma. Lancet 338:1422–1423, 1991

Robey A: Criteria for competency to stand trial: a checklist for psychiatrists. Am J Psychiatry 122:616–623, 1965

Robinson A, Spencer B, White L: Understanding Difficult Behavior—Some Practical Suggestions for Coping With Alzheimer's Disease and Related Illnesses. Ann Arbor, MI, Geriatric Education Center of Michigan, 1988

Robinson DJ, Merskey H, Blume WT, et al: Electroencephalography as an aid in the exclusion of Alzheimer's disease. Arch Neurol 51:280–284, 1994

Robinson DS: Changes in monoamine oxidase and monoamines in human development and aging. Federation Proceedings 34:103–107, 1975

Robinson DS, Davis JN, Nies A, et al: Aging, monoamines and MAO levels. Lancet 1:290–291, 1972

Robinson RG, Forrester AW: Neuropsychiatric aspects of cerebrovascular disease, in The American Psychiatric Press Textbook of Neuropsychiatry. Edited by Hales RE, Yudofsky SC. Washington, DC, American Psychiatric Press, 1987, pp 191–208

Robinson RG, Price TR: Post-stroke depressive disorders: a follow-up study of 103 stroke out-patients. Stroke 13:635–641, 1982

Robinson RG, Starr LB, Kubos KL, et al: Mood changes in stroke patients: relationship to lesion location. Compr Psychiatry 24:555–566, 1983

Robinson RG, Starr LB, Price TR: A two year longitudinal study of mood disorders following stroke: prevalence and duration at six months follow up. Br J Psychiatry 144:256–262, 1984

Robinson RG, Bolla-Wilson K, Kaplan E, et al: Depression influences intellectual impairment in stroke patients. Br J Psychiatry 148:541–547, 1986

Rogers J, Cooper NR, Webster S, et al. Complement activation by β-amyloid in Alzheimer disease. Proc Natl Acad Sci U S A 89:10016–10020, 1992a

Rogers J, Civin WH, Styren SD, et al: Immune-related mechanisms of Alzheimer's disease pathogenesis, in Alzheimer's Disease: New Treatment Strategies. Edited by Khachaturian ZS, Blass JB. New York, Marcel Dekker, 1992b, pp 147–163

Rogers J, Kirby LC, Hempelman SR, et al: Clinical trial of indomethacin in Alzheimer's disease. Neurology 43:1609–1611, 1993

Rohde K, Peskind ER, Raskind MA: Suicide in two patients with Alzheimer's disease. J Am Geriatr Soc 43:187–189, 1995

Román GC: Senile dementia of the Binswanger type: a vascular form of dementia in the elderly. JAMA 258:1782–1788, 1987

Román GC, Tatemichi TK, Erkinjuntti T, et al: Vascular dementia: diagnostic criteria for research studies: report of the NINDS-AIREN International Workshop. Neurology 43:250–260, 1993

Roose SP, Glassman AH, Giardina E-GV, et al: Nortriptyline in depressed patients with left ventricular impairment. JAMA 256:3253–3257, 1986

Rosci MA, Pigorini F, Bernabei A, et al: Methods for detecting early signs of AIDS dementia complex in asymptomatic HIV-1-infected subjects. AIDS 6:1309–1316, 1992

Rosen WG, Mohs RC, Davis KL: A new rating scale for Alzheimer's disease. Am J Psychiatry 14:1356–1364, 1984

Rosenberg MB, Friedmann T, Robertson RO, et al: Grafting genetically modified cells to the damaged brain: restorative effects of NGF expression. Science 242:1575–1577, 1988

Roses AD, Strittmatter WJ, Pericak-Vance MA, et al: Clinical application of apolipoprotein E genotyping to Alheimer's disease. Lancet 343:1564–1565, 1994

Ross ED, Rush AJ: Diagnosis and neuroanatomical correlates of depression in brain-damaged patients. Arch Gen Psychiatry 38:1344–1354, 1981

Rossor M, Iverson LL: Non-cholinergic neurotransmitter abnormalities in Alzheimer's disease. Br Med Bull 42:70–74, 1986

Rovner BW, Edelman BA, Cox MP, Schmuely Y: The impact of antipsychotic drug regulations on psychotropic prescribing practices in nursing homes. Am J Psychiatry 149:1390–1392, 1992

Rowe JW, Katzman R: Principles of geriatrics as applied to neurology, in Principles of Geriatric Neurology. Edited by Katzman R, Rowe JW. Philadelphia, PA, FA Davis, 1992, pp 3–14

Royce S, Rosenberg J: Chelation therapy in workers with lead exposure. West J Med 158:372–375, 1993

Rubin EH, Kinscherf DA: Psychopathology of very mild dementia of the Alzheimer type. Am J Psychiatry 146:1017–1021, 1989

Rubin EH, Drevets WC, Burke WJ: The nature of psychotic symptoms in senile dementia of the Alzheimer type. J Geriatr Psychiatry Neurol 1:16–20, 1988

Rubin RT, Poland RE: The dexamethasone suppression test in depression: advantages and limitations, in Biological Psychiatry: Recent Studies. Edited by Burrows GD, Norman TR, Maguire KP. London, John Libbey, 1984, pp 77–83

Rush B: Medical Inquiries and Observations Upon the Diseases of the Mind. Philadelphia, PA, Kimber & Richardson, 1812

Russell EW: The pathology and clinical examination of memory, in Handbook of Clinical Neuropsychology. Edited by Filskov S, Boll T. New York, Wiley, 1981, pp 287–319

Ryden MB: Aggressive behavior in persons with dementia who live in the community. Alzheimer Dis Assoc Disord 2:342–355, 1988

Ryden MB: Alternatives to restraints and psychotropics in the care of aggressive, cognitively impaired elderly persons, in Geriatric Mental Health Nursing: Current and Future Challenges. Edited by Buckwalter KC. Thorofare, NJ, Slack, 1992, pp 84–93

Sachs E Jr: Meningiomas with dementia as the first presenting feature. Journal of Mental Science 96:998–1007, 1950

Sack GH: Acute intermittent porphyria. JAMA 264:1290–1293, 1990

Sadler JZ, Hulgus YF: Clinical problem solving and the biopsychosocial model. Am J Psychiatry 149:1315–1323, 1992

St. George-Hyslop PH: The molecular genetics of Alzheimer disease, in Alzheimer Disease. Edited by Terry RD, Katzman R, Bick KL. New York, Raven, 1994, pp 345–367

St. George-Hyslop PH, Tanzi RE, Polinsky RJ, et al. The genetic defect causing familial Alzheimer's disease maps on chromosome 21. Science 235:885–890, 1987

Salmon DP, Butters N, Heindel WC: Alcoholic dementia and related disorders, in Neuropsychology of Alzheimer's Disease and Other Dementias. Edited by Parks RW, Zec RF, Wilson RS. New York, Oxford University Press, 1993, pp 186–209

Salthouse T: A Theory of Cognitive Aging. Amsterdam, Elsevier, 1985

Salthouse T, Babcock R: Decomposing adult age differences in working memory. Developmental Psychology 27:763–776, 1991

Salthouse T, Babcock R, Shaw R: Effects of adult age on structural and operational capacities in working memory. Psychol Aging 6:118–127, 1991

Salzman C: Clinical Geriatric Psychopharmacology. New York, McGraw-Hill, 1984

Salzman C: Geriatric psychopharmacology. J Geriatr Psychiatry 20:11–27, 1987

Salzman C: Treatment of the agitated demented elderly patient. Hosp Community Psychiatry 39:1143–1144, 1988

Salzman C: Treatment of anxiety, in Clinical Geriatric Psychopharmacology, 2nd Edition. Edited by Salzman C. Baltimore, MD, Williams & Wilkins, 1992, pp 189–212

Salzman C, van der Kolk B: Treatment of depression, in Clinical Geriatric Psychopharmacology. Edited by Salzman C. New York, McGraw-Hill, 1984, pp 77–115

Sand T, Bovim G, Grimse R, et al: Idiopathic normal pressure hydrocephalus: the CSF tap-test may predict the clinical response to shunting. Acta Neurol Scand 89:311–316, 1994

Sano M, Bell K, Cote L., et al: Double-blind parallel design pilot study of acetyl levocarnitine in patients with Alzheimer's disease. Arch Neurol 49:1137–1141, 1992

Sapolsky RM: Stress, the Aging Brain, and the Mechanisms of Neuron Death. Cambridge, MA, MIT Press, 1992

Satel SL, Nelson JC: Stimulants in the treatment of depression: a critical overview. J Clin Psychiatry 50:241–249, 1989

Satlin A, Teicher MH, Liberman HR, et al: Circadian locomotor activity rhythms in Alzheimer's disease. Neuropsychopharmacology 5:22–25, 1991

Satlin A, Volicer L, Ross V, et al: Bright light treatment of behavioral and sleep disturbance in Alzheimer's disease. Am J Psychiatry 149:1028–1032, 1992

Saxton J, McGonigle-Gibsons KL, Swihart AA: Description and validation of a new neuropsychological test battery; psychological assessment. J Consult Clin Psychol 2:298–303, 1990

Schaffer G, Poon L: Individual variability in memory training with the elderly. Educ Gerontol 8:217–229, 1982

Schaie KW: The Seattle longitudinal study: a 21-year exploration of psychometric intelligence in adulthood, in Longitudinal Studies of Adult Psychological Development. Edited by Schaie KW. New York, Guilford, 1983, pp 64–135

Scheck DN, Hook EW III: Neurosyphilis. Inf Dis Clin North Am 8:769–795, 1994

Scheff SW, Price DA: Synapse loss in the temporal lobe in Alzheimer's disease. Ann Neurol 33:190–199, 1993

Scheff SW, DeKosky ST, Price DA: Quantitative assessment of cortical synaptic density in Alzheimer's disease. Neurobiol Aging 11:29–37, 1990

Scheinberg P: Dementia due to vascular disease—a multifactorial disorder. Stroke 19:1291–1298, 1988

Schellenberg GD, Bird TD, Wijsman EM, et al: Genetic linkage evidence for a familial Alzheimer's disease locus on chromosome 14. Science 258:668–671, 1992

Schildkraut J, Kety S: Biogenic amines and emotion. Science 156:21–30, 1967

Schlegel J, Mohr E, Williams J, et al: Guanfacine treatment of Alzheimer's disease. Clin Neuropharmacol 12:124–128, 1989

Schludermann EH, Schludermann SM, Merryman PW, et al. Halstead's studies in the neuropsychology of aging. Arch Geriatr 2:49–172, 1983

Schmidt RM, Neumann V: CSF-oligoclonal bands in multiple sclerosis, in Progress in Multiple Sclerosis Research. Edited by Bauer HJ, Poser S, Ritter G. New York, Springer-Verlag, 1978, pp 123–128

Schneck MK: Nootropics, in Alzheimer's Disease. Edited by Reisberg B. New York, Free Press, 1983, pp 362–368

Schneider LS: Clinical pharmacology af aminoacridines in Alzheimer's disease. Neurology 43 (suppl 4):S64–S79, 1993

Schneider LS, Olin JT: Overview of clinical trials of Hydergine in dementia. Arch Neurol 51:787–798, 1994

Schneider LS, Sobin P: Treatments for psychiatric symptoms and behavioral disturbances in dementia, in Dementia. Edited by Burns A, Levy R. London, Chapman & Hall, 1994, pp 517–538

Schneider LS, Cooper TB, Severson JA, et al: Electrocardiographic changes with nortriptyline and 10-hydroxytriptyline in elderly depressed outpatients. J Clin Psychopharm 8:402–408, 1988

Schneider LS, Pollock VE, Lyness SA: A metaanalysis of controlled trials of neuroleptic treatment in dementia. J Am Geriatr Soc 38:553–563, 1990

Schneider LS, Olin JT, Pawluczyk S: A double-blind crossover pilot study of l-deprenyl (selegiline) combined with cholinesterase inhibitor in Alzheimer's disease. Am J Psychiatry 150:321–323, 1993

Schnelle JF: Treatment of urinary incontinence in nursing home patients by prompted voiding. J Am Geriatr Soc 38:356–360, 1990

Schwartz JA, Speed NM, Brunberg JA, et al: Depression in stroke rehabilitation. Biol Psychiatry 33:694–699, 1993

Schwarzman AL, Gregori L, Vitek MP, et al: Transthyretin sequesters amyloid β protein and prevents amyloid formation. Proc Natl Acad Sci USA 91:8368–8372, 1994

Schweizer E, Case WG, Rickels K: Benzodiazepine dependence and withdrawal in elderly patients. Am J Psychiatry 146:529–531, 1989

Scinto LFM, Daffner KR, Dressler D, et al: A potential noninvasive neurobiological test for Alzheimer's disease. Science 266:1051–1054, 1994

Scott RB: Extraneuronal manifestations of Alzheimer's disease. J Am Geriatr Soc 41:268–276, 1993

Scoville WB, Milner B: Loss of recent memory after bilateral hippocampal lesions. J Neurol Neurosurg Psychiatry 20:11–21, 1957

Scremin OU, Scremin AM, Heuser D, et al: Prolonged effects of cholinesterase inhibition with eptastigmine on the cerebral blood flow-metabolism ratio of normal rats. J Cereb Blood Flow Metab 13:702–711, 1993

Segre G, Cerretani D, Baldi A, et al: Pharmacokinetics of heptastigmine in rats. Pharmacol Res 25:139–146, 1992

Selkoe DJ: Deciphering Alzheimer's disease: the amyloid precursor protein yields new clues. Science 248:1058–1060, 1990

Selkoe D: Amyloid protein and Alzheimer's disease. Sci Am 265:68–78, 1991

Selkoe DJ: Physiological production of the β-amyloid protein and the mechanism of Alzheimer's disease. Trends Neurosci 16:403–409, 1993

Seltzer HS: Drug-induced hypoglycemia: a review based on 473 cases. Diabetes 21:955–266, 1972

Selye H: The stress concept today, in Handbook on Stress and Anxiety. Edited by Kutash I, Schlesinger L. San Francisco, CA, Jossey Bass, 1980, pp 124–144

Settle EC Jr: Rapid neuroleptization, in Manual of Psychiatric Consultation and Emergency Care. Edited by Guggenheim FG, Weiner MF. New York, Jason Aronson, 1984, pp 43–48

Senin U, Abate G, Fieschi C, et al: Aniracetam (Ro 13-5057) in the treatment of senile dementia of Alzheimer type (SDAT): results of a placebo controlled multicentre clinical study. Eur Neuropsychopharmacol 1:511–517, 1991

Serban D, Taraboulos A, DeArmond SJ, et al: Rapid detection of Creutzfeldt-Jakob disease and scrapie prion proteins. Neurology 40:110–117, 1990

Settle EC Jr: Rapid neuroleptization, in Manual of Psychiatric Consultation and Emergency Care. Edited by Guggenheim FG, Weiner MF. New York, Jason Aronson, 1984, pp 43–48

Seubert P, Vigo-Pelphrey C, Esch F, et al: Isolation and quantification of soluble Alzheimer's β-peptide from biological fluids. Nature 359:325–327, 1992

Sevush S, Leve N: Denial of memory deficit in Alzheimer's disease. Am J Psychiatry 150:748–751, 1993

Sevush S, Guterman A, Villalon AV: Improved verbal learning after outpatient oral physostigmine therapy in patients with dementia of the Alzheimer type. J Clin Psychiatry 52:300–303, 1991

Shader RI, Greenblatt DJ: Clinical implications of benzodiazepine pharmacokinetics. Am J Psychiatry 134:652–655, 1977

Shader RI, Harmatz JS, Salzman C: A new scale for clinical assessment in geriatric populations: Sandoz Clinical Assessment Geriatric (SCAG). J Am Geriatr Soc 22:107–113, 1974

Sharp P, Gemmell H, Cherryman G, et al: Application of iodine-123-labeled isopropylamphetamine imaging to the study of dementia. J Nucl Med 27:769–774, 1986

Sherrington R, Rogaev EI, Liang Y, et al: Cloning of a gene bearing missense mutations in early-onset familial Alzheimer's disease. Nature 375:754–760, 1995

Shoji M, Golde TE, Ghiso J, et al: Production of the Alzheimer amyloid beta protein by normal proteolytic processing. Science 258:126–129, 1992

Shroyer JL: New concepts in environmental design. Presented at the meeting Emerging Concepts in Alzheimer Care, San Antonio, TX, October 6–8, 1988

Shroyer JL, Hutton JT, Anderson GM: The Alzheimer patient: interior design considerations. Tex Med 83:54–57, 1987

Shroyer JL, Anderson GM, Dobbs MN, et al: Environmental design factors impacting individuals with Alzheimer's disease. Housing and Society 16:91–97, 1988

Shuman DS: Psychiatric and Psychological Evidence. New York, McGraw-Hill, 1986

Shutske GM, Pierrat FA, Cornfeldt ML, et al: (+)-9-Amino-1,2,3,4-tetrahydroacridin-1-ol: a potential Alzheimer's disease therapeutic of low toxicity. J Med Chem 31:1278–1279, 1988

Shutske GM, Pierrat FA, Kapples KJ, et al: 9-Amino-1,2,3,4-tetrahydroacridin-1-ol: synthesis and evaluation as potential Alzheimer's disease therapeutics. J Med Chem 32:1805–1813, 1989

Sibley WA: Diagnosis and course of multiple sclerosis, in Neurobehavioral Aspects of Multiple Sclerosis. Edited by Rao SM. New York, Oxford University Press, 1990, pp 5–14

Siebens H, Trupe E, Siebens H, et al: Correlates and consequences of eating dependency in institutionalized elderly. J Am Geriatr Soc 34:192–197, 1986

Siegfried KR: First clinical impressions with an ACTH analog (HOE 427) in the treatment of Alzheimer's disease. Ann N Y Acad Sci 640:281–283, 1991

Sier HC, Hartnell J, Morley JE, et al: Primary hyperparathyroidism and delirium in the elderly. J Am Geriatr Soc 36:157–170, 1984

Siever LJ, Davis KL: Overview: toward a dysregulation hypothesis of depression. Am J Psychiatry 142:1017–1031, 1985

Silverman JM, Breitner JCS, Mohs RC, et al: Reliability of the family history method in genetic studies of Alzheimer's disease and related dementias. Am J Psychiatry 143:1279–1282, 1986

Simard D, Oleson OB, Paulson OB, et al: Regional cerebral blood flow and its regulation in dementia. Brain 94:273–288, 1971

Simpson DM, Tagliati M: Neurologic manifestations of HIV infection. Ann Intern Med 121:769–785, 1994

Skoldenberg B: Herpes simplex encephalitis. Scand J Inf Dis 80:40–46, 1991

Sloane P, Mathew L: Dementia Units in Long-Term Care. Baltimore, MD, Johns Hopkins University Press, 1991

Smith CD, Carney JM, Starke-Reed PE, et al: Excess brain protein oxidation and enzyme dysfunction in normal aging and Alzheimer's disease. Proc Natl Acad Sci U S A 88:10540–10543, 1991

Smith G, Ivnik RJ, Petersen RC, et al: Age-associated memory impairment diagnoses: problems of reliability and concerns for terminology. Psychol Aging 6:551–558, 1991

Smith JM, Kocen RS: A Creutzfeldt-Jakob-like syndrome due to lithium toxicity. J Neurol Neurosurg Psychiatry 51:120–123, 1988

Smith M, Buckwalter KC, Mitchell S: Geriatric Mental Health Training Series. New York, Spring Publishing Company, 1993

Smith MA, Sayre LM, Monnier V, et al: Radical AGEing in Alzheimer's disease. Trends Neurosci 18:172–176, 1995

Smith RC, Vroulis G, Johnson R, et al: Comparison of the therapeutic response to long-term treatment with lecithin versus piracetam plus lecithin in patients with Alzheimer's disease. Psychopharmacol Bull 20:542–545, 1984

So YT, Choucair A, Davis RL, et al: Neoplasms of the central nervous system in acquired immunodeficiency syndrome, in AIDS and the Nervous System. Edited by Rosenblum ML, Levy RM, Bredesen DE. New York, Raven, 1988, pp 285–300

Sommer R, Ross H: Social interaction on a geriatric ward. Int J Soc Psychol 4:128–133, 1958

Sourander LB, Portin R, Molsa P, et al: Senile dementia of the Alzheimer's type treated with aniracetam. Psychopharmacology 91:90–95, 1987

Spagnoli A, Tognoni G: "Cerebroactive" drugs: clinical pharmacology and therapeutic role in cerebrovascular disorders. Drugs 26:44–69, 1983

Squire LR: Memory and Brain. New York, Oxford University Press, 1987

Squire LR: Memory and the hippocampus: a synthesis from findings with rats, monkeys, and humans. Psychol Rev 99:195–231, 1992

Stahl HD, Ettlin TH, Plohmann A, et al: Central nervous system lupus: concomitant occurrence of myelopathy and cognitive dysfunction. Clin Rheum 13:273–279, 1994

Starkstein SE, Robinson RG (eds): Depression in Neurologic Disease. Baltimore, MD, Johns Hopkins University Press, 1993

Stern Y, Gurland B, Tatemichi T, et al: Influence of education and occupation on the incidence of Alzheimer's disease. JAMA 271:1004–1010, 1994

Stern Y, Tang MX, Denaro J, et al: Increased risk of mortality in Alzheimer's disease patients with more advanced educational and occupational attainment. Ann Neurol 37:590–595, 1995

Sternbach H: Danger of fluoxetine therapy after MAOI withdrawal. Lancet 2:850–851, 1988

Sternberg DE, Jarvik ME: Memory functions in depression: improvement with antidepressant medication. Arch Gen Psychiatry 33:219–224, 1976

Stokely EM, Sveinsdottir E, Lassen NA, et al: A single photon dynamic computer assisted tomograph (DCAT) for imaging brain function in multiple cross-sections. Journal of Computer Assisted Tomography 4:230–240, 1980

Stokely EM, Totah J, Homan R, et al: Interactive graphics methods for regional quantification of tomographic blood flow images. Proceedings of the MED-COMP Symposium. New York, Insitute of Electrical and Electronic Engineers, 1982

Stolley JM: Fall risk for elderly Alzheimer's patients, in Geriatric Mental Health Nursing: Current and Future Challenges. Edited by Buckwalter KC. Thorofare, NJ, Slack, 1992, pp 94–102

Storey PL, Harell LE, Duke LW, et al: Does chronic oral physostigmine alter the course of Alzheimer's disease? in Alzheimer's Disease: Advances in Clinical and Basic Research. Edited by Corain B, Iqbal K, Nicolini M, et al. New York, Wiley, 1993, pp 563–568

Strachan RW, Henderson JG: Dementia and folate deficiency. Q J Med 36:189–204, 1967

Strittmatter WJ, Saunders AM, Schmechel DE, et al: Apolipoprotein E: high avidity binding by β-amyloid and increased frequency of type 4 allele in late onset familial Alzheimer disease. Proc Natl Acad Sci U S A 90:1977–1981, 1993

Strittmatter WJ, Weisgraber KH, Goedert M, et al: Hypothesis: microtubule instability and paired helical filament formation in the Alzheimer disease brain are related to apolipoprotein E genotype. Exp Neurol 125:163–171, 1994

Strub RL, Black FW: The Mental Status Examination in Neurology, 3rd Edition. Philadelphia, PA, FA Davis, 1993

Strub RL, Black FW: Neurobehavioral Disorders: A Clinical Approach. Philadelphia, PA, FA Davis, 1988

Strumpf NE, Evans LK: The ethical problems of prolonged physical restraint. J Gerontol Nurs 17:27–33, 1991

Styren SD, DeKosky ST, Rogers J, et al: Epidermal growth factor receptor expression in demented elderly: localization to vascular endothelial cells of brain, pituitary and skin. Brain Res 615:181–190, 1990

Styren SD, Civin HW, Rogers J: Molecular, cellular, and pathologic characterization of HLA-DR immunoreactivity in normal elderly and Alzheimer's diseased brain. Exp Neurol 110:93–104, 1990

Sugaya K, Takahshi M, Kojima K, et al: SUT-8701, a CCK8 analogue, as a possible anti-dementia drug, in Alzheimer's Disease: Advances in Clinical and Basic Research. Edited by Corain B, Iqbal K, Nicolini M, et al. New York, Wiley, 1993 pp 577–587

Sullivan M: Atrophy and exercise. J Gerontol Nurs 13:26–31, 1987

Summers WK, Viesselman JO, Marsh GM, et al: Use of THA in treatment of Alzheimer-like dementia: pilot study in twelve patients. Biol Psychiatry 16:145–153, 1981

Summers WK, Majovski LV, Marsh GM, et al: Oral tetrahydro-aminoacridine in long-term treatment of senile dementia, Alzheimer's type. N Engl J Med 315:1241–1245, 1986

Sunderland T, Tariot PN, Newhouse PA: Differential responsivity of mood, behavior and cognition to cholinergic agents in elderly neuropsychiatric populations. Brain Res 472:371–389, 1988

Sunderland T, Hill JL, Mellow AM, et al: Clock drawing in Alzheimer's disease: a novel measure of dementia severity. J Am Geriatr Soc 37:725–729, 1989

Sunderland T, Molchan S, Lawlor B, et al: A strategy of "combination chemotherapy" in Alzheimer's disease: rationale and preliminary results with physostigmine plus deprenyl. Internat Psychogeriatrics 4 (suppl 2):291–309, 1992

Sungaila P, Crockett DJ: Dementia and the frontal lobes, in Neuropsychology of Alzheimer's Disease and Other Dementias. Edited by Parks RW, Zec RF, Wilson RS. New York, Oxford University Press, 1993, pp 235–264

Suzuki T, Nairn AC, Gandy SE, et al: Phosphorylation of Alzheimer amyloid precursor protein by protein kinase C. Neuroscience 48:755–761, 1992

Suzuki N, Cheung T, Cai XD, et al: An increasedpercentage of long amyloid *a* protein secreted by familial amyloid a protein precursor (*a* APP 717) mutants. Science 264:1336–1340, 1994

Svejdova M, Rektor I, Silva Barrat C, et al: Unexpected potentializing effect of a tacrine derivative (9-amino-7-methoxy-1,2,3,4 tetrahydroacridine) upon the non-epileptic myoclonus in baboons *Papio papio*. Prog Neuropsychopharmacol Biol Psychiatry 14:961–966, 1990

Swartzbeck E: The problems of falls in the elderly. Nursing Management 14:34–38, 1983

Swearer JM, Drachman DA, O'Donnell BF, et al: Troublesome and disruptive behaviors in dementia: relationships to diagnosis and disease severity. J Am Geriatr Soc 36:784–790, 1988

Swedish Cooperative Study Group: High dose acetylsalicylic acid after cerebral infarction. Stroke 18:325–334, 1987

Talbot C, Lendon C, Craddock N, et al: Protection against Alzheimer's disease with apoE 2. Lancet 343:1432–1434, 1994

Tanaka K, Ogawa N, Asanuma M, et al: Effects of the acetylcholinesterase inhibitor ENA 713 on ischemia induced changes in acetylcholine and aromatic amine levels in the gerbil brain. Arch Int Pharmacodyn Ther 323:85–96, 1993

Tanzi RE, Bird ED, Latt SA, et al: The amyloid β protein gene is not duplicated in brains from patients with Alzheimer's disease. Science 238:666–669, 1987

Tariot PN, Sunderland T, Weingartner H, et al: Cognitive effects of L-deprenyl in Alzheimer's disease. Psychopharmacology 91:489–495, 1987a

Tariot PN, Cohen RM, Sunderland T, et al: L-deprenyl in Alzheimer's disease. Arch Gen Psychiatry 44:427–433, 1987b

Tariot PN, Cohen RM, Welkowitz JA, et al: Multiple-dose arecoline infusions in Alzheimer's disease. Arch Gen Psychiatry 45:901–905, 1988a

Tariot PN, Sunderland T, Cohen RM, et al: Tranylcypromine compared with L-deprenyl in Alzheimer's disease. J Clin Psychopharmacol 8:23–27, 1988b

Tariot PN, Mack JL, Patterson MB, et al: The CERAD Rating Behavior Rating Scale for Dementia (BPRS) (abstract). Gerontologist 32:160, 1992

Taulbee LR, Folsom JC: Reality orientation for geriatric patients. Hosp Community Psychiatry 17:133–135, 1966

Teri L: Common problems and how to deal with them, in Alzheimer's Disease and the Nursing Home: A Staff Manual. Edited by Feifler BV, Orr NK. Tacoma, WA, Westprint Division of Hillhaven Corp, 1985, pp 57–66

Teri L: Behavioral treatment of depression in patients with dementia. Alzheimer Dis Assoc Disord 8 (suppl 3):66–74, 1994

Teri L, Gallagher-Thompson D: Cognitive-behavioral interventions for treatment of depression in Alzheimer's patients. Gerontologist 31:413–416, 1991

Teri L, Logsdon R: Identifying pleasant activities for individuals with Alzheimer's disease: the pleasant events schedule—AD. Gerontologist 31:124–127, 1991

Teri L, Rabins P, Whitehouse P, et al: Management of behavior disturbance in Alzheimer's disease: current knowledge and future directions. Alzheimer Dis Assoc Disord 6:77–88, 1992

Terry RD, Katzman R: Senile dementia of the Alzheimer type: defining a disease, in The Neurology of Aging. Edited by Katzman R, Terry RD. Philadelphia, PA, FA Davis, 1983, pp 51–84

Terry RD, Peck A, De Teresa R, et al: Some morphometric aspects of the brain in senile dementia of the Alzheimer type. Ann Neurol 1010:184–192, 1981

Terry RD, Masliah E, Salmon DP, et al: Physical basis of cognitive alterations in Alzheimer's disease: synapse loss is the major correlate of cognitive impairment. Ann Neurol 30:572–580, 1991

Terry RD, Masliah E, Hansen LA: Structural basis of the cognitive alterations in Alzheimer disease, in Alzheimer Disease. Edited by Terry RD, Katzman R, Bick KL. New York, Raven, 1994, pp 179–196

Thomas J: A Complete Pronouncing Medical Dictionary. Philadelphia, PA, JB Lippincott, 1889

Thomas JE, Waluchow WJ: Well and Good: Case Studies in Biomedical Ethics. Lewiston, NY, Broadview Press, 1987

Thompson LW, Wagner B, Zeiss A, et al: Cognitive/behavioral therapy with early stage Alzheimer's patients: an exploratory view of the utility of this approach, in Alzheimer's Disease Treatment and Family Stress: Directions for Research. Edited by Light E, Lebowitz BD. Washington, DC, U.S. Dept of Health and Human Services, 1989, pp 383–397

Thompson T, Filley C, Mitchell D, et al: Lack of efficacy of Hydergine in patients with Alzheimer's disease. N Engl J Med 323:445–448, 1990

Tiller JWG, Dakis JA, Shaw JM: Short-term buspirone treatment in disinhibition with dementia (letter). Lancet 2:510, 1988

Tinetti ME, Liu W, Marottoli RA, et al: Mechanical restraint use among residents of skilled nursing facilities. JAMA 265:468–471, 1991

Tison F, Dartigues JF, Auriacombe S, et al: Dementia in Parkinson's disease: a population-based study in ambulatory and institutionalized individuals. Neurology 45:705–708, 1995

Tomlinson BE: The pathology of dementia, in Dementia. Edited by Wells CE. Philadelphia, PA, FA Davis, 1977, pp 113–154

Tomlinson BE, Blessed G, Roth M: Observations on the brains of demented old people. J Neurol Sci 11:205–242, 1970

Traynelis VC: Chronic subdural hematoma in the elderly. Clin Geritr Med 7:583–598, 1991

Treloar A, Assin M, Macdonald A: Detecting Alzheimer's disease (letter). Science 267:1578, 1995

Tucek S, Dolezal V: Negative effects of tacrine (tetrahydroaminoacridine) and methoxytacrine on the metabolism of acetylcholine in brain slices incubated under conditions stimulating neurotransmitter release. J Neurochem 56:1216–1221, 1991

Tulving E: Episodic and semantic memory, in Organization of Memory. Edited by Tulving E, Donaldson W. New York, Academic Press, 1972, pp 381–403

Tupin J, Smith DB, Classon TL, et al: Long-term use of lithium in aggressive prisoners. Compr Psychiatry 14:311–317, 1973

Tuszynski MH, Gage FH: Neurotrophic factors and neuronal loss—potential relevance to Alzheimer disease, in Alzheimer Disease. Edited by Terry RD, Katzman R, Bick KL. New York, Raven, 1994, pp 405–417

U.S. Congress Office of Technology Assessment: Special Care Units for People with Alzheimer's and Other Dementias: Consumer Education, Research, Regulatory and Reimbursement Issues, #OTA-H-543. Washington DC, U.S. Government Printing Office, 1992

U.S. Department of Health and Human Services: Final Regulations Amending Basic HHS Policy for the Protection of Human Research Subjects: Final Rule 45CFR46. Federal Register: Rules and Regulations 46:9814–9820, 1981

U.S. Department of Health and Human Services: Alzheimer's Disease: Report of the Secretary's Task Force on Alzheimer's Disease (DHHS Publ No ADM-84-1323). Washington, DC, U.S. Department of Health and Human Services, 1984

U.S. Food and Drug Administration: FDA Safety Alert: Potential Hazards With Restraint Devices. Rockville, MD, U.S. Department of Health and Human Services, 1992

Vago L, Trabattoni G, Lechi A, et al: Neuropathology of AIDS dementia: a review after 205 postmortem examinations. Acta Neurol 12:32–35, 1990

Vaillant GE: Adaptation to Life. Boston, MA, Little, Brown, 1977

Van Broeckhoven C, Backhovens H, Cruts M, et al: Mapping of a gene predisposing to early onset Alzheimer's disease to chromosome 14q24.3. Nature Genet 2:335–339, 1992

van Duijn CM, de Knifff P, Wehnert A, et al: The apolipoprotein E $n2$ allele is associated with an increased risk of early-onset Alzheimer's disease and reduced survival. Ann Neurol 37:6055–610, 1995

van Gool WA, Schenk DB, Bolhuis PA: Concentrations of amyloid-β protein in cerebrospinal fluid increase with age in patients free from neurodegenerative disease. Neurosci Lett 172:122–124, 1994

van Gool WA, Kuiper MA, Walstra GJM, et al: Concentrations of amyloid a protein in cerebrospinal fluid of patients with Alzheimer's disease. Ann Neurol 37:277–279, 1995

Van Gorp WG, Mandelkern MA, Gee M, et al: Cerebral metabolic dysfunction in AIDS: findings in a sample with and without dmentia. J Neuropsychiatr Clin Neurosci 4:280–287, 1992

Van Gorp WG, Hinkin C, Satz P, et al: Neuropsychological findings in HIV infection, encephalopathy, and dementia, in Neuropsychology of Alzheimer's Disease and Other Dementias. Edited by Parks RW, Zec RF, Wilson RS. New York, Oxford University Press, 1993, pp 153–185

Van Gorp WG, Hinken C, Satz P, et al: Subtypes of HIV-related neuropsychological functioning: a cluster analysis approach. Neuropsychology 7:62–72, 1993

Van Nostrand WE, Wagner SL, Shankle WR, et al: Decreased levels of soluble amyloid β-protein precursor in cerebrospinal fluid of live Alzheimer's disease patients. Proc Natl Acad Sci U S A 89:2551–2555, 1992

Vanneste JA: Three decades of normal pressure hydrocephalus: are we wiser now? J Neurol Neurosurg Psychiatry 57:1021–1025, 1994

Van Ort S, Phillips L: Feeding nursing home residents with Alzheimer's disease. Geriatr Nurs 13:249–253, 1992

van Zomeren AH, Brouwer WH, Minderhoud JM: Acquired brain damage and driving: a review. Arch Phys Med Rehabil 68:697–705, 1987

Varga E, Sugerman AA, Varga V, et al: Prevalence of spontaneous oral dyskinesia in the elderly. Am J Psychiatry 139:329–331, 1982

Veatch RM: The Patient as Partner: A Theory of Human-Experimentation Ethics. Bloomington, IN, University of Indiana Press, 1987

Vestal RE, Wood AJ: Influence of age and smoking on drug kinetics in man: studies using model compounds. Clin Pharmacokinet 5:309–319, 1980

Vestergaard P, Amdisen A, Schou M: Clinically significant side effects of lithium treatment: a survey of 237 patients in long-term treatment. Acta Psychiatr Scand 62:193–200, 1980

Victor M: Persistent altered mentation due to ethanol. Neurol Clin N Am 11:639–661, 1993

Victor M: Alcoholic dementia. Can J Neurol Sci 21:88–99, 1994

Victor M, Adams RD, Collins GH: The Wernicke-Korsakoff Syndrome: A Clinical and Pathological Study of 245 Patients, 82 With Post-Mortem Examinations. Philadelphia, PA, FA Davis, 1971

Vieweg V, Glick JL, Herring S, et al: Absence of carbamazepine-induced hyponatremia among patients also given lithium. Am J Psychiatry 144:943–947, 1987

Vieweg V, Lombana A, Lewis R: Hyper- and hyponatremia among geropsychiatric inpatients. In J Geriatr Psychiatr Neurol 7:148–152, 1994

Vigo-Pelfrey C, Seubert P, Barbour R, et al: Elevation of microtubule-associated protein tau in the cerebrospinal fluid of patients with Alzheimer's disease. Neurology 45:788–793, 1995

Vijayashankar N, Brody H: A quantitative study of the pigmental neurons in the nuclei locus coeruleus and subcoeruleus in man as related to aging. J Neuropathol Exp Neurol 38:490–497, 1979

Vishwanath BM, Navalgund AA, Cusano W, et al: Fluoxetine as a cause of SIADH. Am J Psychiatry 148:542–543, 1991

Visser RSH: Manual of the Complex Figure Test. Amsterdam, Swets & Zeitlinger, 1985

Volicer L, Fabiszewski K, Rheaume Y, et al: Clinical Management of Alzheimer's Disease. Rockville, MD, Aspen Publishers, 1988

Volicer L, Seltzer B, Rheaume Y, et al: Eating difficulties in patients with probable dementia of the Alzheimer's type. J Geriatr Psychiatr Neurol 2:188–195, 1989

von Einsiedel RW, Fife TD, Aksamit AJ, et al: Progressive multifocal leukencephalopathy in AIDS: a clinicopathologic study and review of the literature. J Neurol 240:391–406, 1993

Wallace W, Haroutunian V: Using the subcortically lesioned rat cortex to understand the physiological role of amyloid precursor protein. Behav Brain Res 57:199–206, 1993

Wang YE, Yue DX, Tang XC: Anti-cholinesterase activity of Huperzine A. Acta Pharmacologica Sinensis 7:110–113, 1986

Warrington EK: Recognition Memory Test Manual. Windsor, UK, NFER-Nelson Company, 1984

Watkins PB, Zimmerman HJ, Knapp MJ, et al: Hepatotoxic effects of tacrine adminstration in patients with Alzheimer's disease. JAMA 271:992–998, 1994

Weber C: Design of the physical environment: modifications and adaptations for dementia care, in Alzheimer Care Strategies: Practical Approaches, Professional Alliances. Chicago, IL, National Alzheimer's Association, 1992, pp 98–99

Wechsler D: The Measurement and Appraisal of Adult Intelligence, 4th Edition. Baltimore, MD, Williams & Wilkins, 1958

Wechsler D: Wechsler Adult Intelligence Scale—Revised. New York, The Psychological Corporation, 1981

Wechsler D: Wechsler Memory Scale—Revised: Manual. San Antonio, TX, The Psychological Corporation, 1987

Weiler PG, Mungas D, Pomerantz S: AIDS as a cause of dementia in the elderly. J Am Geriatr Soc 36:139–141, 1988

Weiner MF: Hallucinations in children. Arch Gen Psychiatry 5:54–63, 1961

Weiner MF: Beyond the presenting complaint. Psychosomatics 10:310–313, 1969

Weiner MF: Coping styles and behaviors of medical/surgical patients, in Manual of Psychiatric Consultation and Emergency Care. Edited by Guggenheim FG, Weiner MF. New York, Jason Aronson, 1984, pp 124–134

Weiner MF: Practical Psychotherapy. New York, Brunner/Mazel, 1986

Weiner MF: Group therapy in a public sector psychiatric clinic. Int J Group Psychother 38:355–365, 1988

Weiner MF, Crowder JD: Psychotherapy and cognitive style. Am J Psychother 40:17–25, 1986

Weiner MF, Davis KL: Anticholinergic drugs, in Drugs in Psychiatry, Vol 4. Edited by Burrows GD, Norman TR, Davies B. Amsterdam, Elsevier, 1986, pp 191–205

Weiner MF, Lovitt R: Conservation-withdrawal versus depression. Gen Hosp Psychiatry 1:347–349, 1979

Weiner MF, Fitzpatrick MC: Treating depression in elderly patients. Compr Ther 13:65–70, 1987

Weiner MF, Lovitt R: An examination of patients' understanding of information from health care providers. Hosp Community Psychiatry 35:619–620, 1984

Weiner MF, Bruhn M, Svetlik DS, et al: Experiences with depression in a dementia clinic. J Clin Psychiatry 52:234–238, 1991

Weiner MF, Denke M, Williams K, et al: Intramuscular medroxyprogesterone acetate for sexual aggression in elderly men. Lancet 339:1121–1122, 1992

Weiner MF, Vobach S, Svetlik D, et al: Cortisol secretion and Alzheimer's disease progression: a preliminary report. Biol Psychiatry 34:158–161, 1993

Weiner MF, Edland SD, Luszczynska H: Prevalence and incidence of major depression in Alzheimer's disease. Am J Psychiatry 151:1006–1009, 1994

Weingartner H, Cohen RM, Murphy DL, et al: Cognitive processes in depression. Arch Gen Psychiatry 38:42–47, 1981

Weingartner H, Grafman J, Boutelle W, et al: Forms of memory failure. Science 221:380–382, 1983

Weisman GD: Wayfinding and architectural legibility: design considerations in housing environments for the elderly, in Housing the Aged: Design Directives and Policy Implications. Edited by Regnier V, Pynoos J. New York, Elsevier, 1987, pp 441–464

Weisman GD, Cohen U, Ray K, et al: Architectural planning and design for dementia care, in Specialized dementia care units, Edited by Coons D. Baltimore, MD, Johns Hopkins University Press, 1991, pp 83–105

Wells CE: Pseudodementia. Am J Psychiatry 136:895–900, 1979

Wengel SP, Burke WJ, Ranno AE, et al: Use of benzodiazepines in the elderly. Psychiatr Ann 23:325–331, 1992

Wenk GL: A primate model of Alzheimer's disease. Behav Brain Res 57:117–122, 1993

Wesseling H, Agoston S, Van Dam GBP, et al: Effects of 4-aminopyridine in elderly patients with Alzheimer's disease. N Engl J Med 310:988–989, 1984

Wettstein A, Spiegal R: Clinical studies with the cholinergic drug RS-86 in Alzheimer's disease (AD) and senile dementia of the Alzheimer type (SDAT). Psychopharmacology 84:572–573, 1984

Whelan TB, Schteingart DE, Starkman MN, et al: Neuropsychological deficts in Cushing's syndrome. J Nerv Ment Dis 168:753–757, 1980

White MH, Armstrong D: Cryptococcosis. Inf Dis Clin North Am 8:383–398, 1994

Whitehouse PJ (ed): The Dementias. Philadelphia, PA, FA Davis, 1993

Whitehouse P, Price DL, Struble RG, et al: Alzheimer's disease and senile dementia: loss of neurons in the basal forebrain. Science 215:1237–1239, 1982

Whitley RJ, Alford CA, Hirsch MS, et al: Vidarabine versus acyclovir therapy in herpes simplex encephalitis. N Engl J Med 314:144–149, 1986

Whitson JS, Selkoe DJ, Cotman CW: Amyloid β protein enhances survival of hippocampal neurons in vitro. Science 243:1488–1490, 1989

Wilcock GK, Esiri MM, Bowen DM, et al: Alzheimer's disease: correlation of cortical choline acetyltransferase activity with the severity of dementia and histological abnormalities. J Neurol Sci 57:407–417, 1982

Wilcock GK, Surnom DJ, Scott M, et al: An evaluation of the efficacy and safety of tetrahydroaminoacridine (THA) without lecithin in the treatment of Alzheimer's disease. Age Ageing 22:316–324, 1993

Wilcox SM, Himmelstein DU, Woolhandler S: Inappropriate drug prescribing for the community-dwelling elderly. JAMA 272:292–296, 1994

Wilkins AJ, Shallice T, McCarthy R: Frontal lesions and sustained attention. Neuropsychologia 25:359–365, 1987

Wilkinson DA: CT scan and neuropsychological assessments of alcoholism, in Neuropsychology of Alcoholism: Implications for Diagnosis and Treatment. Edited by Parsons OA, Butters N, Nathan PA. New York, Guilford, 1987, pp 76–98

Will B, Hefti F: Behavioral and neurochemical effects of chronic intraventricular injections of nerve growth factor in adult rats with fimbria lesions. Brain Res 17:17–24, 1985

Williams KH, Goldstein G: Cognitive and affective response to lithium in patients with organic brain syndrome. Am J Psychiatry 136:800–803, 1979

Williams ME, Pannill FC III: Urinary incontinence in the elderly: pathophysiology, diagnosis, and treatment. Ann Intern Med 97:895–907, 1982

Wilson BA: Rehabilitation of Memory. New York, Guilford, 1987

Winograd CH: The physician and the Alzheimer patient, in Treatments for the Alzheimer Patient. Edited by Jarvik LF, Winograd CH. New York Springer Publishing Company, 1988, pp 3–38

Wisner E, Green M: Treatment of a demented patient's anger with cognitive-behavioral strategies. Psychol Rep 59:447–450, 1986

Wisniewski HM: Neuritic (senile) and amyloid plaques, in Alzheimer's Disease. Edited by Reisberg B. New York, Free Press, 1983, pp 57–61

Wisniewski K, Howe J, Williams DG: Precocious aging and dementia in patients with Down's syndrome. Biol Psychiatry 13:619, 1978

Wisniewski KE, Wisniewski HM, Wen GY: Occurrence of neuropathological cahanges and dementia of Alzheimer's disease in Down's syndrome. Ann Neurol 17:278–282, 1985

Wittenborn JR: Pharmacotherapy for age-related behavioral deficiencies. J Nerv Ment Dis 169:139–156, 1981

Wojcieszek JM, Lang AE: Hyperkinetic movement disorders, in The American Psychiatric Press Textbook of Geriatric Neuropsychiatry. Edited by Coffey CE, Cummings JL. Washington, DC, American Psychiatric Press, 1994, pp 404–431

Wolanin MO, Phillips L: Confusion: Prevention and Care. St. Louis, MO, Mosby, 1981

Wolfson LI, Katzman R: The neurological consultation at age 80, in The Neurology of Aging. Edited by Katzman R, Terry RD. Philadelphia, PA, FA Davis, 1983, pp 221–244

Wood PL, Nair NP, Etienne P, et al: A lack of cholinergic deficit in the neocortex in Pick's disease. Prog Neuropsychopharmacol Biol Psychiatry 7:725–727, 1983

Woods SW, Tesar GE, Murray GB, et al: Psychostimulant treatment of depressive disorders secondary to medical illness. J Clin Psychiatry 47:12–15, 1986

Wragg RE, Jeste DV: Neuroleptics and alternative treatments: management of behavioral symptoms and psychosis in Alzheimer's disease and related conditions. Psychiatr Clin North Am 11:195–213, 1988

Wragg RE, Jeste DV: Overview of depression and psychosis in Alzheimer's disease. Am J Psychiatry 146:577–587, 1989

Yamaguchi H, Yamazaki T, Ishiguro K, et al: Ultrastructural localization of Alzheimer amyloid-beta/A4 protein precursor in the cytoplasm of neurons and senile plaque-associated astrocytes. Acta Neuropathol 85:15–22, 1992

Yamaguchi MD, Meyer JS, Yamamoto M, et al: Noninvasive regional cerebral blood flow measurements in dementia. Arch Neurol 7:410–418, 1980

Yamamoto T, Hirano A: Nucleus raphe dorsalis in Alzheimer's disease: neurofibrillary tangles and loss of large neurons. Ann Neurol 17:573–577, 1985

Yamamoto T, Ohno M, Kitajima I, et al: Ameliorative effects of the centrally active cholinesterase inhibitor, NIK 247, on impairment of working memory in rats. Physiol Behav 53:5–10, 1993a

Yamamoto T, Ohno M, Sugimachi K, et al: Discriminative stimulus properties of NIK 247 and tetrahydroaminoacridine, centrally active cholinesterase inhibitors in rats. Pharmacol Biochem Behav 44:769–75, 1993b

Yankner BA, Dawes LR, Fisher S, et al: Neurotoxicity of a fragment of the amyloid precursor associated with Alzheimer's disease. Science 245:417–420, 1989

Yankner BA, Duffy LK, Kirschner DA: Neurotrophic and neurotoxic effects of amyloid β protein: reversal by tachyleinin neuropeptides. Science 250:279–282, 1990

Yesavage J, Brink T, Rose T: Development and validation of a geriatric depression screening scale: a preliminary report. J Psychiatr Res 17:37–49, 1983

Yesavage J, Sheikh J, Tank ED, et al: Response to memory training and individual differences in verbal intelligence and state anxiety. Am J Psychiatry 145:635–639, 1988

Yudofsky S, Williams D, Gorman J: Propranolol in the treatment of rage and violent behavior in patients with organic brain syndrome. Am J Psychiatry 138:218–220, 1981

Zarit SH: Do we need another "stress and caregiving" study? Gerontologist 29:147–148, 1989

Zarit SH, Teri L: Interventions and services for family caregivers, in Annual Review of Gerontology and Geriatrics. Edited by Schaie K, Lawton MP. New York, Springer, 1992, pp 287–310

Zarit SH, Reever K, Bach-Peterson J: Relatives of the impaired elderly: correlates of feelings of burden. Gerontologist 20:649–655, 1980

Zarit SH, Orr NK, Zarit JM: The Hidden Victims of Alzheimer's Disease: Families Under Stress. New York, New York University Press, 1985

Zec RF: Neuropsychological functioning in Alzheimer's disease, in Neuropsychology of Alzheimer's Disease and Other Dementias. Edited by Parks RW, Zec RF, Wilson RS. New York, Oxford University Press, 1993, pp 3–80

Zhan S, Beyreuther K, Schmitt H: Quantitative assessment of the synaptophysin immuno-reactivity of the cortical neuropil in various neurodegenerative disorders with dementia. Dementia 4:66–74, 1993

Zhang RW, Tang XC, Han YY, et al: Drug evaluation of huperzine A in the treatment of senile memory disorders (English abstract). Chung Kuo Yao Li Hsueh Pao 12:250–252, 1991

Zola-Morgan S, Squire LR, Amaral DG: Human amnesia and the medical temporal region: enduring memory impairment following a bilateral lesion limited to field CA1 of the hippocampus. J Neurosci 6:2950–2967, 1986

Zubenko GS, Moosy J: Major depression in primary dementia: clinical and neuropathologic. Arch Neurol 45:1182–1186, 1988

Zweig RM, Ross CA, Hedreen JC, et al: The neuropathology of aminergic nuclei in Alzheimer's disease. Ann Neurol 24:233–242, 1988

Index

Lecithin, 207, 333
Legal issues
    competence, 252–254
    durable powers of attorney for
        health care, 258–259
    fiduciaries, 259–261
    guardianship, 259–260
    informed consent, 254–256
    powers of attorney, 257–259
    testamentary capacity, 256
    undue influence, 257–258
    wills, 262–263
Leigh's disease, 137
Leukoaraiosis, 78
Lewy body, 123
Lewy body variant of Alzheimer's
    disease, 130
Limbic encephalitis, 136
Lithium carbonate, 195–197
Lithium intoxication, 105
Living wills, 262–263
Locus coeruleus, 54, 126, 314, 315,
    319–320
Lorazepam, 19, 187, 189
Loxapine, 192
Lumbar puncture, 74, 113, 115–117
Lupus cerebritis, 67
Luria-Nebraska Neuropsychological
    Battery, 215

Magnetic resonance imaging, 78–80
Magnetic resonance spectroscopy,
    80–83
Major depression, 25–27, 52–55
Malingering, 28
Manganese poisoning, 105
MAO inhibitors. See Monoamine
    oxidase inhibitors
Mattis Dementia Rating Scale, 71, 223
Medical illness considerations,
    169–170
Medical workup, 65–99
Medroxyprogesterone, 203
Memory
    episodic, 218

measurement, 217–219
primary, 31, 217
retrieval, 218
secondary, 31, 217
semantic, 218
tertiary, 217
training, 167–168
types, 217–218
Mental retardation, 16–17
Mental status examination, 31–33
Mercury poisoning, 105
Metabolic disorders as dementia
    causes, 106–109
Metabolic enhancers, 205–206
Metachromatic leukodystrophy, 137
Metal poisoning, 105
    aluminum toxicity, 105
Methoxytacrine, 335
Methylphenidate
    apathy and withdrawal
        treatment, 202–203
    depression treatment, 186
Metrifonate, 337
MID. See multi-infarct dementia
Milacemide, 345–346
Mini-Mental State Exam, 26, 39, 71,
    222–223, 377–378
Minnesota Multiphasic Personality
    Inventory, 224
Mixed dementia, 131
MMSE. See Mini-Mental State Exam
Molindone, 192
Monoamine oxidase inhibitors
    Alzheimer's disease treatment,
        343
    depression treatment, 185–186
Motor function measurement, 221
MRI. See Magnetic resonance
    imaging
MS. See Multiple sclerosis
Multiple cuing, 155
Multiple sclerosis, 24, 69, 119–120
Music, 33